Metchnikoff
and the Origins of
Immunology

Monographs on the History and Philosophy of Biology

RICHARD BURIAN, RICHARD BURKHARDT, JR.,
RICHARD LEWONTIN, JOHN MAYNARD SMITH
EDITORS

The Cuvier-Geoffroy Debate: French Biology in the Decades Before Darwin
TOBY A. APPEL

Controlling Life: Jacques Loeb and the Engineering Ideal in Biology
PHILIP J. PAULY

Beyond the Gene: Cytoplasmic Inheritance and the Struggle for
Authority in Genetics
JAN SAPP

The Heritage of Experimental Embryology: Hans Spemann and the Organizer
VIKTOR HAMBURGER

The Evolutionary Dynamics of Complex Systems:
A Study in Biosocial Complexity
C. DYKE

The Wellborn Science: Eugenics in Germany, France, Brazil, and Russia
Edited by MARK B. ADAMS

Darwin without Malthus: The Struggle for Existence in Russian
Evolutionary Thought
DANIEL P. TODES

Theory Change in Science: Strategies from Mendelian Genetics
LINDLEY DARDEN

Metchnikoff and the Origins of Immunology: From Metaphor to Theory
ALFRED I. TAUBER AND LEON CHERNYAK

Metchnikoff and the Origins of Immunology

From Metaphor to Theory

ALFRED I. TAUBER
LEON CHERNYAK

Boston University School of Medicine

New York   Oxford
OXFORD UNIVERSITY PRESS
1991

Oxford University Press

Oxford   New York   Toronto
Delhi   Bombay   Calcutta   Madras   Karachi
Petaling Jaya   Singapore   Hong Kong   Tokyo
Nairobi   Dar es Salaam   Cape Town
Melbourne   Auckland

and associated companies in
Berlin   Ibadan

Library of Congress Cataloging-in-Publication Data
Tauber, Alfred I.
Metchnikoff and the origins of immunology:
from metaphor to theory /
Alfred I. Tauber, Leon Chernyak.
p. cm. Includes bibliographical references and index.
ISBN 0-19-506447-X
1. Metchnikoff, Elie, 1845–1916. 2. Immunologists—Ukraine—Biography.
3. Immunologists—France—Biography.
4. Immunology—History.
I. Chernyak, Leon. II. Title.
QR180.72.M48T38 1991 591.2′9′092—dc20 [B] 90-26245

9 8 7 6 5 4 3 2 1

Printed in the United States of America
on acid-free paper

TO OUR CHILDREN

Foreword

Thank goodness someone has written a new biography of Elie Metchnikoff! Rather, it took two people: Metchnikoff's scientific career was so incredible and his personal life so interesting that you can't really expect one person to encompass it all. Moreover, Metchnikoff was such a complex and, at times, contradictory person that two authors' viewpoints are actually more appropriate to have than one. The richness of this book is due to a most fruitful interaction between the American immunologist Alfred Tauber and the Russian philosopher Leon Chernyak. Those of us who have enjoyed their series of historical articles in *Cellular Immunology* already know the vitality of their scholarship; but those articles were only the embryonic form of this book.

I expect that many immunologists reading those initial papers were surprised to discover that Metchnikoff's discipline-creating theory of "active host immunity" originated within the matrix of comparative embryology. For although Metchnikoff is considered the founder of the notion of active host immunity against disease and, hence, the founder of the field of immunology, he did not do so out of an interest in medicine. Rather, Tauber and Chernyak have traced these roots of immunology back to the revolution in embryology when traditional comparative embryology began incorporating evolutionary concepts in the late 1860s.

This evolutionary embryology was a remarkably rich mulch, and the embryonic shoots of many of our most successful disciplines have their roots in this strange soil. Thomas Hunt Morgan and E. B. Wilson, the principal founders of modern genetics, did their original research in this area and so did Hans Spemann, Wilhelm Roux, and many of the other founders of experimental embryology. In this volume, Tauber and Chernyak demonstrate that modern immunology is also deeply rooted in evolutionary embryology. It should be noted that comparative and evolutionary embryology were extremely strong in Russia and the Baltic region, and historian Fred Churchill has recently shown that modern comparative embryology originated there. Christian Pander (1794–1865), the discoverer of the germ layers, was born in Riga; Karl Ernst Baer (1792–1876), the discoverer of the mammalian egg and the process of neurulation, was born in Dorpat (now Tartu, Estonia); and Heinrich Rathke (1793–1860), the preeminent comparative embryologist who discovered the mammalian gill clefts and who focused most of his research on vertebrate urogenital systems, was born in Danzig (now Gdansk). These three embryologists knew each other well and had interests in comparing the embryogenesis of different animals. These investigators inspired a second generation of embryologists in Russia, a group that included Elie Metchnikoff, Nicolaus Kleinenberg, and Alexander Kowalevsky. All three of these investigators sought to link animal development with evolutionary biology.

Metchnikoff was a comparative embryologist, and a very good one. One of the first comparative embryologists to study invertebrates, Metchnikoff was ideally situated to discuss the origins of metazoans. In combatting the competing theories of Ernst Haeckel, Metchnikoff created a hypothesis for the origin of metazoans that is still the basis for our current theories. Libby Hyman explicitly linked her theories to those of Metchnikoff, and much of Leo Buss's current hypothesis on the origin of metazoans is based on Metchnikoff's principles and examples. As Tauber and Chernyak document, Metchnikoff entered into immunology through his attempt to prove that embryonic mesodermal cells had an intrinsic capacity for phagocytosis and that the earliest metazoans, like the earliest embryonic stages, had a solely intracellular mode of digestion. This digestion was accomplished, Metchnikoff asserted, by the amoeboid cells of the mesoderm. He would later frame the hypothesis that this primitive digestive function became a property of specialized phagocytes (i.e., macrophages) that would engulf and digest foreign objects such as pathogenic bacteria. This notion that the intracellular digestion found in protists would eventually give rise to the properties of immunocompetent cells is still a basic concept in modern immunology. Throughout his scientific career, Metchnikoff productively linked digestion, immunology, and evolution.

Metchnikoff is usually remembered neither for his hypothesis of metazoan origins nor for his assertion that phagocytosis is the function by which one can trace the mesodermal cell lineage. He is mostly known for his concept of active host resistance to infection. Tauber and Chernyak demonstrate that Metchnikoff's theory of active host resistance—that the body had cells that provided innate immunity to infectious agents—was the result of both his embryological theories and a particular philosophical view of the body that grew out of them. This philosophy saw the body not as the product of harmonious interactions beginning with the fertilized egg, but as a struggle within the body between potentially disharmonious parts. What created this whole out of such parts? What harmonized the potentially competitive lineages? One of these harmonizing whole-making functions belonged, according to Metchnikoff, to the mesodermal phagocytic cells. These cells were essential for providing nutrition for the developing organism and would later defend the organism against external pathogens. Believing (as did his mentor Louis Pasteur and his adversary Paul Ehrlich) that immunity was linked to nutrition, Metchnikoff brought the first yogurt cultures into France to counter the putatively deleterious effects of toxin-producing colonic bacteria and thereby to promote longevity.

Metchnikoff was a scientist in the Romantic tradition. Like Pasteur, he saw science as the cure for the evils that have plagued humankind. Metchnikoff saw the scientist as savior to the world, and he put his religious faith and fervor into science. He was also a scientist who would survive two suicide attempts, engage in vitriolic polemics against his rivals, and who would become a leader of that most French establishment, the Pasteur Institute, even though he was a half-Jewish Russian immigrant. Although Metchnikoff received a Nobel Prize (with Ehrlich) in 1908, his immunological theories were eclipsed soon afterwards. Ehrlich and his school had formulated a humoral antibody theory of immune responsiveness upon the scaffold of Metchnikoff's theory of active host response. Only recently, after acknowledging macrophage activity in the generation of the humoral immune response and in the innate immunity to specific pathogens, can we see the importance of this scaffold that underlies and supports all subsequent theories of immunity.

The story of Metchnikoff's life and science is a story of arguments; for Metchnikoff had an uncanny ability to bring out the polarities present at any given time. Therefore, in documenting the origin, acceptance, and eclipse of Metchnikoff's theory, Tauber and Chernyak provide a view into the larger story of the changes occurring in embryology as it attempted to incorporate notions of evolution and the changes in pathology and medicine as they met the sciences of bacteriology and cytology. The story of Metchnikoff becomes our vantage point to see how a science became accepted by medicine during an era when medicine was just beginning to find its scientific bases. We see biology and medicine as each group reacted to Metchnikoff's central hypotheses. There were the arguments with Kowalevsky (over the nature of homology), the arguments with Haeckel (over the origins of phyla), the arguments with Baumgarten and Ziegler (over the nature of inflammation and the host response), and the well-known arguments with Ehrlich and the humoralist immunologists over the nature of that host response. Throughout these debates and polemics, Metchnikoff maintains his hypothesis that phagocytosis is the fundamental integrating activity of the organism, first for its role in embryonic digestion and then for its role in protecting the body from infection.

This volume is, therefore, a history of that fascinating era when embryology had to integrate evolutionary biology and when medicine had to integrate cellular science. That Metchnikoff played critical roles in *both* transformations is remarkable and understandable only in the light of his ideas on phagocytosis. Tauber and Chernyak meticulously trace this intellectual odyssey from its origins in the germ-layer controversies of Russian embryology to the immunological laboratories of Paris.

We are extremely fortunate to have this excellent volume, and I expect that this is but the first and seminal volume of an entire library of new Metchnikoff studies. What this book does is to pare away a great deal of Metchnikoff mythology (much of it promulgated by Metchnikoff himself) and to document the turbulent origins and reception of one of the most important biomedical concepts of our times. In so doing, Tauber and Chernyak also show how evolutionary biology and comparative embryology converged with medical interests to formulate a new view of the organism and gave rise to the science of immunology.

Swarthmore College   SCOTT GILBERT
July 1990

As the whisper perhaps evolved before lips,
And leaves spun and circled long before there were trees,
So those, it may be, whom our experience endows,
Before such experience have acquired their traits.

O. MANDEL'SHTAM, *Ottave VII*

Preface

This book examines the intellectual genesis of immunology. Although a chronicle of scientific events, it is truly a history of an idea, an intellectual adventure of the late nineteenth century, that quickly witnessed the emergence of a biochemically based biology from an observational science. The immunology of today was clearly defined in its theoretical progression by 1900, a scant eighteen years after Elie Metchnikoff, a Russian embryologist, first presented his phagocytosis theory of host defense. The idea of immunity is thus a modern concept. Certainly, the phenomenon of nonrecurrent disease in those previously infected, or the resistance of certain members of a population subject to an epidemic, was well recognized since recorded history, but we have reserved the term *immunity* in its specific modern meaning to those activities that confer protection to a host based on an *active* response of a specialized system. It is the central notion of active, purposeful reaction to infection that was novel in Metchnikoff's formulation, and the birth of immunology as a discipline resides securely in the establishment of his theoretical edifice. We are thus committed to tracing how his studies in comparative zoology led to the novel recognition of phagocytic function, its extrapolation to a new understanding of the inflammatory reaction, and the presentation of a new theory of health and disease based on these studies. We will also examine the mixed reaction of Metchnikoff's colleagues—who reflect the countercurrents of biological theory of the time—and attempt to dissect the dynamics of that debate and its resolution.

This chapter of modern biology might appear like others, as a product of two conflicting ideologies—teleology and mechanoreductionism; the former was subsumed under holistic reductionism, a still-struggling and dissenting voice, whereas the latter grew to dominate molecular biology and biochemistry in the twentieth century. However, as Metchnikoff's case demonstrates, this controversy presents a superficial interpretation of a fundamental reorientation in biological thinking, and reflects the inertial dependence of modern biology's intellectual framework. Metchnikoff was to overcome this traditional opposition and to assert a radically new orientation. However, both alternatives of this traditional conflict are still active in modern immunology, which most clearly illustrates the importance of each perspective: the power of molecular biological definition of the immune system on a componential level is self-apparent, whereas the integration and ordering of immune reactions still requires formalization in an encompassing hierarchical or dialogical theory. But it is here that the historical record warrants careful inspection, for in the genesis of the immune theory, the precision of the original formulation offers insight into the bewildering complexity of our modern construction. For the logic of Metchnikoff's theory makes explicit that the birth of the very idea of immunity was provided by a new perspective, deeper than the traditional alternative—organism versus mechanism. The importance of assessing Metchnikoff's opus is, in part, accounted for by our belief that his research has direct relevance to current understanding of the scientific and metaphysical concept of organism as defined by immunity.

In the early reception of Darwin's natural selection theory, a profound alteration in the concept of organism took place: no longer was the organism a preset balance of forces (humors/elements of any kind), but rather the organism was intrinsically a product of evolved, potentially imbalanced structures/functions harmonized by evolutionary forces and biological needs that yielded functional units more adaptive in a competitive, hostile environment. Explicit appreciation of this basic shift in the metaphysical structure of the organism was made by Metchnikoff, who presented the phagocytosis theory—the basic conceptual notion of immunity—in response to how the organism was defined by such evolutionary challenges; in the process, he established a modern definition of selfhood. The Self emerged as the result of dynamic processes; in Metchnikoff's vision, these were those activities that constituted—in fact, established—organismic integrity. Only by secondary phenomena was this integrity, or selfhood, protected (i.e., defended) against pathogens. From the immunological process, mediated by immune cells (i.e., phagocytes), Self was defined; this radical view of the organism arose from Metchnikoff's notions of the evolutionary dynamic and formed the metaphysical basis of his diverse research.

A new formulation of the relationship between host and contagious disease was established in 1883 by Metchnikoff's convergence of three disparate and up to then unrelated theoretical streams: (a) bacteria as etiologic agents of infection, (b) the nature and role of inflammation, and (c) the place of evolutionary principles as applied to physiology. The germ theory of disease was established by Louis Pasteur and Robert Koch by the mid-1870s, but there was no theory akin to our modern notion of immunological defense. Pasteur as late as 1880, while developing vaccines, believed that immunity was conferred by the exhaustion of essential nutrients—a theory analogous to the test-tube model systems of bacterial growth. Koch was not even interested in the host response, confining himself to the establishment of bacterial etiology. Inflammation was generally viewed as a deleterious process whose various components were regarded as reactive, not defensive. The white cells (some of which were already identified as amoeboid phagocytes), with purposeful movement and containing bacteria, were dismissed as transport vehicles for the pathogens, with no protective function hypothesized. In short, how bacteria might cause disease, and more fundamentally, the relation of host and pathogen from a physiological (organism) or evolutionary (species) perspective was left mute.

On these themes, Metchnikoff, an embryologist, applied lessons learned from his debate with Darwinians and other morphologists as to the relation of evolutionary principles to ontogeny. He proposed that mesodermal phagocytic cells in primitive organisms served a nutritive function, but in higher animals with a digestive cavity, they assumed new activities devoid of their original digestive purpose. He extended the metaphor of "eat or be eaten" to a dedicated function of these cells that, wandering beneath epithelial surfaces and various interstices, recognized nonself elements and devoured them. Originally, he viewed the process as a general physiological mechanism he called "physiological inflammation," for the phagocytes in protecting the host recognized nonself in every form—from senescent, malignant, damaged, or otherwise diseased cells to foreign invaders. The latter became Metchnikoff's focus only as he was initially drawn into vociferous debate with microbiologists (who first opposed him because they misunderstood the theory and could not engage him within the same intellectual framework), and soon thereafter with the early humoral immunologists (who opposed him on the basis of specific mechanisms). The cardinal point to be elucidated is how Metchnikoff established an entirely new vision of the organism, one that arose from a potentially disharmonious evolved self made up of elements that had to be harmonized. For Metchnikoff, the phagocytes served as the principal harmonizing element; from that formulation, the basis of Self emerged and immunological defense and surveillance were born. More broadly, the idea of selfhood was revolutionized.

The nature of discovery represents a central issue of current discussion, and the case of Metchnikoff is fascinating from several points of view in this regard. First, he left an easily followed trail. Metchnikoff was truly a remarkably innovative scientist whose creativity was recurrently exhibited. He also exposed his naivete and dogged narrow defensiveness during the repeated cycles of attack and defense throughout his career. His personality markedly defined both his professional scientific postures, but it also clearly illustrated his metaphysical horizons. Metchnikoff is easily accessible for analysis. The events of his career and the extensive published record of his philosophical writings offer a rich mine of exploration. Second, the development of immunology represents the convergence of several fields: microbiology, pathology, embryology, evolutionary biology, and biochemistry. Metchnikoff's theory is held as a beacon for orienting potentially divergent trends in these disciplines; thus, his research serves as a framework by which the various contributory currents may be analyzed and assigned their respective roles. Third, Metchnikoff was frankly intellectual and was comfortable with acknowledging the metaphysical basis of his thinking. His scientific construct was an intellectual endeavor that organized observations into a schema with a theoretical basis both explicitly formulated and implicitly resting upon a novel metaphysical foundation. In respect to his scientific development, the axis of disharmony striving toward functional harmony represented a rich resource. At the same time, he was simplistic in his reliance on those biological concepts to dictate explanations of more complex organization and to serve as a philosophy of human behavior and a program of health. For our purposes, however, the conscious philosophy is a useful probe to understanding the dynamics of his mind and the metaphysical basis of his thinking. Finally, Metchnikoff's scientific logic may be viewed from the perspective of a century. The outline of his scientific construction still serves as a useful map of the current posture that attempts to understand our own concept of modern immunology, the nature of an organism, and the logic of our molecular-based biology. Although study of Metchnikoff is of interest in its own right, we believe the examination of his discovery reveals our own endeavor. In many respects, we still reflect in his insights, and the lessons of submerging metaphysics in our scientific programs are yet to be satisfactorily revealed.

Metchnikoff construed biology in a dynamic model, which was immediately criticized as teleological and vitalistic. Today he would have found a happy harbor in epigenetic posturing against hard-line genetic determinism and thrived, even in severely reductionistic models that allowed for interplay and competition of various cellular lineages in development. Metchnikoff's vision of the phagocyte was the epiphany of the striving organism seeking its advantage in competition with its environment to establish hegemony in one sense, harmony in another. A consummate observer, his elegant descriptive powers, both graphically illustrative and logicodeductive, were oriented by a particular vision of life processes. In many facets, the development of the phagocytosis theory, its defense, and broad extrapolation were born out of Metchnikoff's personality—his dynamism and basic spirituality. The science can but reflect the man. In this case, to know Metchnikoff is to glimpse the workings of a mind that constructed an objective science around an underlying vision of biological processes. Upon that vague and largely undefined matrix, the foundation of a new biological and philosophical concept emerged along the axis of ancient opposition of harmony/disharmony. Only thereafter was the foundation of his research realized: the phagocytosis hypothesis, the resultant theory of immunity, and the modern concepts of inflammation. We may only tentatively claim such insight. Certainly, he could not enunciate this construction, but we have come to know Metchnikoff, the scientist and the man, and in the process have had the opportunity to peer into his mind from a vantage he never possessed and over time to focus our sights on his intellectual and ultimately spiritual struggle. It is a romantic chronicle (as Joseph Lister had already noted in 1896), for Metchnikoff was truly a man of his time and lived its ideal successfully. But his professional triumph more saliently reflected a personal resolution of a conflicted soul: a tempestuous, striving personality who still believed in the salvation of science and the domination of Nature. Perhaps it is under the guise as the author of modern immunology that the true romanticism is exposed, for it is in his naivete that nineteenth-century science most revealingly bases its limits. Alfred North Whitehead warned of misplaced concreteness, but Metchnikoff never could gain the perspective between goal and endeavor. In this sense, he truly was a nineteenth-century romantic whose identity was immersed in his science. In this narcissistic trap, Metchnikoff defined selfhood in a novel formulation and created a new science.

The story is well-defined chronologically, the sources readily available, the preceding scholarship, for our purpose, scant. This is not a biography in the usual sense; a comprehensive analysis of Metchnikoff's life is yet to be written, with careful examination of his unpublished correspondence and an assembly of the multitudinous historical record. The Russian archives, including his personal papers, have not been opened to recent scrutiny, and his position as national hero has not subjected him to a critical assessment. There are numerous chronicles of Metchnikoff's life, including an (auto)biography of his wife Olga. These are generally superficial treatments, and there has been no attempt to show how the theory of immunity was established as an intellectual endeavor. We have assigned ourselves only this last task. This endeavor required supplementation of the scientific record with analysis of scientific logic, interpersonal dynamics, and sympathetic scrutiny of the philosophical orientation of the researcher. We believe our collaboration has constructively complemented our respective analyses and thus is a synergistic product, one unlikely to have been developed independently of the enriched exchange of scientific and philosophical perspectives. Neither of us held exclusive domain over his own discipline, for only a sympathetic ear could have allowed this dialogue to thrive rather than turn into cacophony. We thus share equally in the result.

We are the first to admit that our exposition is potentially difficult, for it cannot rest in the individual fields of biology, history, or philosophy of science, but the book has been enriched by that ambiguity. Second, we have not been shy in focusing on either Metchnikoff's science or theory from a modern perspective, invoking insights from our vantage that not only serve to delineate Metchnikoff's thought but that potentially empower our own thinking with a new dimension. Finally, we have attempted to weave various themes into a coherent message by (a) tracing the embryological research of the period, (b) outlining Metchnikoff's relationship to the Darwinian debate, (c) reconstructing theories of inflammation and microbiology, and (d) synthesizing issues of teleology and vitalism into the ensuing scientific polemic. The book is organized in three general parts: the embryology of Metchnikoff's prephagocyte research serves as the scientific and metaphysical foundation of his entire career, and it is that work—divided roughly by 1872—that comprises the foundation of this study. It is in Metchnikoff's early research that we perceive the origin and development of his thinking concerning Darwinism, disharmony, selfhood, and the broad construct of his conception of organism. Following a brief biographical sketch and an introduction to his intellectual orientation (chap. 1), chapters 2 and 3 are devoted to an explication of Metchnikoff's early and mature embryological studies. A separate essay (chap. 4) discusses his evolutionary concepts *in toto;* then we proceed to set the stage for the phagocytosis theory with a description of Metchnikoff's concept of inflammation (chap. 5) in the context of his earlier, seemingly unrelated research. The difficulty pathologists of the 1880s had in accepting the phagocytosis theory is documented in chapter 6; in chapter 7, a discussion of Metchnikoff's hypothesis in the debate with other immunologists in the 1890s allows us the opportunity to explore his scientific eclipse. We have left to the notes and references—in places with quite extensive discussion—Metchnikoff's scientific legacy in various modern research areas and to two appendixes a modern perspective on the Darwinian debate and the science of the phagocyte, respectively.

The metaphysical infrastructure appears several times as we deal with Metchnikoff both as a scientist and as a philosopher of biology. He always maintained a strong theoretical orientation, but only in the retrospective treatment of his scientific development did that theoretician attain a degree of order and consistency. In fact, his career from its early beginnings was continuously influenced by his metaphysical orientation; this posture changed and in following the detail of his scientific development we are then offered an approach toward a more complete appreciation of Metchnikoff's contribution. Our concluding chapter attempts to summarize and extend the philosophical basis of Metchnikoff's science and to integrate the various avenues of his lifework around the theme of his novel conception of integrity. The epilogue (chap. 8) crystalizes what we concede is a radical interpretation of Metchnikoff's thesis, its scientific origins, and its metaphysical structure.

This book, of course, is our responsibility and in many respects represents an almost private dialogue with each other. We profited by publishing five articles (1–5) that were reviewed and revised according to the constructive criticisms offered by anonymous readers—to them we offer our sincere gratitude for the scholarly appraisal they offered. We also thank the editors, Sherwood Laurence *(Cellular Immunology)* and Everett Mendelsohn *(Journal of the History of Biology)* who kindly allowed major portions of the essays that first appeared in their journals to be included herein. We were generously supported by the Boston University School of Medicine, whose department chairpersons, Alan Cohen and Leonard Gottlieb, as well as successive deans, John Sandson and Aram Chobanian, collectively thought our academic mission might profitably be extended into the history and philosophy of biology. Further gratitude is extended to our co-workers at the Boston City Hospital who good-naturedly tolerated our rambling musings on this topic and knew that our frequent distractions were due to a good cause. Of these friends, Ann Marie Happnie, our secretary, deserves accolades for her tireless and expert efforts in preparing the manuscript. The assistance given by the Boston University School of Medicine Library in obtaining materials by interlibrary loan was invaluable, as were the translations by Anne Dubitzky. We appreciate the thoughtful discussions of Sahotra Sarkar, Daniel Todes, and Arthur Silverstein, and the useful comments by Jan Bibel, Gerald Weissmann, Bernard Babior, Manfred Karnovsky, Ilana Lowy, and Ann Marie Moulin, and especially Scott Gilbert's perspective, offered in the foreword. Needless to say, the good offices of Bill Curtis, our editor, and his staff at Oxford University Press, have made the process of obtaining the published product both highly professional and personally satisfying. Finally, and most important, we thank our families, whose love always sustained our endeavors and who served as our best, albeit uncritical, judges; thanks, also, to friends Isadore Twersky, Steve Levisohn, and David Kahzdan, whose enthusiastic support buoyed us throughout this venture. Of special note, we acknowledge that without the multitudinous support of Laszlo Tauber this project would never have been contemplated, for only by his generosity could we fulfill our ambition; we are most pleased to share our satisfaction with him.

Boston   A.I.T.
July 1990   L. C.

Contents

**Metchnikoff
and the Origins of
Immunology**

CHAPTER 1

Introduction

Immunology began as a biological discipline in the 1880s. It arose from convergence of several disciplines, principally microbiology, pathology, and embryology. The emergence of the germ theory of infectious diseases was well established by the mid-1870s. The studies by Robert Koch and Louis Pasteur of anthrax in 1876–1877, where each claimed to first establish the etiology of the disease (1), served as the experimental basis of a new discipline. Koch's postulates (although he never formally so presented them [2]) were quickly applied to human diseases, so that by the mid-1880s the basis of infectious diseases was firmly established as the science of microbiology. But how anthrax or mycobacteria caused disease was not Koch's original purpose. The nature of the inflammatory reaction at the end of the 1870s had still not attained its modern orientation. The function of leukocytes, the mediators involved, and the beneficial and deleterious aspects of inflammation as a reparative process were yet to be formulated into a coherent scheme. The key observations had been made, but the theoretical structure remained to be established. The third tributary to the birth of immunology was the formal discipline of comparative embryology. We can only attribute this research as seminal because the central theme of immunity was discovered by Elie Metchnikoff, who at the time of his discovery, was attempting to establish genealogical relationships of invertebrates based on the function of mesoderm-derived amoeboid phagocytic cells. Thus embryological research, an unlikely source for a new concept of immunity, served as the framework by which a new foundation of health and disease was erected. This book is devoted to charting the basis of Metchnikoff's work as it led to his theory, which has served as the foundation of twentieth-century immunology. Metchnikoff's novel insight that the host mounts an *active* response to invading pathogens was the first to propose such a reaction and arose from both his scientific observation and a new metaphysical concept of the organism. The theory of immunity was derived from an idea that organized well-known scientific facts into a novel concept of health and disease. Metchnikoff's seminal hypothesis has had repercussive effects on fields other than medicine, for example, evolutionary biology and embryology, but the theory has yielded its best harvest in immunology.

This book is not so much a history of immunology as an attempt to define the history of its basic idea. We will explore in detail the embryology of Metchnikoff's

3

research, for it is here that the biological concepts became enunciated. Metchnikoff, in retrospect, clearly saw the scientific line of his development, but that is only the sage rationalizing his adventure. The nature of his discovery is far more complex than he could acknowledge. The insight we might obtain in reconstructing his research logic reveals an intellectual portrait of a brilliant and creative scientist dogged in his pursuit of an ordered concept of organism, an idea that was fully integrated into his vision of selfhood and purpose. Metchnikoff was possessed to discover his own nature through his science, and he revealed that endeavor clearly in his published writings. The record is extraordinarily rich. We are fortunate to possess the materials to explore the nature of discovery and examine the inner workings of personality, logic, and observations on a scaffold so plainly exposed (3).

In the sense that Metchnikoff is an "interesting" scientist, the story has rich drama and offers insight into the process of discovery. But the history of Metchnikoff's phagocyte theory has broader importance, for it not only established the discipline of immunology but also formed the conceptual horizon of its scientific purpose. The struggle between Metchnikoff and the newly emerging biochemists who wished to measure and quantitate the immune reaction, and thereby define its mechanism, shifted the focus of primary interest from Metchnikoff's domain of cellular biology to that of immunochemistry. This deviation had enormous impact on the development of immunology, and it is only in relatively recent years that new consideration has focused on the nature of immunity that more closely corresponds to Metchnikoff's original hypothesis. We will explore new conceptual notions concerning the nature of the immunological reaction and will thus recognize that Metchnikoff's original broad concept of immunity must be resurrected in order to adequately assemble the divergent and varied roles of the immune system. The vision of immunity as reactive to pathogens is obviously an important aspect of leukocyte function, but endogenous self-recognition and integrative functions are emerging and declaring that what we have long-recognized as an immune reaction is but a specialized by-product of more fundamental self-regulatory processes.

Before dealing with our central purpose, a brief chronological sketch of our protagonist is offered prior to immersing ourselves in the details of his research. This biographical orientation is required to place in the contextual framework of his life's work the sequence of his discoveries and to understand the nature of the scientific debate that swirled around Metchnikoff.

A Biographical Note

Metchnikoff's life has been well documented because he was a celebrated and well-known biologist by the 1890s. He became a popular figure in France in the first decade of the century through his efforts to apply his scientific theories to health. With the Nobel Prize for physiology or medicine coawarded in 1908 to him and Paul Ehrlich, Metchnikoff's prominence was assured. The publication by his wife Olga of *The Life of Elie Metchnikoff* (1919) shortly after his death primarily contained autobiographical material, and it has served as the official rendition of his career. The account is simply offered with a minimum of psychological and scientific complexity.

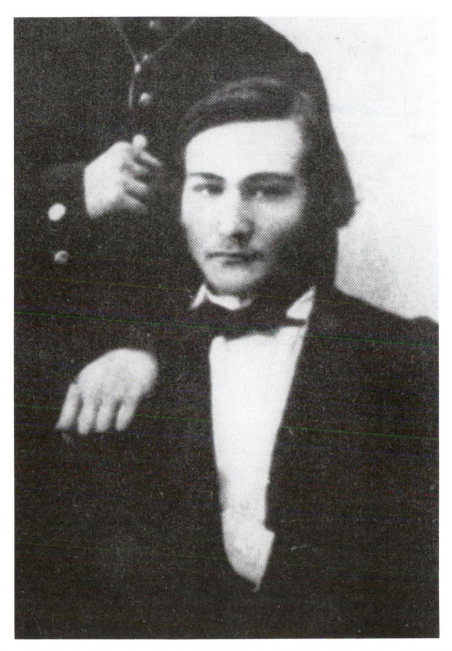

Figure 1. Metchnikoff, the student. Reprinted from P. Lepine, *Elie Metchnikoff et l'immunologie.* Vichy: Seghers, 1966.

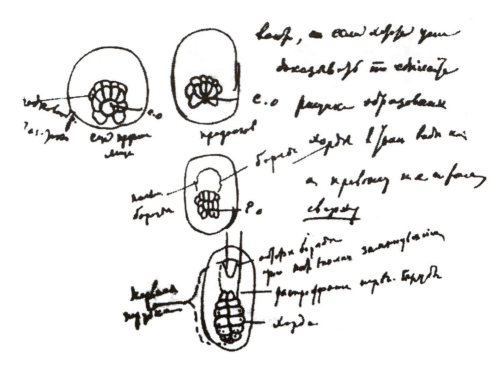

Figure 2. Letter fragment from A.O. Kowalevsky to Metchnikoff. Metchnikoff based his model of the primordial metazoan, *parenchymella,* as a colonial flagellate developed from a gastrulalike structure. His version differed from Haeckel's model primarily in noting that lower invertebrates gastrulate by introgression, not emboly, as do vertebrates. This distinction was made by another Russian embryologist, Kowalevsky, who in this letter fragment, diagrams the introgression process.

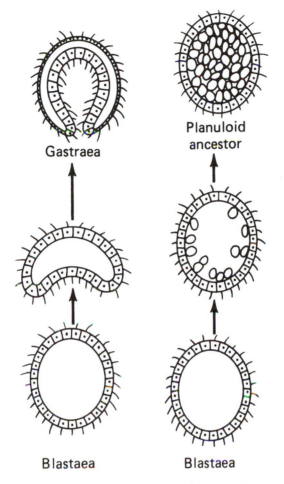

Gastraea

Planuloid
ancestor

Blastaea

Blastaea

Figure 3. The hypothetical development of Haeckel's *gastraea (left)* and the introgressive development of Metchnikoff's *parenchymella* modeled after planuloid development.

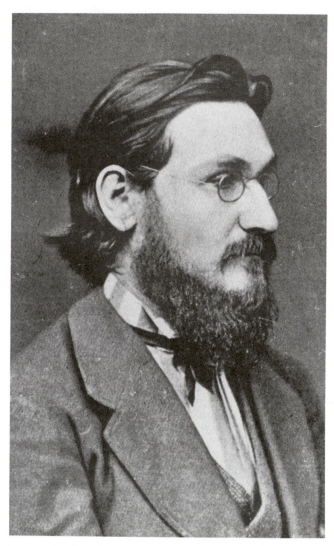

Figure 4. Elie Metchnikoff, 1875, O.N. Metchnikoff. *Life of Ilya Ilyitch Metchnikoff.* Moscow and Leningrad: State Publishing House, 1926.

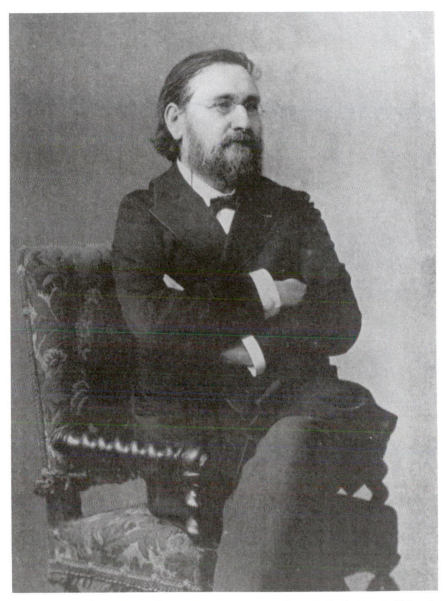

Figure 5. Metchnikoff in his forties. Reprinted frontispiece of E. Metchnikoff, *The Nature of Man: Studies in Optimistic Philosophy.* New York: Putnam, 1903.

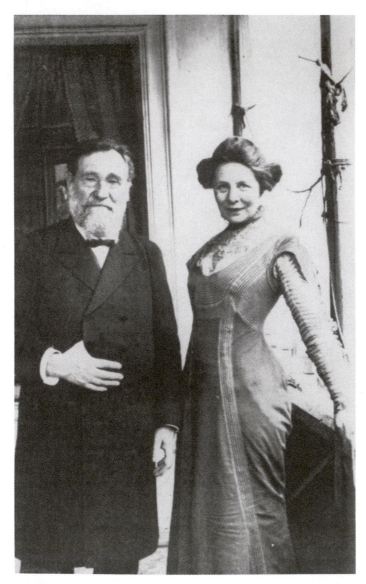

Figure 6. Elie and Olga Metchnikoff, approximately 1906. Reprinted from P. Lepine, *Elie Metchnikoff et l'immunologie.* Vichy: Seghers, 1966.

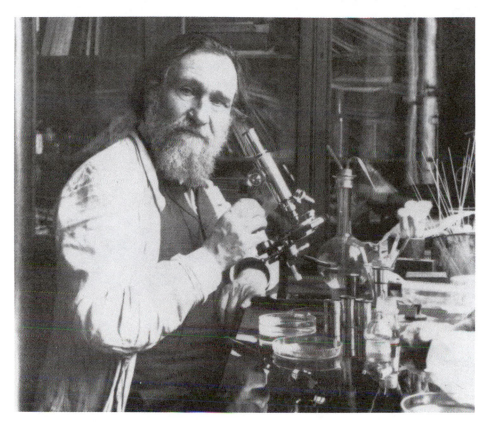

Figure 7. Metchnikoff at the Pasteur Institute, approximately 1906. Reprinted from P. Lepine, *Elie Metchnikoff et l'immunologie.* Vichy: Seghers, 1966.

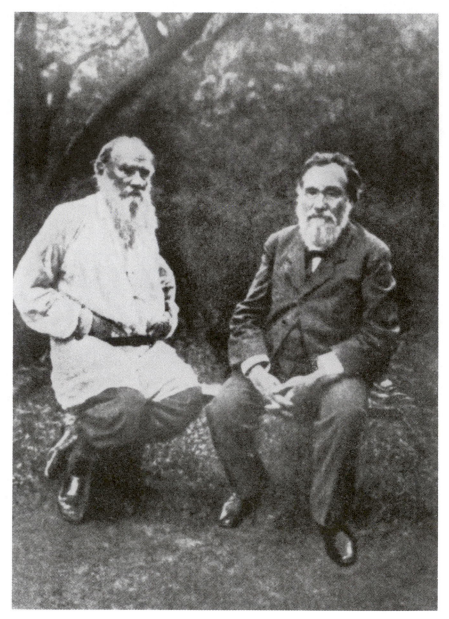

Figure 8. Leo Tolstoy and Elie Metchnikoff at Yasnay Polyana, May 30, 1909. Reprinted from S. Resnik, *Metchnikoff*. Moscow: Molodaya guardiya, 1973.

Written as a personal retrospective, the logical development of the research that led to the phagocytosis theory is defined, and the thread of its subsequent defense is given with self-righteous zeal. In this sense, the biography presents an insightful glimpse as to how Metchnikoff viewed himself: a figure whose logical approach, masterful defense, and honest intelligence attempted to devour the opposition and establish the primacy of his research. It is a sympathetic portrait and, in fact, deservedly so.

Elie Metchnikoff was born May 16, 1845, in Ivanovka, Kharkov Province, Russia, the youngest of five children. His father, Ilia Ivanovitch, an Imperial Guards' officer (eventually promoted to the rank of general) was a landowner who held serfs; for our purposes, he seems to have had little impact on his children, remaining aloof and seemingly indifferent to their development, which he left to his wife. Elie's mother, Emilia Lvovna, was the daughter of a converted Jewish entrepreneur (later a writer), Leo Nevahovitch; she apparently had a close and loving relationship with her children. Metchnikoff, in 1909, cited his Jewish roots as the source of his scientific genius (4), and clearly identified with a nebulous and assimilated Jewish heritage. There is no clear record that he was professionally restricted in Russia because of his lineage, but he sympathized with the problem his Jewish colleagues suffered owing to Russian anti-Semitism; his personal religious commitment was to atheism (4), although he received strict Christian religious training at home. However, Metchnikoff's atheism smacked of religious fervor in the embrace of rationalism and science. We may fairly argue that Metchnikoff's religion was based on the belief that rational scientific discourse was the solution for human suffering. His enthusiasm for the Pasteur Institute, where he arrived almost as a refugee in 1888, echoed the prevalent cloistered attitude of the staff, who ventured out into the world to combat epidemics but otherwise remained huddled in study like medieval monks devoted in a singular fashion to obtaining insight and revelation. Metchnikoff found a true home in this secularized seminary.

As a child he was tutored at home, where his volatile nature was hardly contained. He was nicknamed Quicksilver, which might well have been retained in his later years during the highly defensive and impassioned defense of his scientific views—first as an embryologist, later as an immunologist. He was energetic, highly intelligent, and manipulative. Given the diagnosis of frailty and poor eyes, he often rubbed them, invoking irritation in order to combat restrictions on his whims. Although indulged, his mother viewed him as neurotic and his older sister called him "a little beast." We catch glimpses of this personality throughout his public career and most dramatically on the occasions of his suicide attempts, when frustration was dealt with in the most extreme form of denial. Elie was pampered throughout his life by mother and wife, and he poorly tolerated scientific criticism or academic restrictions.

The romance of the developing biologist seems almost a story of a child with possessed purpose. In a comic account, Olga narrates how at age eight, Elie began collecting flowers and writing descriptions; he offered his pocket money to his siblings to listen to his botanical discourses! By age eleven, he had begun his natural history library and almost drowned by falling into a pond while collecting hydrae. In 1856, he enrolled in the Kharkov Lycée, where he was an excellent student. He pursued his interest in science aggressively, attending supplemental lectures at the university and beginning his microscopic studies of infusoria. At this time, being attracted by

Rudolf Virchow's cellular theory, he already envisioned the prospect of creating a grand theory of medicine. A hastily written paper was accepted by the *Bulletin of the Moscow Society of Naturalists,* but Metchnikoff withdrew it because of erroneous conclusions (5). The first acknowledged publication was a critical review of a geology textbook published in the *Journal de Moscow.* Metchnikoff was sixteen years old. The facts point to singular purpose, precocious intelligence, and highly energized motivation. But sensitivity and naivete took its toll for the wunderkind. Attracted to Germany, he wished to enroll at the University of Wuerzburg and study with Rudolf Koelliker, but Metchnikoff arrived six weeks prior to the beginning of the term. Received with hostility by other Russian students (Paul de Kruif says because of his Jewishness [6]), Metchnikoff quickly returned to Kharkov and enrolled at the university there. The most important result of his visit to Germany was the acquisition of Charles Darwin's *Origin of Species,* a seminal work for Metchnikoff's personal scientific career. His formal reviews of this work will be studied in detail later; each review reflects a step in Metchnikoff's scientific and philosophical development.

Originally, Metchnikoff wished to study medicine, but his mother dissuaded him, arguing that he was too sensitive to witness suffering. We suspect that this rationalization played a role, but the detemined young scientist seems to have already defined his interests. He thus embarked on zoological studies under the tutelage of Ivan Petrovich Tschelkoff, one of the few Kharkov professors Metchnikoff respected. Not content with attending lectures, Metchnikoff began his own research with a study of the mobile stalk of a ciliated infusorian, the *Vorticella,* to characterize whether it was analogous to muscle in higher organisms. His paper, published in 1863 in *Muellers Archives* (7) was severely criticized by Wilhelm Kuhne, and after Metchnikoff confirmed his original conclusions (8), Kuhne aggressively rebutted. The bitterness of this first encounter repeatedly punctuated Metchnikoff's career.

Metchnikoff's university career lasted only two years, condensing the usual period by half. He aborted his research activities, intensified his studies with minimal social distractions, and thus passed his qualifying exams. Metchnikoff still required a thesis, so in 1864, he went to the North Sea island of Heligoland where the botanist Ferdinand Cohn guided him to Rudolf Leuckart of Giessen University. Metchnikoff read two papers at the Naturalists Congress held in Giessen; struck by his precociousness, Leuckart immediately accepted him into his laboratory. The two key events of this period were reading Fritz Mueller's *Fuer Darwin* and discovering the alternation of sexual and asexual generations in nematodes wherein parasitic hermaphroditic worms give birth to a free bisexual generation. According to Olga Metchnikoff, Mueller's book had a profound influence because it was the first to purportedly confirm Darwin's theory by tracing genealogies through embryonic structures. However, we view the true basis of Metchnikoff's research prior to the mid-1870s with some skepticism in regard to this grand scheme. We have not been convinced that "an uninterrupted thread can be followed right through his life-work, from the beginning to the end" ([3] *Life,* p. 52). Although there is obvious continuity of Metchnikoff's research, the underlying rationale does not necessarily follow this simple quest for evolution's structure. This issue will be discussed in detail later, but it suffices to simply note here that because of eyestrain, Metchnikoff took a vacation (visiting his brother in Geneva) and discovered that Leuckart had stolen his results and published them independently. Metchnikoff publicly denounced the theft (in DuBois-Rey-mond's journal, *Arch. Anat. Physiol. wiss. Med.*) (9) and in 1865 went off to Naples with a grant from the Russian Ministry of Public Instruction. His singleness of pur-pose must have insulated him from both professional frustrations and ill health. In Italy, he began a systematic study of germ layers in invertebrate embryos, sharing common interests with another Russian zoologist, Alexander O. Kowalevsky, with whom he had a long-standing and productive (at times acrimonious) collaboration.

Metchnikoff found time to delve into philosophical writings that reflected his sci-entific orientation. He first focused on educational issues (begun in 1868 but pub-lished three years later) (10), but soon extended his musings to broad cultural and biological issues. In summary, Metchnikoff began with a new metaphysical con-struct: the organism began not as a totality of harmonious elements that when dis-rupted by disease or environmental factors then strove to regain its harmonious bal-ance; instead, the organism was intrinsically disharmonious and its biology was based on the endeavor of integrating the disharmonious elements by active processes. From early adulthood until the end of his life, Metchnikoff wrote extensively on this subject and applied it to the fields of social and natural philosophy. In such works as *The Nature of Man: Studies in Optimistic Philosophy* (11) and *The Prolongation of Life: Optimistic Studies* (12), he extrapolated his embryological (and later immunological) studies to broad generalizations of the biological basis of human behavior, aging, and social organization. We will explore these issues in terms of Metchnikoff's early sci-entific development in order to establish the broad construct of his Weltanschauung. We believe this offers fascinating insight into scientific discovery and also leads to a broader study of his conceptual framework.

In the autumn of 1865, Metchnikoff continued his formal embryological studies in Goettingen and then Munich independent of his faculty mentors; once again, he returned to Naples in 1867, where he and Kowalevsky finished their studies. They returned to Saint Petersburg to receive their doctorates and shared in the prestigious von Baer Prize. Metchnikoff's early work, in a sense, predicted his scientific devel-opment, and we may well appreciate the inner dynamics of his thinking from this period. Much of our purpose will be to examine in detail the concrete research and underlying embryological studies pursued until the 1882 phagocyte experiments. We must note here that Metchnikoff's later (after the mid-1870s) evolutionary approach to embryology excluded the assumption that in an ontogenetic development there was some universal, predetermined scheme of evolution realized. This was in direct conflict with Ernst Haeckel and other prominent embryologists of the time. In con-trast, Metchnikoff projected embryological data to offer a powerful means for a reconstruction of some particular, not general, phylogenetic development (13).

At age twenty-two, Metchnikoff was appointed *docent* at the new University of Odessa. Soon after his arrival, the hot-tempered young man was so incensed that he had not been initially chosen to represent the university at a congress of Russian naturalists that he incited his students to protest and thus won a place at the meeting. This incident of academic intrigue—one of many that was to plague him until he found a happy home with Pasteur in 1888—and the prospect of better working con-ditions at Saint Petersburg (which proved illusionary), prompted his transfer in 1868. His scientific research of this period was conducted on sponges and echinoderms; but he was bitterly disappointed with his working conditions, salary, and general disposition of life in Saint Petersburg, which reinforced his growing melancholy and pessimism. At this time, he turned to Ludmilla Federovitch for succor, and they fell in ‚ love during an illness in which she nursed him. They were married in 1869, but the bride, suffering from "bronchitis," was carried to the church in a chair and ultimately died of tuberculosis in April 1873. Metchnikoff attended her compassionately (contemplating leaving science and opening a bookshop in the more salubrious climate of Madeira to be with her); and upon her death, he became so depressed that he attempted suicide. One of the most bizarre incidents narrated by Olga is the description of Metchnikoff awakening from a morphine stupor and, dismayed at his failure to successfully commit suicide, resolving on the need to contract a grave illness that would

> save him, either by ending in death or by awaking the vital instinct in him. In order to attain his object, he took a very hot bath and then exposed himself to cold. As he was coming back by the Rhone bridge [in Geneva], he suddenly saw a cloud of winged insects flying around the flame of a lantern. They were Phryganidae, but in the distance he took them for Ephemeridae, and the sight of them suggested the following reflection: "How can the theory of natural selection be applied to these insects? They do not feed and only live a few hours; they are therefore not subject to the struggle for existence, they do not have time to adapt themselves to surrounding conditions." His thoughts turned towards Science; he was saved; the link with life was re-established. ([3] *Life,* p. 81)

Science as religion was a recurrent theme of Metchnikoff's life, ordering his passions, resolving his pessimism, focusing his ambition.

> His dominating point was his passionate vocation; his worship of Science and of Reason made of him an inspired apostle. He had the faults and qualities of a rich and powerful nature. Vibrating through all the fibres of his being, he shed life and light around him. His temper was violent and passionate; he could bear no attack on the ideas which were dear to him, and became combative as soon as he thought them threatened. His was a wrestler's temperament; obstacles exasperated his energy and he went straight for them, pursuing his object with an invincible tenacity; he never gave up a problem, however difficult, and never hesitated to face any sacrifice or any privation if he thought them necessary. ([3] *Life,* p. 96)

Metchnikoff returned to Odessa in 1872 (and remained on the university faculty until 1882). With the personal tragedy of Ludmilla's death in Madeira, his eyesight worsened (psychosomatic [?]), and he joined an anthropological expedition to the Kalmuk steppes. On his return from the expedition, he met Olga Belokopitova in Odessa. Olga fulfilled the requisites of his original idea of a wife: young, impressionable, and susceptible to "training . . . according to his own ideas" ([3] *Life,* p. 87). Olga, in turn, felt "terror that he must be mistaken about me; I felt as if I were going up for an examination without any previous study" ([3] *Life,* p. 88). Olga passed admirably, and they were married in February 1875; she served as Metchnikoff's close confidante, assistant, and (later) collaborator throughout his life. They never had children. Truly, only an extraordinary devotee could have admired Metchnikoff so completely as to tolerate such a volatile and narcissistic man. Her infatuation was complete: she described him "not unlike a figure of Christ" ([3] *Life,* p. 89).

Metchnikoff's Odessa period (1872–1882) was marked by an active teaching schedule and involvement in academic politics. There was feuding between the Ukrainian and Moscow faculty along liberal–conservative ideologies. Metchnikoff attempted to remain aloof, but with the assassination of Tsar Alexander II in 1881, reactionaries gained control, limited the independence of the university, and made political appointments to the faculty. Matters worsened and Metchnikoff was active in the attempt to restore academic integrity; in the process, he witnessed the collapse of academic freedom and resigned. The combination of political unrest, Olga's infection with typhoid in 1880, and the difficulty of pursuing his science led Metchnikoff to a second suicide attempt after his resignation. He injected himself with the spirochete *(Borrelia)* of relapsing fever; after a long illness, he recovered. It is noteworthy that this volatile, yet resilient man, had a renaissance of vitality. His eye problems never recurred again. We believe this was coincident with a general reorientation of his pessimistic philosophy to an optimism that was reflected in his phagocytosis theory and his later philosophical writings. For it was out of this period that Metchnikoff made his most important discovery: the defensive function of leukocytes. That insight totally reoriented his scientific career from embryologist to that of the first immunologist and, concomitantly, turned his pessimistic philosophy of life into an optimistic one.

As early as 1865 in Giessen, Metchnikoff studied the terrestrial flatworm (planarian) *Geodesmus bilineatus,* which lacked a gut and whose digestion he compared to the digestive process of protozoans (14). Between that study and his extensive research begun around 1877 on intracellular digestion of invertebrates, he was primarily occupied with the search for fundamental principles to establish a theoretical basis for comparative embryology. This line of inquiry was translated into a predominant interest in inflammation and infectious diseases. By 1882, while he was in Messina, having escaped from the political turmoil of Odessa, Metchnikoff concentrated his scientific efforts on establishing the basic function of mesodermal amoeboid cells through the phyla, thus merging his interest in embryology with a newly acquired commitment to inflammation. With the death of Olga's parents in 1881, Metchnikoff was endowed with financial resources that allowed him to move to Italy to conduct his research free of academic and political encumbrances. The laboratory was set up in the drawing room of an apartment convenient to fishermen who provided the required specimens. It was an idyllic time and his seminal discovery is described in a romantic and highly contrived manner:

One day when the whole family had gone to a circus to see some extraordinary performing apes, I remained alone with my microscope, observing the life in the mobile cells of a transparent star-fish larva, when a new thought suddenly flashed across my brain. It struck me that similar cells might serve in the defence of the organism against intruders. Feeling that there was in this something of surpassing interest, I felt so excited that I began striding up and down the room and even went to the seashore in order to collect my thoughts. I said to myself that, if my supposition was true, a splinter introduced into the body of a star-fish larva, devoid of blood vessels or of a nervous system, should soon be surrounded by mobile cells as is to be observed in a man who runs a splinter into his finger. This was no sooner said than done.

There was a small garden to our dwelling, in which we had a few days previously organized a "Christmas tree" for the children [in-laws] on a little tangerine tree; I fetched from it a few rose thorns and introduced them at once under the skin of some beautiful star-fish larvae as transparent as water.

I was too excited to sleep that night in the expectation of the result of my experiment, and very early the next morning I ascertained that it had fully succeeded.

That experiment formed the basis of the phagocyte theory, to the development of which I devoted the next twenty-five years of my life. ([3] *Life,* pp. 116–117)

Why Metchnikoff viewed this discovery as a flash of insight and not the product of a deliberate and exhaustive research program is a problem we must address.

The presentation of his theory to Rudolf Virchow and Nicholaus Kleinenberg who were in Messina that summer of 1883, was well received; Karl Claus in Vienna helped coin the term *phagocyte* (from the Greek *phagos* [to eat] and *cyte* [cell]). The first publication in 1883 did not arouse much interest, but when applied as the mechanism of host defense, Metchnikoff came under intense criticism. The opponents did not offer an alternative theory, and it was not until the humoralists established their position (1888–1892) that a true debate ensued. It is of interest that Metchnikoff initially carried out his experiments in the realm of physiological inflammation and continued his embryological research with the formal presentation of the *phagocytella* primal metazoan (earlier called *parenchymella*) in 1886. But Metchnikoff soon became a pathologist, abandoning his zoological orientation by the early 1890s. It is of particular interest that this career shift coincided with the emergence of experimental embryology in the same period. This is hardly an accident in that, strictly from a methodological perspective, it was quite simple for Metchnikoff to apply his extraordinary observational skills to the newly developed field of immunology. He probably did not anticipate that this nascent science would also soon turn to a reductionistic approach in its research program. Chemistry, not observation, would serve as the primary tool of the emerging discipline.

By 1886, Metchnikoff had become an international scientific celebrity. He was invited back to Odessa to head a research institute (similar in design to the Pasteur Institute) devoted to bacteriological studies. This was his last Russian appointment. His desire to emigrate was sealed by his frustration owing to internal political and administrative intrigue, by his inability to conduct a human immunization program because he was not a physician, and by a disastrous inoculation of sheep. Metchnikoff visited Germany, looking for refuge, but was either received with hostility or otherwise found his options limited. Fortuitously, he visited Pasteur, who greeted him warmly. The Pasteur Institute opened in November 1888, and Metchnikoff was given an entire floor for his cellular immunology school. He retained two rooms for his own use, which he kept until his death on July 16, 1916. The first half of this period in his career was devoted to a ferocious defense of the phagocytosis theory and is conveniently bracketed by two summary texts: *Lectures on the Comparative Pathology of Inflammation,* derived from lectures he delivered at the Pasteur Institute in April and May 1891 (15), and his consummate opus, *Immunity in Infective Diseases,* published in 1901 (16). These works present fair and comprehensive statements of Metchnikoff's scientific posture of this period: the phagocyte was the defensive moiety of immunity, with humoral factors but elaborated leukocyte products. His steadfast and restricted posture reflected his personality: although mellowed,

Metchnikoff lost none of his vociferous nature. For our purposes, the relevant bio-graphical orientation is complete. He continued to work in his laboratory, collabo-rating with Émile Roux on syphilis studies (showing both its transference to monkeys and the efficacy of treatment with mercurials), but his primary attention now turned to applying his biological theories to health and longevity.

Metchnikoff, after completing *Immunity in Infective Diseases* turned almost exclu-sively to the problem of how to extend his notions of harmony/disharmony and, more specifically, the role of the phagocyte in the problem of senility—the natural deterioration of the body. The genesis of this work can be traced to his reply to the humoralists, who had shown by the mid-1890s that bacterial toxins elicited an immune response. Metchnikoff, of course, believed the phagocytes played a direct role in the neutralization of toxins; in 1897 at a congress held in Moscow, he pre-sented a paper on the phagocytosis reaction against toxins (17). His position arose, naturally, out of a defense of the phagocytosis theory. At this time, Metchnikoff's health was deteriorating: recurrent tachycardia, insomnia, and mild kidney dysfunc-tion. His response in light of the potential to establish "harmony" (i.e., cure his ailing and aging body) was to interject corrective (balancing) factors, and he decided that a hygienic diet would correct a chronic poisoning by intestinal microbes. Soon after completing *Immunity in Infective Diseases,* he delivered a lecture in Manchester (1901) entitled "Flora of the Human Body." This was the formal presentation of a theory he expounded in several books (11,12) and extended essays (e.g., *The New Hygiene,* 18), which became a crusade that preoccupied him for the rest of his life. Basically, he believed that the large intestine, a supposed atavistic organ in man, housed deleterious bacteria whose elaborated toxins diffused into the body, thus damaging normal tissue. The cumulative damage was then detected by the phago-cytes, which in mounting a scavenging attack caused further tissue damage that might not be repaired. The result was bodily deterioration. With the replacement of the colon's natural bacteria with *lactobacilli,* Metchnikoff hoped to reverse the senile process by limiting the elaboration of damaging toxins. He suggested a diet that con-tained curdled milk or yogurt, thus promoting a new industry in France. *The Nature of Man* (1903) (11) and *Prolongation of Life* (1907) (12) extended this scientific phi-losophy, and he continued to dabble in the laboratory to verify his hypothesis relating senility and intestinal flora, but with little success.

In 1908, Metchnikoff went to Sweden to accept the Nobel Prize (shared with Paul Ehrlich) and then made a triumphant tour of Russia. He met Leo Tolstoy in 1909. The famous interchange of the apostles of Science and Spirituality was reported as cordial and polite. Metchnikoff was enthralled with Tolstoy; Tolstoy thought Metch-nikoff a bit naive. Metchnikoff fulfilled the role of elder scientific statesman until his death. He led an expedition in 1911 to study tuberculosis susceptibility in the same Kalmuk steppes that he had visited as a young man, and he continued to maintain his laboratory in Paris. With the outbreak of hostilities in 1914, the Pasteur Institute was essentially closed; the men went off to war, the animals used in experiments were killed, and Metchnikoff was left depressed at the irrationality and futility of this col-lapse of civilization. Olga makes the emphatic point that Metchnikoff's demise was closely related to the overwhelming sense of loss the Great War personified, both in terms of the young lives lost and the awful challenge to his hard-won optimism. In a profound sense, Metchnikoff's optimistic ideology was assaulted by the trauma of the war. Bedridden with prolonged cardiac failure for several months, he finally died shortly after his seventy-first birthday. To the very end, however, he defended his views of orthobiosis, believing that heredity and the belated introduction of a rational diet at age fifty-three limited the interventions he had applied. His optimism triumphed, as Olga quotes him two days before his death:

> Everything which troubled me, everything that seemed so disturbing, so terrible, like this war for instance, seems so transitory now, such a small thing by the side of the great problems of existence! . . . Science will solve them some day. ([3] *Life,* p. 270)

Metchnikoff's Autobiographical Retrospection of His Phagocytosis Hypothesis

Dealing with the history of the phagocytosis hypothesis, one must be cautious concerning Metchnikoff's retrospective attempts to reconstruct its history. A complete account is found in the biography written by his wife, but the true coauthor of this work was Elie Metchnikoff himself:

> Often [recalls Olga Metchnikoff], when he was not too tired, he would sit comfortably in his armchair and recount to me with his usual spirit and animation some period or episode of his past. I read to him a sketch of the first part of this biography and a few chapters only of the second, which was hardly begun. Thus we spent many evenings, never to be forgotten.

> He wanted this biography written, for he held that the evolution of mind, of a character, of a human life is always an interesting psychological document. (19, pp. xxii–xxiii)

As if this statement were insufficient to convince us of Metchnikoff's authorship, in works published after 1883 (the year the phagocytosis hypothesis was presented), he often reviewed the theoretical controversies of the theory's prehistory, always outlining them in a similar manner to Olga's account. Relative to current scientific publications, memoirs make an essential contribution in reconstructing the history of ideas. We expect to find not only an outline that formulates the idea in question but, more important, a personal testament of how the idea was born; we are less interested in a satisfactory solution of the problem than in an account of the true circumstances under which the problem was formulated. We hope to find that very "subjective" factor whose creative effort was responsible for the genesis of the idea. No wonder the different aspects of Metchnikoff's theoretical development, as they are presented in Olga Metchnikoff's account as well as in the few short memoirs written by Elie Metchnikoff himself (collected in *The Pages of Memory* [20]), dominate most works devoted to the history of the phagocytosis idea. The factual history of Metchnikoff's scientific results, arguments with his opponents, and the temporal order of his intellectual development have been well studied. But such recounts that represent themselves as history of ideas appear to be only repetitions of Metchnikoff's own renditions (e.g., V. A. Dogel and A. E. Gaisinovich [21]), despite the apparent contradictions in these reconstructions with the factual history. On the other hand, in works that follow more closely the factual history (as in the serious papers of A. D. Nekrasov, "Metchnikoff's Works in Embryology" [22]; and in R. I. Belkin, "Metchnikoff's Embryological Studies as Evaluated by His Contemporaries" [23]), there is no attempt to understand theoretical development as history in a broad intellectual context.

Our memory is not a mere record of the history of our thoughts but an intrinsic component of that history. We imperil the veracity of our understanding by replacing the history of a thought with our thoughts about the history; thus, we replace the true development of the problem with our final, refined, and filtered appraisal. Olga Metchnikoff writes, "In his life, as in his work, everything was so closely knitted that it was impossible to understand the whole without knowledge of every link of his evolution" (19, p. xxii). To trace Metchnikoff's general idea of active immunological defense requires that we first establish the most crucial links in his research development. And here we meet with some apparent difficulties and inconsistencies. First, there are contradictions between the factual history of Metchnikoff's scientific development and his retrospective account of that history. He would like to believe that "an uninterrupted thread can be followed right through his life work, from the beginning until the end" (19, p. 51). The autobiographical version of this thread may be summarized:

> At age eighteen (1863), Metchnikoff read Darwin's *Origin of Species:* The theory of evolution deeply struck the boy's mind and his thoughts immediately turned in that direction. He said to himself that isolated forms which had found no place in definite animal or vegetable orders might perhaps serve as a bond between those orders and elucidate their genetic relationships. (19, p. 41)

Devotion to Darwin's idea focused Metchnikoff's interest in zoology. Sometime around 1865, he read Fritz Mueller's *Fuer Darwin,* a book that "had a decisive influence on the future direction of his researches" (19, p. 50). Working with crustaceans, Fritz Mueller had demonstrated that the most important information concerning the genealogy of creatures was to be found in their embryology. It was the basic result that supported the future formulation of the so-called Mueller–Haeckel biogenetic law. Olga Metchnikoff states, "Under influence of this work, Elie . . . resolved to concentrate all his efforts on the comparative embryology of animals" (19, p. 50).

In the 1860s, extensive knowledge of the three primary embryonic layers in vertebrates had been accumulated but correspondingly little was known about invertebrates. To establish the evolutionary unity of animals and thus support Darwinism, Metchnikoff began his studies in the neglected field of invertebrate embryology. Over the next several years, Metchnikoff and his friend A. O. Kowalevsky created a new field of biology: comparative embryology of invertebrates. They also demonstrated that the individual development of invertebrates begins with the same three embryonic layers as found in vertebrates. In 1865, Kowalevsky discovered the development of two embryonic layers in *Amphioxus* (lancelet) larvae. He observed a division of the lancelet's fertilized ovule into a set of new cell segments. The division had turned the ovule into a multicellular sphere (the blastula). Then, one-half of the blastula was observed to sink into the other (invagination), thus forming a two-layered creature— the gastrula. Soon thereafter, the surface of the embryo was covered with cilia, and the oval embryo ruptured the ovule's membrane and freed the gastrula to begin its free-swimming phase. Lancelet, a Chordata, has larvae that are similar to those of invertebrates, and Kowalevsky extended these observations to other lower metazoans, obtaining similar results. Metchnikoff first met Kowalevsky during the summer of 1865 in Naples. He recalled, "In Naples I was able to be convinced with my own eyes in the truth and importance of the discovery of the lancelet larvae" (20, p. 24). The discovery, according to Metchnikoff's testament, firmly established the fact that "vertebrates and invertebrates are connected by the indissoluble link of wandering by cilia lancelet larvae" (20, p. 26).

Kowalevsky believed that invagination, the forming of two embryonic layers, was characteristic for most, if not all, multicellular organisms. Concurrently, Metchnikoff discovered among sponges, hydroids, and lower medusae a second pattern of embryonic layer formation. He observed that the second layer (the endoderm) was formed not by means of invagination (of the ectoderm), but by migration of a number of flagellated cells from one pole of the blastula wall into the central cavity. These cells drew in their flagellum and became amoeboid and mobile, multiplied by division, filled the cavity of the blastula, and became capable of digestion. Metchnikoff named this stage, *parenchymella.* In the organisms forming a digestive cavity, this parenchymatic mass differentiated further into two layers: the mesoderm and the endoderm. Thus, in these cases, the gastrula formed not by invagination, but by introgression.

In 1872, Haeckel (*Die Kalkschwaemme,* Vol. 2. Berlin: G. Reiner, 1872), using Kowalevsky's discovery of the development of the lancelet larvae, formulated his famous *gastraea* hypothesis in which he proposed that the common metazoan ancestor was similar to the lancelet's gastrula. The hypothetical model was supposed to provide comparative embryology with a phylogenetic basis. Acknowledging the importance of this kind of theoretical reconstruction, Metchnikoff, on the one hand, argued that the true author of the hypothesis was Kowalevsky; on the other hand, he asserted that his own *parenchymella* more closely fitted the role of the embryonic image of the primordial metazoan. Haeckel's model presupposed that extracellular digestion within a digestive cavity was the basic feature of complex organisms, recapitulating the function of the *gastraea* digestive cavity. Metchnikoff's *parenchymella* represented intracellular digestion as the common feature of unicellular organisms and most primitive metazoans. This archaic form of digestion had been preserved in the ability of the amoeboid mesodermal cells of the higher animals to perform intracellular digestion. Thus, the function of the mesodermal cells provided an evolutionary basis for the comparative embryology of animals. The study of the evolutionary fate of this function led Metchnikoff to the idea of phagocytosis as the crucial process in ontogenetic development and as the mechanism for active immunological defense. This is the prehistory of the phagocytosis idea as it was seen by Metchnikoff himself and repeated by many historians of the idea. Thus, according to this version, the most crucial events of Metchnikoff's phagocytosis hypothesis development were:

(a) Metchnikoff's early enthusiasm from the age of eighteen for the Darwinian theory of evolution determined his decision to study zoology in order to prove the evolutionary kinship of different animal groups.

(b) Metchnikoff's early acquaintance with Fritz Mueller's *Fuer Darwin* and the decision to study comparative embryology were the most powerful means for establishing evolutionary kinship.

(c) Metchnikoff recognized the validity of Kowalevsky's description of lancelet larvae.

(d) The lancelet discovery was important to Metchnikoff for reconstruction of evolutionary relationships, and this kind of reconstruction was crucial for the success of comparative embryology itself.

(e) Metchnikoff observed an alternative formation of two-layered fetuses in sponges, hydroids, and lower medusae.

(f) Metchnikoff's polemic with Haeckel's theory of *gastraea*—according to Metchnikoff's view—suffered from a nonscientific naturphilosophical generalization and schematization of Kowalevsky's ideas and added nothing new to Metchnikoff's own opinion on the relationship between evolutionary biology and comparative embryology.

(g) Metchnikoff's formulation of the *parenchymella* theory, with its focus on intracellular digestion, illustrated the evolutionary development of the function of amoeboid mesodermal cells.

This is the reconstructed scheme of how Metchnikoff formulated the general biological background of his phagocytosis hypothesis. But it is astonishing how little this recount, tested by documents of the time (scientific publications, manuscripts, and private correspondence), coincides with the factual history:

(a) Metchnikoff did read Darwin's *Origin of Species* in 1863, but as seen in his essay written in the same year (24), his reaction to the book was highly critical. He did not change his negative position for the next several years.

(b) Metchnikoff did read Fritz Mueller's *Fuer Darwin* around 1865. But in no way did the book determine his approach to comparative embryology. Even in 1869, four years after Kowalevsky's description of the gastrula, when Metchnikoff himself was already deeply involved in comparative embryologic study, he firmly opposed those embryologists he called the Darwinians, and he included Mueller and Haeckel as prominent among them.

(c) In 1902, Metchnikoff wrote that in Naples in 1865 he was able to convince himself of the truth and importance of Kowalevsky's discovery of lancelet larvae development. But later in 1865, during Kowalevsky's defense of his master's thesis about the development of *Amphioxus* (lancelet), it was Metchnikoff who heatedly stated that Kowalevsky's claim was nonsense and that the digestive cavity never, and nowhere, could be formed by invagination. In 1866, Metchnikoff published a paper in which he stated that Kowalevsky's assertion about invagination was in contradiction with all known facts (25). The polemic continued at least until 1873. Thus, it is problematic to refer to parallel and coordinated work of the two friends (26).

(d) In his publications immediately following Kowalevsky's discovery, Metchnikoff did not write about the importance of the discovery for reconstructing evolutionary relationships. He asserted something quite the opposite: morphological similarities of different groups of animals is a well-known fact, but there is no necessity to interpret them as a reflection of "blood relations" (27). There is no evidence that in his early comparative embryological studies, Metchnikoff considered this kind of reconstruction of any significant importance for comparative embryology itself. But opposite evidence exists (27).

(e) Metchnikoff did observe an alternative way of formulating primary embryonic layers in sponges, hydroids, and lower medusae, but those observations do not necessarily indicate that from the very beginning he considered those results as a basis for an alternative in respect to Haeckel's phylogenetic reconstruction.

(f) Metchnikoff in his polemic against the *gastraea* theory did accuse Haeckel of nonscientific naturphilosophical generalizations of some known facts and neglect of others. But it is not true that the theory offered Metchnikoff no lead. Indeed, under the influence of Haeckel's theory, Metchnikoff recognized the importance of phylogenetic reconstruction for studies in comparative embryology. The *gastraea* theory concentrated his attention on the role of intracellular digestion in phylogenetic and ontogenetic development.

(g) The facts Metchnikoff laid down as the basis of his *parenchymella* hypothesis had been discovered by Metchnikoff himself. But the logic that structured the facts into a hypothesis had been elaborated in the arguments with Haeckel. Metchnikoff's hypothesis was the answer to the problems generated by the *gastraea* theory, which had failed to offer a satisfactory solution.

This discrepancy between Metchnikoff's retrospective history of the phagocytosis hypothesis and the actual facts of its development can hardly be explained by Metchnikoff's ambitious unwillingness to recognize his own mistakes or by his intention to affirm his own priority in every step of the process. We know that after the publication of the phagocytosis theory a few pretenders claimed priority, but Metchnikoff was not concerned with that question and focused on the real problems of the theory itself (28). Metchnikoff was the author of a revolutionary idea, and in some sense we concur with Olga Metchnikoff that there was a certain logic in his intellectual development. The discrepancies in his account of the prehistory of the phagocytosis hypothesis do not result from a conscious intention to put his own scientific development in a more attractive light, but rather are the result of an intention to *present* the phagocytosis hypothesis. And from this tidied up retrospection, Metchnikoff presents a refined and altered attitude toward Darwin, Fritz Mueller, Kowalevsky, and Haeckel. Predictably, a retrospection evaluates previous stages by their contributions to the final one. There is nothing "wrong" with this approach to historical reconstruction if only we recognize that it is a biased presentation. A prospective approach should also be considered to test the final formulation of the idea in question. An exclusive retrospective approach that evaluates previous stages of an idea's development by the contribution of each stage to the final theory always has the task of paying debts to the theory's infancy. It is the last effort on the path of perfecting the complete emancipation of the theory from its own intellectual restrictions. This approach reduces the history of the idea to the level of footnotes, depriving the story of its mediating role between the theory itself and its "objective" content. Thus, the approach is just another expression of the desire to establish the objectivity of a theory and, as such, this reflection may be completely justified. On the other hand, depriving the mediating role of history means, at the same time, emancipation of the theory from its own intellectual framework, from its own metaphysical nucleus.

In the course of his intellectual evolution, Metchnikoff changed his attitude toward Darwinism, the scientific significance of the Mueller–Haeckel biogenetic law, and Kowalevsky's early discoveries. Together with Metchnikoff, we can evaluate those changes as constructive because they indicate essential steps in developing the phagocytosis hypothesis. In altering his attitudes, Metchnikoff could not suspect the future birth of the hypothesis and, accordingly, he could not perform those changes for the sake of this final outcome. On the other hand, a change in a theoretical position is not a matter of taste, nor is it an immediate result of recognizing the persuasive power of some facts. A theoretical assimilation of the facts that remain in contradiction to a previously held position indicates reconstruction of initial problematics and elaboration of new intellectual tools. The efforts that were spent for those reconstructions and elaborations provided the true intellectual musculature for the future hypothesis: the intellectual nucleus that supports the entire theoretical structure. But these efforts are only unrecognizable when the history of the theory is considered retrospectively by evaluation of each stage of the history according to its fitness in the final form. What matters in this case is not the effort, but the final integration. Thus, we should not forget that this retrospective approach in the history of ideas must always be correlated with the complementary prospective approach: measuring intellectual power of an idea against its own history. We believe that this complementarity is of great importance for those who are professionally involved in studies in the history of science—but it is not exclusively for them. We will argue further that Metchnikoff's own one-sided retrospective history damaged him when, in the passionate debate of his phagocytosis theory, he attempted to defend it against the most penetrating arguments of a general theoretical nature: (a) accusations of teleology, (b) doubts concerning the right to support his theory by the Darwinian theory of evolution, and (c) skepticism about the very possibility of active host defense.

The Problem of a Metaphor

In 1883, Metchnikoff presented a new hypothesis concerning an active immunological response of leukocytes; he proposed that these cells recognized foreign microorganisms and destroyed them by a process of engulfment, or *phagocytosis,* a term he adopted to express the concept of its "eating" character. This hypothesis, resulting from almost eighteen years of research in embryology and intracellular digestion, remained the focus of his experimental career for the next thirty years in a seemingly ceaseless struggle first with German microbiologists and later the humoral immunologists. Because the first attempts to formulate a scientific humoral theory of immunity was made several years after Metchnikoff's initial proposal, we may fairly argue that Metchnikoff offered the first theory of immunity. But in order to understand the intellectual circumstances of the birth of this theory, it is insufficient to argue that earlier concepts of immunity were speculative in their nature and did not possess a sufficient experimental basis. The characteristic of Metchnikoff's undertaking as a first attempt to create a scientific theory of immunity—one that has proven valid over a century's perspective—conceals a radical difference in the metaphysical orientation between Metchnikoff and his predecessors.

What enables us to consider Metchnikoff's theory and those of his predecessors as belonging to the same chapter of scientific history, namely, the history of immunology, is only the empirical appreciation of acquired immunity and differences in susceptibility to infection. Metchnikoff's understanding of those observations was unique. In order to generate a theory, a fact must be formulated within an intellectual framework that allows meaningful recognition of that fact as a real problem, as a challenge to a theoretical response. Of course, the observation of ingested microorganisms within leukocytes for Metchnikoff and for any of his predecessors proposed the obvious question: What is the nature of the phenomenon? But this question can be addressed to any phenomenon and does not elucidate in what respect Metchnikoff focused the observed facts of ingested microorganisms into the issue that posed immunity as a theoretical problem open to experimental inquiry. We will argue that, although related to commonly known observations, Metchnikoff's theory and those theories of his predecessors are as different from each other as might be two answers to two different questions. Metchnikoff asked, What is the mechanism of the organism's defense? What kind of active response does an organism undertake in order to protect itself against infection? Nothing of this sort can be found in any previous theory of immunity; there is no indication of even the nascent idea of studying a mechanism or a subsystem responsible for host defense.

If we expect that a theory of immunity is to propose an explanation of a defensive mechanism, then Metchnikoff's contribution is not the formulation of the first scientific theory of immunity, but the scientific formulation of the first immunological theory. In other words, we stress not its *scientific* character, but the *novel concept* of immunity itself. We cannot explain Metchnikoff's insight by simply following the development of a serious investigative approach to an old question. Instead, Metchnikoff asked a very different question with a radical shift of meaning.

Theories prior to Metchnikoff's (29) were built on metaphysical assumptions that excluded a mechanism by which an organism actively supports its own integrity. The organism's integrity (consciously or intuitively) was considered as the very basic support of all living processes, as something primary and immediately given. With this metaphysical assumption, any biological function must be related to the given state of the organism as a whole; the integrity of the organism is a priori. Any objective and positive description of the essence of an activity must coincide with a chosen model of the organism's integrity. Correspondingly, although the idea of the self-healing power of the organism was popular in Western medicine, it did not reflect the thought of a subsystem whose special function was to protect (or to restore) the integrity of the organism. The self-healing power was thought of as another expression of integrity: the *nature* of the organism, its *physis* was the self-sustaining selfhood in a Heraclitean flux. In this perspective, nature must be self-protective. Thus, the problem of self-healing processes was discussed as the problem of the *natural* healing power, where *natural* simply refers itself to an expression of nature (30).

The interpretations of *nature* varied, but a widespread concept was embodied in the ancient thesis of harmony between the four humors (31). *Corpus Hippocraticum,* which represents a vast diversity of ancient theoretical approaches to the question of health and disease, reflected a metaphysical unity: a human being as a microcosm, wherein the very nature of life was viewed as the process of representation of a primordial design. There could be different interpretations of that design, but there was no question about its validity. All living processes were but an expression of the primary order. With this metaphysical assumption, the issue is how processes exist that are not in conformity with the balanced scheme. In other words, the question is not how health is derived, but how disease is possible. Because harmony offers the basis of existence, how could the intrusion of disharmony be possible (32)? Indeed, the intuitive apposition harmony/disharmony, which openly followed medical thought until the middle of the nineteenth century, and implicitly until our (presumably) antimetaphysical times, is just a trace of the ancient opposition cosmos/chaos. Thus, in order to understand the intellectual context of Metchnikoff's undertaking, we must recognize his theory as a response to a shift from these metaphysical assumptions.

In the tenth century, the Islamic physician, Rhazes (33) described smallpox and the phenomenon of protection after recovery from infection. In accordance with Hippocratic tradition, Rhazes considered health as the state of harmony, or balance, of the four basic humors—blood, phlegm, yellow bile, and black bile. In disharmony, in respect to quality or changes in quantities, he saw causes of diseases (i.e., smallpox was due to fermentation of blood that took place as a result of excess amounts of that humor). Smallpox, by eliminating excess blood, eliminates disease susceptibility. The theory offers an explanation to the question of the nature of acquired immunity: What is the *nature* of the kind of disease that does not recur? The object is disease, not the host organism. Rhazes' theory is not a singular case of this kind of speculation. Even if a disease was thought to arise from an external intrusion, the necessity of immunity as a defensive process was not appreciated. For instance, the Italian physician of the sixteenth century, Girolamo Fracastoro (34), believed that the cause of all disease results from small germs (seminaria) that spread from one person to another; each germ had a specific affinity for a given organ and humor. In the case of smallpox, the germ purged a specific humor that would provide a site for a second infection. Again, no active host response is suggested. Although Fracastoro's theory presents another explanation of the empirical fact of immunity, it has the same metaphysical structure as that of Rhazes—by answering the question of the nature of a disease that cannot recur, not the question concerning host activity in respect to its own defense.

There is in Fracastoro's theory the idea of depletion of some specific substances that will have broad influence in the eighteenth and nineteenth centuries. In 1880, only three years before Metchnikoff's formulation of the phagocytosis theory, Louis Pasteur, who was soon to become Metchnikoff's mentor, demonstrated that acquired immunity against fowl cholera could be attained by innoculation with attenuated bacteria (35). The explanation Pasteur gave for this phenomenon was constructed by analogy with bacterial growth in vitro, where the initial phase of rapid multiplication is followed by a second phase of abrupt termination of growth. Pasteur explained these observations by the presupposition that abrupt growth termination is due to the depletion (beyond a critical trace) of some substance(s) that is specific and necessary for multiplication of each bacterial species. Acquired immunity, from his point of view, was due to a postulated factor whose depletion arose either from a preceding infection or by an innoculation with attenuated microorganisms.

Pasteur's hypothesis cannot be treated as nonscientific. His belief in the bacteriological nature of disease was not a result of free speculation but appeared out of his experimental bacteriological research. As a reasonable scientific construction, Pasteur's hypothesis provided the possibility of its own refutation (viz., see Sir Karl Popper), which was soon offered by David E. Salmon and Theobold Smith, who demonstrated (36) that an effective vaccination is possible with dead bacteria and even more convincingly when Emil von Behring and Shibasaburo Kitasato showed similar results with bacteria-free supernatants from cultures of diphtheria or tetanus (37).

Pasteur's model had been taken from direct observations of growing bacteria in vitro, but the theory failed because it did not account for the host response, a far more critical parameter of health than his extrapolated test-tube model would allow. Although obviously scientific, Pasteur's hypothesis in its metaphysical orientation is much closer to Fracastoro's speculation than to Metchnikoff's theory—as with his Renaissance predecessor, Pasteur's hypothesis does not pose any questions concerning a defensive mechanism, but it is only concerned with the nature of the infective agent and the mechanism of its development in a given circumstance (38).

This is not to say that the concept of protective responses played no role in the development of medicine. Metchnikoff's theory of immunity implies the idea of a special activity, not simply another manifestation of the organism's underlying integrity, but allegedly of its performance in a distinct fashion, that is, to restore or create the organism's integrity. We will argue that under traditional metaphysical assumptions, this special activity could not be reduced to integrity in an "objective" explanation (e.g., within a theoretical construct) and could only appear metaphorically. Such is the case with the famous metaphor of "warfare against disease." Whatever the role of metaphor in science, by definition, it is a shift from a "natural" (for the phenomenon in question) theoretical language to a linguistic circle pertaining to another phenomenon. Consequently, if a phenomenon receives, within the theoretical tradition, only a metaphorical description, it signifies that the phenomenon did not attain an interpretation in "objective" traditional terms, that is, in terms that are considered within the tradition as pertinent to the very "nature" of the object in question. A metaphor may play an important role as a means of creating an "objective" explanation, but being taken only as a metaphor, it indicates a shift from "objectivity". Thus, by its very nature, a metaphorical explanation of a phenomenon may play a marginal role in a theoretical tradition that seriously claims explanations in "objective" terms. That was the issue with the metaphor of "warfare against disease" in the Hippocratic–Galenic tradition (39). With the development of a positivistic and mechanistic approach toward biomedical problems in the nineteenth century, the issue of organismic integrity was not reformulated immediately. Instead of inquiring, "What is integrity?" a new question was asked, "By what means is organismic integrity realized?" (40) Old metaphysical assumptions were implicitly operative, and with the new mechanoreductive attitude, there was no longer a compelling rationale to accept ideas of a protective mechanism than in the old Hippocratic–Galenic tradition. In spite of the dominance of the old metaphysics in the nineteenth century, the first attempts to overcome that tradition were made during this period, and we wish to argue that Metchnikoff was one of the pioneers of this scientific revolution.

The notion of "warfare against disease" was marginal to the predominant scientific trends of the nineteenth century and could function metaphorically, but not as a rationally formulated program to reconstruct a mechanism of defense. This, on the one hand, accounts for the attractiveness of the concept for practical-minded physicians; on the other hand, we can easily understand why Metchnikoff's critics, who represented the predominant new positivistic trends of science, recognized in his theory the relics of the ancient program. Even in the nineteenth century, the metaphor of organismic protective forces meant the determination and will of the microcosm to oppose the destructive forces of the external chaos (41). Thus, the metaphor did not express any metaphysical alternative either to the Hippocratic–Galenic tradition or to the implicit metaphysical assumptions of the new positivistic approach to the problem of an organism's integrity. Instead, the very presence of the metaphor in the then-current scientific literature signified an inability (or certain limitations) to offer a positive description of an organism's activity. The presence of the metaphor (as anything that *sounded* teleological) compromised the metaphysical premises of the new thinking and roused the indignation of the scientific community (42).

The transformation of the metaphorical "warfare against disease" with a new science demanded creation of a theoretically articulated research program, a task we believe entailed a change in the metaphysical basis of the construct. It is interesting that none of Metchnikoff's so-called predecessors (those few scientists who around the late 1870s and the early 1880s suspected that the leukocyte reaction was potentially a defensive process) proposed an experimental program to justify their "theory." Maybe the most insistent pretender for the title or, at least, cofounder of the phagocytic immunological theory was an American bacteriologist and military physician, George Sternberg, who claimed that he proposed the central idea in 1881, two years before Metchnikoff's first paper on the subject (see chap. 5). But Sternberg neither made any attempt to prove the supposition himself, nor proposed an experimental program that could be performed by others. In this circumstance, his competition with Metchnikoff appears as a matter of priority in regard to the ancient medical-military metaphor, "warfare against disease", in its application to the phagocytosis phenomenon than a matter of priority in regard to a theory of phagocytosis and the first formulation of the idea of immunity. The true question, in regard to the birth of the phagocytosis theory of immunity, is not who was the first to apply the metaphor "warfare against disease" to the phagocytosis phenomenon, but rather in which way had the theoretical (including metaphysical) assumptions (in regard to integrity of organism) been changed so that it became possible to refer to the protective activity of the organism, not in a metaphorical, extratheoretical fashion, but to place the activity within a general biological context and formulate the problem of its investigation in an experimental program. Our goal is to reconstruct that historical process and to trace the revolution in metaphysical assumptions adopted by Metchnikoff.

Harmony and Disharmony—Metchnikoff's Metaphysics

Although Metchnikoff was well read in the contemporary philosophical literature of the mid-nineteenth century, he sought his rational Weltanschauung through scientific research. He did not naively adopt a preconceived metaphysical scheme to a scientific problem, but mutually reformulated his scientific inquiry with his philosophical orientation. His philosophical development mirrored his scientific findings—each helped frame the other. Metchnikoff's explicit statements of philosophical beliefs, omitting the context of his scientific development, leave us groping for the intellectual machinery that gave birth to the phagocytosis theory. The key pillars of Metchnikoff's Weltanschauung, which unexpectedly seem to echo the typical product of earlier metaphysical medical speculation, are the notions of "harmony" and "disharmony".

> Man, having appeared as the result of a long cycle of development, carries in himself obvious traces of animal origin. Having acquired an unknown, in the animal realm, degree of intellectual development, he preserved many signs which happened to be not just needless but directly harmful. The high intellectual development has conditioned awareness of death but his animal nature has shortened life because of the chronic poisoning by toxins elaborated by bacteria of the intestinal flora. (43, p. 21)

Along with the disharmonies in the digestive system, to which Metchnikoff devoted much research, he attempted to define the disharmonies of the reproductive apparatus, which he believed was the basic cause of unrest in family and social life; he studied disharmony in the instinct of self-preservation; and he found disharmony in the relationship of phagocytic mesodermal cells (macrophage) to "higher elements" in the destruction of muscle cells and neurons by phagocytes. He saw this process as the main cause of senility and, more generally,

> human nature, as it is revealed to us by science, does not demonstrate a presence of a special law of harmonious development of different parts. . . . Man appeared as a result of a one-sided, but not total improvement of the organism, by joining not so much adult apes, but rather their unevenly developed fetuses. From the pure nature-historical point of view, it would be possible to recognize man as an ape's "monster", with an enormously developed brain, face and hands. (44, p. 226, 1913)

With these assumptions, a pessimistic conclusion is natural, "[a] human being, in that state in which he has appeared on earth, is an abnormal, sick creature subjected to medicine" (45, p. 274). Thus, Metchnikoff titles one of his important essays "Weltanschauung and Medicine" (1910), although, at first, he intended to call it "Weltanschauung and Biology," but as he attests, medicine held a higher affinity to his general interests. The diverse disharmonies were for him the cause of human pessimism, but with science and scientific "rational hygiene"

> the possibility was offered for man to live a complete and happy cycle of life ending with peaceful and natural death. It was so-called orthobiosis that might be viewed as the goal of rational human existence. ([43], p. 21)

The theme of elusive biological harmonies, which had been the basis of Metchnikoff's early pessimistic Weltanschauung, preoccupied him all his life. In his 1871 essay "Upbringing from the Anthropological Point of View" (46), he attempted to demonstrate that any theory of child rearing had to focus on the inherited disharmony of the child. In the same vein, he writes of sexual disharmony in "Age of Marriage" (47); again, in "Essay of Opinions Concerning Human Nature" (48), the idea of inherited disharmony has reached a level of sui generis, "biological schizophrenia": "Figuratively speaking, we can say that in the human body, a whole lower animal is included." By 1878, in "Struggle for Existence in a Broad Sense," he gave to these meditations a form of biological reason for a general philosophical pessimism, "The most noble qualities of our nature contradict the law of the struggle for existence, because not the best but the most practical people obtain the victory in the struggle" (49). Thirty-five years later, Metchnikoff referred to these essays and their "scientific" motivation quite ironically. He wrote:

> [In] these four essays under a cover of scientific ways and in form which gives the impression of professional pedantry, the young author carries out a pessimistic point of view upon life, which point of view is based on the disharmony of human nature. (43, p. 20)

But Metchnikoff does not put aside the idea of inherited disharmony of organisms in the "optimistic" half of his life. The idea remained fundamental to his worldview. Repeatedly, he reiterates this position in his later studies, for example, *Immunity in Infective Diseases* (1901) (16), *The Nature of Man* (1903) (11), *Prolongation of Life* (1907) (12), and in practically all his works when he makes any attempt to draw general biological conclusions.

Science for Metchnikoff was not just one of several possible professional occupations. Here were rooted his deepest beliefs; conversely he believed that in his scientific life the deepest sources of his existence established their expression. When he wrote that "youthful pessimism is a real disease of youth" (43, p. 20), we hear both the man who made suicide attempts, thus dramatically confirming his own existential disharmony, and the scientist whose understanding of evolution convinced him that natural selection does not provide a perfected organism. Fortunately, for Metchnikoff, he came to view optimism as the first sign of maturity and in his later years expressed the belief that

> in spite of the inexpedient arrangement of the human organism, happy existence and rational ethics are possible. The latter must not be the rules of life conforming to the present imperfect nature of man, but based upon moral deeds of nature changed in accordance with the human ideal of happiness. (43, p. 21)

It is important for us to note here the rejection of the ancient idea of a natural harmony. Harmony could only be possible (if possible at all) as a result of expedient efforts. Metchnikoff frequently returned to this opposition between his own idea of harmony and that of the ancient Greeks. The starting point of his transition to the optimistic phase of his life was the formulation of the phagocytosis theory: its significance was the discovery of inner forces of life that could possibly provide harmonization of conflicting functions. At the same time, in accordance with his existential attitude toward his scientific occupation, he considered the transition to the optimistic phase of his life as an expression of his own biological maturity (12, pp. 183–187). Biological organization offers the opportunity to actively balance disparate function if we follow the rational attitude that can lead life to biological harmonization. As an embryologist, Metchnikoff sought to understand how ontogenetic development represented the process of solving problems inherited from evolutionary development, a theme we explore in detail hereafter.

Metchnikoff sought support of his Weltanschauung not only in the combination of biology with introspective meditations but in the application of the theory to a broad array of cultural phenomena. He analyzed pessimism in poetry (George Gordon, Lord Byron; Giacomo Leopardi, Mikhail Lermontov, Aleksandr Pushkin [11, pp. 172–176]), in pessimistic philosophy (Eduard von Hartmann and Artur Schopenhauer [12, pp. 176–192]), and he was especially attentive to the artistic evolution of Johann Wolfgang von Goethe (12, pp. 193–223). Goethe's poetic development reflected, from Metchnikoff's point of view, the natural biological development of the human organism: the youthful pessimism (the young Werther, the Faust of Part 1) naturally developed into the optimism of maturity (the Faust of Part 2). *Faust* is more than the poet's biography in that it serves as a poetic sublimation of Goethe's biological development.

These literary essays add little to our understanding of the nature of poetry, but more germane, they leave us with unresolved questions concerning Metchnikoff's understanding of the key notions of harmony and disharmony. If orthobiosis (the life that attains a final harmony) is a natural course of development, then, what is the reason of "natural harmony." Maybe the difference is that harmony is a result of development but not its initial stage. But the ancient thinkers also considered the most reasonable development of life as an approach to an ideal state. For them, ideal harmony was primary not because it appeared as the first in sequence, but because life as a result of development reveals its essence as the ideal harmony. Although essence is not a function that is of time, it is revealed as the last stage of development.

In some respects, Metchnikoff's concept of harmony is not a single ideal state, but an "essence" developing and changing in the course of time. Thus, he wishes to correlate essence with a human ideal of happiness that can be formulated in history. But, then, how can orthobiosis be a process of natural development? Perhaps Metchnikoff is expressing that time and history are required to reveal natural biological harmony. Does this then mean that he repeats, in a disguised form, the ancient metaphysical idea of harmony revealed in time? But we have already noted that the ancient construct of harmony does not allow for the idea of immunity as an activity of a defensive mechanism. We must now recognize the full meaning of Metchnikoff's harmony/disharmony opposition, tracing the path of his notions in the development of his scientific inquiry.

There is not much originality in a nineteenth-century intellectual's complaints of creation's imperfections or his preaching of a pessimistic view of life. In an abstract formulation, both ideas of disharmony and a general pessimistic Weltanschauung present a prevalent cultural cliché of the period. In order to understand the role of these concepts in Metchnikoff's intellectual development, we have to comprehend how these commonly held intuitions oriented and ultimately determined his scientific construct. We will argue that the peculiarity and true meaning of disharmony, as the concept appeared in Metchnikoff's studies, must be understood from his embryological research. Metchnikoff's idea of inherited disharmonies is immediately connected with his formulation of the problems pertaining to the relationship between phylogeny and ontogeny, which arose in his studies of invertebrate embryology, the subject to which we now turn.

CHAPTER 2

Metchnikoff's Early Embryology

The Concept of the Embryonic Layers, 1817–1865

As Metchnikoff wrote in 1869, apparently not without some patriotic sentiments, "The first scientific basis of embryology, that is, the history of animals' development was founded by the former St. Petersburg academicians, Pander and von Baer (1, *AC,* p. 254). In 1817, Christian Pander described the trilaminar structure of the earliest incubated chick embryo stage (2). According to his description, at the twelfth hour, the embryo consisted of two separate layers: an outer layer that was thin, smooth, and transparent, which he named the serous layer, and the inner layer that was thicker, granular, and opaque, which he named the mucous layer. Between these two layers appeared a third, where blood vessels were formed, which he named the vessel layer.

> Actually there begins in each of these three layers a particular metamorphosis, and each one strives to achieve its goal; only each is not yet sufficiently independent by itself to produce that for which it is destined. Each one still needs the help of its companions; and therefore all three, until each reached a specific level, work mutually together although destined for different ends. (3, p. 258)

Pander observed that the second layer was formed from the first (4). Pander's teaching about the primary embryonic layers was developed further by Karl Ernst von Baer (5), Pander's friend and colleague.

Von Baer was the true founder of comparative embryology, as Metchnikoff wrote in 1869:

> His discovery of the human and mammal female's ovum connected the most essential moment in development of the viviparous and oviparous Vertebrata. His other discovery, the discovery of the so-called *dorsal string*—the primary basic skeleton of all Vertebrata—offered a similar important fact for establishing the general type of development of the higher animals. (1, *AC,* p. 254)

Von Baer expanded Pander's germ-layer concept for the chicken to all vertebrates. From his own studies, von Baer concluded that every layer contained within itself a germ of a definite set of organs that developed in accordance with a single general

25

plan *(Bauplan)*. According to von Baer, the first layer is the origin of the "animal life" organs (the organs of motions and the nervous system); the second layer, the organs of "vegetative life" (the digestive organs); and the third layer develops the blood vessels. Von Baer observed formation of the digestive and nervous tubes and the somites as the basic elements of primary organ-system development. He described the provisional embryonic membranes and began study of their role in embryonic development.

A new stage in the history of embryology followed after Theodor Schwann's establishment of the cellular theory (1837), which asserted cells as the basic element of living tissue. Once the ovum was recognized as a single cell, fragmentation into a set of embryonic cells (forming the primary layers) was shown to follow fertilization. The prior view of embryonic layers was reconsidered from this new histological vantage, first by Robert Remak in 1850–1855, who recognized the three layers but, at the same time, rejected von Baer's interpretation. He discerned them according to their future histological development instead of the germ carriers of future "animal-life" and "vegetative-life" organs. Remak recognized *two* primary embryonic layers: the upper one subdivided into medullary and epidermic plates; the lower layer, in turn, divided into two sublayers: the trophic layer, which forms the alimentary canal and its derivatives; and the middle layer, which forms muscle, connective tissue, blood vessels, sex glands, and peripheral nerves. The middle layer was thought to further divide into dorsal and ventral somite plates by a cavity, which we know now as the coelom. In his work of 1869, Metchnikoff cites Remak as the most prominent figure in animal embryology of the 1850s (1). It is true that most of the facts established by Remak agree with our current concept of embryonic layers (except for the origin of the peripheral nerves), but what must interest us is a parallel between Remak's concept of the layers and Metchnikoff's ideas developed not in the middle 1860s, but in the 1870s and 1880s.

The debates concerning the evolutionary significance of the layers started in the second half of the 1860s with the work (in 1865) of Alexander Kowalevsky. He argued that the most general pattern of layer formation proceeded (a) through the cleavage of the fertilized ovum, leading to formation of the primary multicellular sphere and (b) through the production of the second layer by invagination. These two steps would then form a two-laminar sac. The third layer was thought then to arise from the cells of the first two layers. From Kowalevsky's (and after him Haeckel's) point of view, this manner of embryonic development reflected the most ancient stage of evolutionary formation of multicellular organisms. Metchnikoff admitted the importance of this kind of genealogical reconstruction only in the 1870s; when he initially participated in the debates, he had already proposed another model for formation of the primary layers. In his original model, the middle layer did not develop *after* formation of the outer and inner layers. According to Metchnikoff, the primary sphere (the blastula) is gradually filled by a parenchymatic mass of cells that are further divided into the inner and middle layers (the endoderm and the mesoderm). Thus, Metchnikoff's concept of the embryonic layers (developed in the 1870s and 1880s) is homological relative to that proposed by Remak who (in the 1850s) also asserted that the inner and middle layers were formed by division of the second layer.

If there was obvious progress in development of vertebrate comparative embryology, the state of invertebrate embryology in the middle 1860s was quite different. Note Metchnikoff's appraisal written in 1869:

> Embryology, in the sense of a science studying gradual formation of the organism and separation of organs out of common germs was mainly cultivated by the specialists in the anatomy and physiology of man (Remak, Reichert, Bischoff, Koelliker) and because of this it related almost exclusively to the higher animals. True, there was some work concerning the development of Invertebrata having as their goal the establishment of the main types of development but they treated very few (comparatively) forms and some of them were erroneous due to preconceived theories.
>
> Meanwhile the elaboration of embryology of lower organisms continued very actively as independent from any comparative-embryological goals.... There was accumulated in science a huge material in the history of the Invertebrata development obtained mainly by Mueller, Krohn, Siebold, Leuckart, Busch, and others. These researchers, having in view mainly the studies of the most external forms of development, paid comparatively very little attention to formation and development of organs, because of all of this, the purely comparative embryological questions have been laid aside, not only without elaboration but even without being formulated. With this state of affairs all the accumulated material could not be put together in a single whole but was destined to exist in the shape of an odd mass. And meanwhile the goal of the history of development as the science which deals with the multitude of changing forms, must exactly establish the general affinity between different animals and the search for the plan of their organization. (1, *AC,* pp. 255–256)

Darwin's *Origin of Species* apparently played the crucial role in changing this situation, offering a new meaning to the program of establishing "a general affinity between separate animals." As Jane Oppenheimer writes:

> By the 1870s the scientific world was flaming with the debate on evolution that was kindled by the publication of Darwin's *Origin of Species....* The decade of the 1870s saw embryology adduced as a complete confirmation of the evolution hypothesis, and the evolution of the race as an explanation *sine qua non* of the course of evolution or development of the individual. (6, p. 266)

We agree with this general view, but place the debate at least six years earlier. Fritz Mueller's *Fuer Darwin* was published in 1864 and Ernst Haeckel's *General Morphology of the Organisms* in 1866. Metchnikoff's intensive work in this field started in 1865; his friend, Kowalevsky, who was five years older, began his research in 1862. These two must be regarded as the cofounders of invertebrate comparative embryology (7). The influence of Darwin and Fritz Mueller on the development of comparative embryology, in general, or comparative embryology of invertebrates, in particular, does not mean that *all* essential contributions in the field between 1865 and the next decade were inspired by the need to confirm or to refute Darwinism; we will argue further that it certainly was not the case for Metchnikoff (8). We simply note that the influence of Darwin, Mueller, and shortly thereafter, Haeckel was crucial in creating the atmosphere in which comparative embryology became a natural focus of scientific attention. And if Darwin's own views on the relationship between evolution and individual development did not much differ from those of von Baer and were in an essential degree speculative in nature, Mueller's *Fuer Darwin* (9) gave rise to a true research program in contrast to the old naturphilosophical idea about isomorphic parallelism between the history of species and individual development. This result was important in establishing the intellectual atmosphere within which the further studies of primary embryonic layers was determined.

Thus, when Metchnikoff started his research in embryology in 1865, the embryonic-layer concept had almost a fifty-year history. Actually, beginning with von Baer's first works on the subject, the concept was viewed as the theoretical foundation of vertebrate comparative embryology. The most influential model of the concept as adapted to the 1860s was that elaborated in the 1850s by Remak. At the same time, although extensive material in embryology of invertebrates had been collected, little was known of their embryonic layers; in fact, the very existence of layers in invertebrates had not been confirmed. Neither a general concept nor a common structure had been established; thus, there was no basis for a comparative approach. In short, there existed no science of invertebrate comparative embryology in 1865. However, we may discern certain attempts to move in this direction as early as the 1840s. In his doctoral dissertation "De Prima Insectorum Genesi" (1842), Koelliker studied the embryology of insects and concluded that there were analogies between the development of arthropods and vertebrates. In 1849, T. H. Huxley noted an essential similarity between the two primary embryonic layers of vertebrates and the two layers structuring the adult forms of Coelenterata (10). We should note that these first attempts to study invertebrate comparative embryology, although appearing from our perspective as purely empirical and descriptive, were supported by specific naturphilosophical speculations. For instance, they were influenced by Étienne Geoffroy Saint-Hilaire's argument that vertebrates and arthropods were designed with a common plan: the dorsum of vertebrates corresponded to the ventral side of arthropods, that is, each realized a single plan in a mutually inverted fashion. In one of his first papers (1866) on insect embryology, Metchnikoff reflected on these views:

> In those times [the 1840s to 1850s] they tried to follow, as strictly as possible, the analogy with typical vertebrate development. The difference in relation of the fetus to the yolk, the difference in the positions of the nerve system they tried to explain by the correspondence of the back side of Vertebrata to the abdominal side of Arthropoda. (11, pp. 389–390)

After Remak's studies in vertebrate embryology, which established the histological approach, Zaddach (1854) undertook new studies in the embryology of insects (12), in which the attempts to draw analogy with vertebrates also played an essential role. He described a split of the so-called embryonic stripe into two layers that corresponded not (as accepted earlier) to the serous layer (the middle layer) of Remak's terminology nor to the mucous layer (Remak's inner layer), but to the horn (external) and muscle layers of vertebrates. Besides this parallel, Zaddach believed that he had also found other similarities, considering as homologous the primary segments of arthropods and the plates of the primary vertebrae. Zaddach's opinions were broadly supported, for example, by Huxley (13) and Leuckart (14). Metchnikoff noted in 1866 how the consensus was inspired by enchantment with the analogy, "Being enthusiastic with Zaddach's ideas these authors found that the ideas were proved even by those facts, which did not correspond to Zaddach's previous observations" (11, p. 390). But in 1864, August Weismann published his work on Diptera development (15), wherein he traced Zaddach's horn layer during Diptera development

and came to the conclusion that it was not homologous to the horn layer of vertebrates. Weismann viewed Zaddach's horn layer as a special formation, which he
named the fold layer, and concluded that nothing in Insecta corresponded to embryonic layers; as a result, he rejected any parallel in the embryology of arthropods with
vertebrates. Although Metchnikoff expressed his skepticism about Huxley and
Leuckart's enthusiastic support of Zaddach's ideas, we may not infer that he totally
rejected the scheme. After all, at the very time when Weismann published his work
on Diptera, Metchnikoff worked in Leuckart's laboratory and believed that in rejecting any similarity of vertebrate and insect development

> Weismann fell into another extreme and in this respect hardly took a more correct
> way. . . . I felt myself now forced to undertake further research in the esoteric sphere
> of insect embryology and to gain footholds which would help somehow to explain
> all these peculiarities. (11, 1866, pp. 391–392)

Metchnikoff's Early Embryological Works, 1865–1872

We have outlined Metchnikoff's general interest in the problem of how to apply (if
at all) the concept of embryonic layers to invertebrates. However, the true origin of
his interest in insect embryology was inspired by Nikolay Wagner's discovery at
Kazan University of the phenomenon that was later defined by von Baer as pedogenesis (parthenogenetic reproduction by insect larvae structurally unable to copulate) (11). Wagner observed that certain Cecidomyiidae larvae spawned new offspring
before attaining adulthood; these juvenile organisms developed within the mother
larva, ultimately destroying it. The larvae are generated in this way in the fall, winter,
and spring, but during the summer, the last larval generation matures into pupae
from which appear the reproduction forms, the small flies. The females lay fertilized
ova and the cycle begins again. Wagner's report was received skeptically. Siebold
initially rejected the paper for *Zeitschrift fuer wissenschaftliche Zoologie,* but the
result was confirmed and the paper was published in 1863.

Metchnikoff's first embryological paper was devoted to the problem of Cecidomyiidae larvae development (16). Wagner argued that the larvae developed from the
fat body cells; others disagreed, thinking that either the larvae developed from germ
cells or from special germ organs. The latter was described by Leuckart as well as
Metchnikoff, who worked in Leuckart's laboratory at this time. As the ovum was
thought not to possess a distinct delimiting membrane, Leuckart called the ova (as
opposed to fertilized, shell-covered ova) the pseudo-ova. Metchnikoff in describing
the development of the larva from the pseudo-ovum, made two important observations: (a) the nuclei of the blastoderm (the single-layered structure formed by the
cleavage of the ovum) are formed out of the germ vacuoli (i.e., the ovum's nucleus)
and (b) Weismann's so-called polar cells gave birth to the sex cells of the next generation. Ganin at Kharkov University also described the germ organs. In contrast to
Leukart and Metchnikoff, he argued that the cells from which the larvae developed
were not pseudo-ova, but true ova; he thus considered Wagner's process as nothing
more than parthenogenesis. Thus arose a controversy that directed Metchnikoff to

continue his studies in Cecidomyiidae. Writing to von Baer, Metchnikoff requested an arbitration of the dispute. Metchnikoff's letter was published (17); and von Baer—in his notes to the letter and in a special paper devoted to the problem (18)—asserted that the true difference between typical parthenogenesis and the reproduction of Cecidomyiidae was not the question of true ova versus pseudo-ova, but rather that in true parthenogenesis the adult female laid ova, whereas Cecidomyiidae ova were laid by its larvae. Von Baer preposed the now-accepted term *pedogenesis.* Metchnikoff considered his Cecidomyiidae paper and the one that followed (19) as preliminary reports, which he intended to include in a later work on insect embryology: "Embryological Research on Insects" was published in 1866 (20). For this research, Metchnikoff shared with Kowalevsky the prestigious von Baer Prize in 1867.

Each of Metchnikoff's predecessors, Zaddach and Weismann, studied only representatives of one order of insects, but Metchnikoff's work encompassed representatives of Diptera, Hemiptera, and Homoptera. Fixed microsections had not yet been developed, and Metchnikoff could only observe living larvae. Therefore, he was limited in his studies to the development of external structures (but only in their early development) and to the emergence of internal organs (but only insofar as transparency allowed). This technical limit was the principal restriction in the studies of the role of embryonic layers in organogenesis. In fact, the very existence of invertebrate embryonic layers was unresolved for the same reason. Despite the methodological restrictions, Metchnikoff came to a number of important conclusions. We noted, for example, his observation that pole cells (discovered by Weismann) give rise to sex cells. In addition, the issue of blastoderm development into a more complex structure had not yet been defined, and Weismann, who had proposed two lines of maturation—one involving a rupture of the blastoderm and the other leaving the blastoderm intact—was refuted by Metchnikoff. Erroneous observations by Weismann and Zaddach were corrected in Metchnikoff's description, but most noticeably, we must ask how this research allows us to trace the development of Metchnikoff's concept of primary embryonic layers: Which facts immediately relate to the problem?

1. At this time, only living ova were studied. Their nuclei are discernible only in a resting state and are invisible in the period of karyokinesis, thus explaining why Weismann concluded that Diptera ova lacked nuclei (the germ vacuoles). The blastoderm in Diptera development (according to Weismann) is formed by a shrinking yolk, leaving the external rim of the protoplasm (the blastema). The nuclei are then formed in the blastema and cleavage begins, forming cells—one around each nucleus. Thus the development of the blastoderm from insects' ova (from Weismann's point of view) is quite different from previously described cleavage patterns.

Metchnikoff was successful in observing the nuclei (the germ vacuoles) in the ova of Cecidomyiidae and aphids. In addition, he observed the multiplication of the nuclei inside the yolk before formation of the blastoderm. Thus, he came to the conclusion that the new nuclei that formed in the division of the ovum's nucleus had migrated to the ovum's periphery when deprived of yolk. Metchnikoff established superficial cleavage as a special mode of a common process to create multicellularity. This does not mean that he was convinced that in all cases the new nuclei of the blastoderm arise out of division of the primary nucleus of the egg (out of the germ vacuole) (1).

2. Weismann came to the conclusion that those insect structures that had previously been viewed as similar to the primary embryonic layers of vertebrates had actually nothing in common. He described this embryonic structure of insects as "the fold layer." Metchnikoff in his Hemiptera paper asserted that the fold layer gave rise to the insects' extremities and proposed to name the layer, the extremities layer. In his next paper, he corrected this mistake and established that out of the fold layer, the fetus membrane (the amnion) developed. We may consider the important result of Metchnikoff's rejection of the fold layer in its role as a basic embryonic structure, that is, the alternative to the primary layers of vertebrates. In other words, the result established certain similarities between insects and vertebrates in respect to the embryonic membrane; at the same time, it was a refutation of Weismann's important argument against existing commonality in the development of insects and vertebrates in respect to the vertebrate embryonic layers. But in no way can Metchnikoff's conclusions be accepted as a positive confirmation of such commonality. Can we find anything confirming the universality of the embryonic layers in Metchnikoff's work of this period? The only statement concerning the layers was his description of bilaminarity in formation of the extremities: one layer was called "the horn layer," the other, "the nerve-muscle layer."

A certain mythology has arisen in the evaluation of these Metchnikovian studies. V. A. Dogel and H. E. Gaisinovich state that while "Weismann (in 1864) had failed in understanding the developmental stages of the embryonic layers in insects" Metchnikoff in his studies of Hemiptera and Diptera "*perfectly* [emphasis added] demonstrated the differentiation of the two primary embryonic layers" (7). The assertion is a strange one, the more so because in 1886 Metchnikoff himself, in recalling the events that took place twenty years earlier, wrote quite openly, "Among Arthropoda I failed to discover with sufficient clarity the embryonic layers in insects" (21, p. 421, 1950). The two quotes are found in the same book but the discrepancy can be explained by the impression created (at least partially) by Metchnikoff himself. In 1866, Metchnikoff asserted that Huxley and Leuckart were too careless in projecting the analogy from vertebrates onto invertebrates and that Weismann was wrong in the opposite extreme, that is, disallowing any similarity between the development of arthropods and vertebrates (20). Twenty years later, Metchnikoff expressed his opinion on the same issue (having by then formulated his phagocytosis hypothesis) and projected the potential carrier of his future theoretically constructed Weltanschauung. From this view, he recognized (in retrospect) not just two poles of possible theoretical exaggerations, but rather an ideological opposition of two (English and German) schools, only with one of which he was allegedly sympathetic from the very beginning. He reconstructs the situation:

> While on the one hand, they were looking for similarity between the embryonic stages of animals and the adult forms, on the other hand, they tried to establish the same similarities between the embryos and the extinct forms. Huxley, in 1849, performed a comparison of the embryonic layers of Vertebrata and the main layers of Coelenterata's body, which he named the ectoderm and the entoderm. (21, p. 418, 1950)

Metchnikoff continues, this notion (not unnoticed in England) was later popularized and further generalized by Herbert Spencer in "The Social Organism." The English philosopher wrote:

Throughout the whole animal kingdom, from the Coelenterata upwards, the first stage of evolution is the same. Equally in the germ of a polyp and in the human ovum, the aggregated mass of cells out of which the creature is to arise, gives origin to a peripheral layer of cells, slightly differing from the rest which they include; and this layer subsequently divides into two—the inner, lying in contact with the included yolk, being called the mucous layer, and the outer, exposed to surrounding agencies, being called the serous layer: or, in the terms used by Professor Huxley, in describing the development of the Hydrozoa—the endoderm and ectoderm [see n. 22]. This primary division marks out a fundamental contrast of parts in the future organism. (23, p. 408)

Following Spencer's quotation, Metchnikoff states, without any hint of skepticism or irony, that Spencer further establishes the analogy of the ectoderm with the highest levels of human society, the entoderm with the lowest ones, and the middle layer with the third estate (21, p. 418, 1950). Twenty years earlier, in 1866, Metchnikoff's criticism was provoked not by this metaphor, but by a much more modest extrapolation from vertebrates to invertebrates. The extrapolation was then further extended (as Metchnikoff wrote in 1866) by Zaddach, Huxley, and Leuckart. But in 1886, Metchnikoff continues:

In Germany, Huxley's teaching did not find, for a long time, its adherents. This was related with the known reaction taking place here [Germany] against the general application of germ-layers. The reaction found its highest expression in Weismann's description of Diptera embryology. This direction corresponded completely to the dominate theory of types, accordingly to which all morphological comparisons were possible only to the limits of one and the same type of animals. (21, p. 419, 1950)

Why does Metchnikoff now oppose the English and German traditions so radically? Why does he not recall that in 1866 he united the Germans [Zaddach and Leuckart] with Huxley in their approach to the problem of the embryonic layers in invertebrates? And even in 1886, one page after the one quoted above, he wrote about another German, Koelliker (24), "Completely independently from this direction [the direction determined by Fritz Mueller] Koelliker in 1865 . . . came to conclusions which mainly coincide with Huxley's opinions" (21, p. 420, 1950). These discrepancies may be explained, in part, by Metchnikoff's rivalry with the Germans after 1883 (owing to the hostility of most German scientists to his phagocytosis hypothesis) and the largely favorable acceptance of his theory in England and France. Beyond the political and national evocations, there was a serious scientific reorientation in Metchnikoff's thinking. In 1886, Metchnikoff considered himself a Darwinist (although, as we will discuss further, a very peculiar one). He recognized, at that time, the radical importance of Fritz Mueller's ideas for his own embryological research and the phagocytosis theory. He also recognized, as a fact of greater importance, that in Kowalevsky's studies of the lancelet larvae there had been traced not just the histological and organological fate of the embryonic layers as a ready, presented structure, but the very *process* of forming the layers themselves. Thus, his theoretical position was now radically different from the one held twenty years previously. Now he viewed the German tradition of the 1850s and 1860s as dominated by George Cuvier's ideas, and he wished to separate them from his own theoretical ideology:

During the long period in establishing resemblance between animals in their anatomy and stages of development, an expression of a general plan was appreciated in an ideal meaning. In the following decades, it was recognized with Darwin's help that in the basis of the resemblance lay the genealogic kinship. (21, p. 419, 1950)

The new theoretical framework of the embryonic-layer problem is for Metchnikoff now of crucial importance. It was not Metchnikoff, but his friend Kowalevsky, who studied the problem of layer formation in 1865. In Metchnikoff's works of that time, he had dealt with the question of the universal presence of layers in different animal groups and the histological-organological perspectives of development of those layers, but without dealing with their formation. Thus, at least in his research methodology, Metchnikoff began with presupposing the possible existence of an "ideal plan" without concern for its origin or genealogy. And we will demonstrate further that it was not solely a question of practical methodology but that Metchnikoff had explicitly rejected the theoretical genealogical approach in embryology at that time. However, he inadvertantly revealed that the genealogical approach was not his own. In 1902, in his essay "Alexandr Onufrievich Kowalevsky . . . ," Metchnikoff wrote of his experience in Leuckart's laboratory (1865):

At Leuckart's laboratory, which was often visited by German and foreign scientists, many scientific questions were discussed and among them Darwin's theory was in the foreground; comparative embryology was not mentioned in any serious way. Even if questions in history of animal development [i.e., in embryology] were touched upon, it was not in any other way but for the sake of some special issue. For instance, at that time the fact, discovered by Professor N. Wagner in Kazan concerning reproduction of larvae of some *Diptera* [sic] was of a particular interest. (25, p. 23, 1946)

Metchnikoff does not mention here that he played the main role in the debate concerning those larvae, an argument that pushed him to study comparative insect embryology.

Twenty years later, Metchnikoff recognized the radical importance for his own theoretical position in separating two naturphilosophical traditions: one descending from Cuvier (and partially from von Baer), another originating with Geoffroy Saint-Hilaire, whose influence was still discernable in Huxley and Herbert Spencer. Metchnikoff viewed the latter tradition (in 1886) as the immediate predecessor of Darwinism and thus the predecessor of his own newly adopted position. From this perspective, he distributed his preferences and attempted to reinterpret his earlier role. In the 1880s, German scientists were highly critical of the phagocytosis theory, whose prehistory was rooted in the problem of the embryonic layers. But in the 1860s, they, too, were unable to correctly appreciate the problem of embryonic layers, yet Metchnikoff wished to radically dissociate himself from his critics. After all, his research in invertebrate embryology refuted Weismann's intention (based on Cuvier's ideas) to establish the profound difference in embryology of insects and vertebrates. Metchnikoff rejected evidence considered as favorable for Cuvier's ideas and, at least negatively, this early (1865) work contributed to his later theoretical development. Metchnikoff certainly had the right to defend the importance of his contribution: he had established (how clearly is another question) the presence of layers in *Sepiola* (1867), in crustaceans (1868), and in the scorpion (1868). Thus in 1886, Metchnikoff was sensitive to his historic role, principally because those musings ultimately led to the phagocytosis theory (26).

Speaking in 1886 about the situation of invertebrate embryology in the mid-1860s, Metchnikoff stated that Leuckart's laboratory was not concerned with problems of comparative embryology. Because he later viewed this account as the prehistory of his special interest in mesodermal cells and, more broadly, in the comparative roles of the embryonic layers, we get the impression that Metchnikoff (at least after his studies of insect embryology) was primarily concerned with the problem of embryonic layers. Dogel and Gaisinovich write:

> In the first decade of his scientific activity, Metchnikoff mainly worked (in parallel with Kowalevsky) in confirming the homology of the primary layers in all invertebrates. From this followed the establishment of general patterns of animals' development and proof of the historical unity of the whole animal realm on the basis of the comparative-embryological material. . . . However, from the moment Metchnikoff . . . turned to sponges (1874) and returned to coelenterates . . . he became interested not so much in the question about the embryonic layers as in the question of identifying the most primitive pattern of multicellular development [which layers were most primitive] . . . and what conclusions could be made on the basis of the research in the early stages of animals' development about the genesis of the multicellular animals. (7, pp. 693–694)

This interpretation corresponds closely with Metchnikoff's own version of his scientific development. But the facts belie this story. Leaving aside the collaborative work with Kowalevsky, (this reflected, in fact, continuous and bitter argument rather than a coordinated research program), we note that Metchnikoff's work in the 1860s was not inspired by the desire to establish "(on the basis of the comparative-embryological material) proof of the historical unity of the whole animal realm." Dogel and Gaisinovich write about Metchnikoff's two goals as if there was just one or at least two closely related and simultaneously performed goals of his research program: (a) the establishment of general animal development patterns and (b) the proof of animal genealogical unity. But the second issue was in no instance Metchnikoff's goal during the 1860s. On the contrary, in the 1860s, he strictly opposed those embryologists who attempted to study the general patterns of development and those who saw in the establishment of genealogical relations the primary goal of comparative embryology. And Metchnikoff identified himself quite explicitly and decisively with the first group. We will demonstrate that precisely because he considered these two goals at that time as independent of each other, the true difficulties in achieving the first forced him to recognize the second issue as important. The shift was not a careless one; he did not simply abandon the failed first ideology and then adopt another. He viewed the new ideology, and its representatives (Darwin, Fritz Mueller, Kowalevsky, Haeckel) through the concrete problems of his own previous position, and he attemped to inscribe them into the content of his concrete research. This explains the peculiarities of his Darwinism and his interpretation of Fritz Mueller's "biogenetical" idea. Further, recognition of this ideological shift allows us to understand his attitude toward Haeckel and Kowalevsky.

With this state of affairs, the issue of Metchnikoff's allegedly predominate preoccupation with the primary layers is closely connected. Is it true that in the first decade of his scientific life Metchnikoff worked mainly with the problem of homology of the embryonic layers in all invertebrates? His scientific career began with studies of protozoans and then turned to metazoans. He studied between 1865 and 1869 annelids (Polychaeta), Gastrotricha (he was the first to establish the class of primitive worms), Turbellaria (Rhabdocoela, Tricladida), roundworms, *myzostoma,* crustaceans, mollusks, nemertine worms, trematodes, cestodes, insects, lower chordates *(Balanoglossus),* and Echinodermata, which resulted in about thirty published works on morphology and embryology of invertebrates. This is the same diversity of research we note in Metchnikoff's published papers during the next five years, until 1874. From that year, new goals were addressed to establish the most primitive development of embryonic layers and the origin of metazoans. These goals limited the range of his research mainly to two organisms: medusae and sponges.

Reading these works, we cannot conclude that they were primarily inspired by the problem of embryonic layers. Even those publications in which he dealt with that problem (and they are far from being the majority of his works) more often had other foci of interest. Working in 1865 in Leuckart's laboratory (devoted mainly to parasitology), Metchnikoff in parallel to his studies in insect embryology initiated a second theme of research: the development of *Ascaris nigro* (a nematode), a parasite of frogs, that has alternating parasitic and free generations (27). (This was the first project involving parasites, an interest Metchnikoff returned to throughout his life.) In 1865, he studied the development and morphology of a crustacean, *Nebalia,* concluding that it was closer to the highest crustacean, Malacostraca, then to Phyllopoda as thought before. The studies of *Nebalia* were the theme of his doctorial dissertation (1868). Also in 1865, Metchnikoff discovered the larvae of *Balanoglossus* and in 1869 returned to this topic and proved that the earliest known tornaria larva was one of the earlier stages of the larvae of *Balanoglossus.* In 1869, Metchnikoff and Édouard Claparède (the naturalist) published work on the larvae of Chaetopoda. Their goal was to determine whether the classification of the diverse larvae proposed by Johannes Peter Mueller corresponded to the classification of adult forms; Metchnikoff continued related research until 1871. In 1869, Metchnikoff published his extant work on the development of echinoderma and Nemertinea (his first publication on the topic appeared in 1868), an opus some specialists have considered especially important in the field (28). Metchnikoff correctly described each of the basic problems of echinoderm development (enterocaelom, metamerism, metamorphosis), and was the first to observe formation of the coelom in animals without metamerism in adult states. (Note that this 1869 description of the coelom's development was long before the studies of Oskar and Richard Hertwig and presented in their *Coelomtheorie* [1881].) Metchnikoff's works on insects (as we noted earlier) were initiated by the question of pedogenesis; although he derived important results on insect development (including his observation of nuclear reproduction in the egg and superficial cleavage), the primary layers were only part of his concern. For instance, in this work (and in some others), he paid no less attention to the problem of embryonic membranes, apparently viewing these structures as highly important for establishing a similarity in the development of vertebrates and invertebrates.

In the 1866 paper "About Development of Lower Crustaceans in the Egg" (29), the public polemic with Kowalevsky began. Metchnikoff doubted Kowalevsky's observation that the digestive cavity formed through invagination. From Kowalevsky's point of view, cleavage in this case results in the formation of the blastula as a monolaminar structure and following invagination leads to formation of a bilaminar creature. Metchnikoff argued that between these two stages, Kowalevsky omitted an unnoticed interval of four hours when, before any trace of invagination (!) the segmentation cavity was surrounded not by one, but by two layers of cells. He writes:

> Kowalevsky asserts that the intestinal cavity in Amphioxus is formed by invagination. . . . But where are the facts speaking for this? In all studied animals the intestinal cavity (of course, providing its front and back parts) *never is formed through such an invagination but always through formation of walls around the nutritious yolk or around the segmentation cavity.* (29, *AC,* p. 41)

Nekrasov explained the discrepancy between Metchnikoff and Kowalevsky by a typical mistake of a young scientist:

> The basic facts of development [of *Balanus, Sacculina, Cyclops*] given by Metchnikoff are accepted now. But Metchnikoff's reasoning about the origin of the intestinal cavity out of the segmentation cavity is an erroneous one and demonstrates how little invertebrate embryology had been elaborated at that time. In the given case, Metchnikoff's mistake was the usual mistake of young naturalists having well studied some forms, they try to extend by analogy their conclusions upon other forms. Because Metchnikoff's first works were devoted to the embryology of insects and crustaceans which develop usually with incomplete cleavage, because of a large amount of yolk, he tried to find in *Cyclops's* egg the embryonic stripe which he knew so well from insect development. The same explains the erroneous parallel between the segmentation cavity and the intestinal cavity. Metchnikoff reasoned in this way: the blastoderm in development of *Sacculina* and *Balanus* surrounds the yolk. In *Cyclops* the blastula's wall surrounds not the yolk but the segmentation cavity with a liquid inside of it. Because in the first case [in *Sacculina* and *Balanus*] the wall of the middle intestine used the yolk and inside of the intestine the intestinal cavity is formed, then the segmentation cavity (surrounded by the cells homological to the blastoderm) was thought to produce the cavity of the middle intestine. (28, p. 409)

We might add that beyond this logical mistake there was a speculative reason pushing Metchnikoff toward the search for a general scheme of development. He believed at that time that the very

> goal of the history of development as science [i.e., the very goal of embryology], which deals with the multitude of changing forms, must exactly establish the general affinity between different animals and discovering the plan of their organization. (1, *AC,* p. 256)

Metchnikoff criticized Kowalevsky, but relied on the original drawings without any attempt to repeat the studies. Kowalevsky wrote in reply to Metchnikoff:

> I have been awfully surprised that you had concluded out of my own drawings that the invagination did not occur. . . . Anyway, during the last week, I repeated again my observations, spending the whole night, and omitted no step, and so from the egg until the fetus my observation is perfectly complete now. All other intervals in further development I will try to add also and then to write in German. Now, I think my drawings will be more convincing. (30, p. 27)

Kowalevsky published his findings (31), which finally convinced Metchnikoff.

In Metchnikoff's introduction to his paper (1867) on Cephalopoda *(Sepiola)* (32), he stated that the subject of his first concern in the work was "rather the primary formation of organs than their further development." He continued, "The essential meaning of history of the organs' origin and that of the germ layers for comparative embryology is alone sufficient to explain my intention" (32, *AC,* pp. 145–146). But he made little progress in defining primary layer formation, at least as compared to Kowalevsky's observation of invagination in the lancelet. Metchnikoff could only make a modest statement concerning the separation of the germ into two layers:

> The formation was realized quite gradually. At first it is possible to see in the mon-ocellular layer a bulge located on the periphery of the germ. . . . Then two layers of cells appear only in the bulged site (probably, they have come out of a cross-division of the primary cells). (32, *AC,* p. 151)

Thus, although Metchnikoff observed that two layers appeared at a certain stage, the process of layer formation was not determined, and his contribution had little correspondence to later embryological concepts. There is no mention concerning an inner layer (entoderm); thus his restricted information limited his main research query: the alleged homology of the layers in vertebrates and mollusks.

In his doctorial dissertation (1868) on the crustacean *Nebalia* (33), Metchnikoff wrote little of the embryonic layers. As mentioned, the technology of the time limited discernment of layers in eggs that contained an extensive amount of yolk. Seeing two layers, he believed that the inner one was the serous layer (i.e., the entoderm). But beginning in 1868, with the studies of scorpion embryology, Metchnikoff applied the new technique of fixation and cross sections. He stated, "The main result of this research is that in the scorpion's fetus the three layers develop which are in some aspects strikingly similar to the Remak [notion of] vertebrate layers." (34, 1871, p. 229) Nekrasov comments:

> It was hardly possible to solve the question concerning early developmental stages of embryonic layers of the scorpion using optical sections as Metchnikoff did, because with this methodology it is impossible to establish the boundaries of the layers. But Metchnikoff is undoubtedly correct in concluding from his optical sections [that] there actually were three embryonic layers. There was a disagreement between the data of the further research [of the question]. (35, *AC,* p. 492)

Kowalevsky's 1866 paper on the development of *Ascidia* evoked general excitement (36). For the first time, a connection between vertebrates and invertebrates was established. Kowalevsky discovered the similarities in development of lancelet (Chordata) and the tunicates (previously considered mollusks) by showing that, as in vertebrates, the nervous system of tunicates developed from the dorsal ectodermal folds, which then formed the dorsal neural tube. Metchnikoff utterly rejected this model (37, 1869, n. 37 herein). He thought that *Ascidia*'s nervous system was formed from a special part of the entoderm, whereas Kowalevsky argued (correctly) that the dorsal evagination of the entoderm formed the chorda and had no role in neural-tube development. Later (1872), Metchnikoff concurred concerning chorda formation (38), but he persisted for several years in believing that the ventral portion of the neural tube derived from entodermal elements. Eventually, he abandoned his model in favor of Kowalevsky's.

Metchnikoff's accurate 1873 description (39) of myriapod (Diplopoda) development (both the external body form and many internal structures) still conflicted with that of Kowalevsky regarding the embryonic layers. Metchnikoff was inclined to observe a differentiation of only two embryonic layers—the ectoderm and the mesoderm; he refused to admit that the origin of the middle intestine was entodermal, though at that time, Kowalevsky had demonstrated it in several animal species. As Oppenheimer asserts:

The first voices were raised against the germ-layer doctrine during the 1870s. . . . Koelliker (1879, 1884, 1889) questioned the validity of the doctrine principally from the histologist's point of view. While some of his reasoning now seems quaint, and some has since been invalidated by modification of the doctrine, some is still cogent. (6, p. 271)

And Oppenheimer explains that the difficult point for Koelliker to understand was the ability of the same embryonic layer to author so many diverse cell types. Specifically, epithelium, nervous cells, neuroglia, and eye-pigmented epithelium derived from the outer layer; but this layer could also give rise to smooth musculature, for example, in sweat glands. Similar diversity is found in the middle layer, but regarding the entoderm, Koelliker erroneously claimed that in *Amphioxus* it formed somites, muscle, and connective tissue; and in many lower forms, it was the origin of chorda. Criticism of the primacy of the germ layers was soon raised:

In 1878, the Hertwigs raised their first question about the application of the germ-layer theory in a small monograph dealing with the histology of the Medusae. . . . [T]hey concluded that what they consider mesoderm in the Medusae is simply a product of the histological differentiation of ectoderm and endoderm. In their monograph on the Actinians, published a year later (1879) as the first of their definitive "Studies on the Germ-layer Theory," they continue their discussion, questioning the precise relationship of the two layers of the Coelenterates to the three of higher forms. On evidence that in some coelenterate groups germ-cells or musculature are derived from ectoderm and in others from endoderm, they conclude that "within particular animal groups the germ-layers have differentiated organologically inequivalently." (6, pp. 272–273)

Finally, the Hertwigs came to the following conclusion:

The germ-layers are neither organological nor histological entities. It is not possible, if one knows the origin of an organ in one animal group, to carry over the result to all other animal groups. (Quoted from 6, p. 273)

We would add that this kind of criticism against the germ-layer doctrine should actually be predated to the first attempts in the 1860s to extend the concept to invertebrates. We have noted both Weismann's assertion that he saw no similarity between the embryology of vertebrates and insects and summarized Metchnikoff's work in insect comparative embryology. But more germane to criticism of Koelliker and the Hertwigs (1879) is Metchnikoff's position formulated as early as 1869:

Out of these data it is possible to conclude that although the formation of the layers is a quite widespread phenomenon among invertebrates, it is similar not to such a degree that it would be possible to lay the similarity as foundation for some morphological conclusions. The formation of the layers being different in different animals at the same time does not present definite relations to groups of tissues; thus, for example, the middle layer of Cephalopoda can give rise to both epithelial and connective tissues, it can also [generate] nerve cells and fibers of different kinds. (1, *AC*, p. 270)

From this review of Metchnikoff's works, it is clear that in 1872 Metchnikoff was still comfortable with the opinions he developed in the 1860s. Only in the late 1870s, especially after his formulation of the phagocytosis hypothesis in 1883, did Metchnikoff alter the version of his scientific opinions and achievements of this period. According to Metchnikoff's revised version of this scientific development (until 1872), he was inspired by the idea of establishing evolutionary relations between different groups of animals. Pursuing this goal and firmly believing in basic evolutionary unity, Metchnikoff's revisionism saw him defining in different groups of animals the same pattern of basic structure—the three embryonic layers. This account is broadly accepted in the Metchnikovian literature. (We will leave until chap. 4 the question as to how the theory of evolution inspired his research.) But what is the concrete record in respect to the role of the primary layers? During that period, Metchnikoff understood the concept as Remak had elaborated it for vertebrates. In his own studies of invertebrates, Metchnikoff sought similar structures. In some cases, he was successful enough to establish a trilaminarity, in others he found only bilaminar structures; in both cases, he was not always sure of the correspondence between these structures and Remak's layers. Occasionally, he failed to establish the presence of these types of structures at all. In these circumstances, it was impossible to assert the universal presence of the layers and the validity of Remak's concept as applied to invertebrates. Metchnikoff was cautious and spoke only of "a quite widespread phenomenon." But because the phenomenon did not have, in his opinion, any clearly established morphological characteristics, it was natural to ask how the phenomenon might be identified. What kind of phenomena is asserted as widespread? Is there such a phenomenon at all? The likeliest answer was the widespread presence of laminarity in embryonic development (note: laminarity not *the layers*). Remak's concept of the embryonic layers provides, beside the morphological criterion, a histological standard: each of the layers has its own histological future. But we saw Metchnikoff's conclusion in this respect, "Formation of the layers being different in different animals at the same time does not present definite relation to groups of tissues." Thus, if the laminarity has neither morphological nor histological identifications, how is it possible to refer to *the layers?* This indefiniteness in respect to the problem of the identification of the embryonic layers was explicitly formulated by Metchnikoff in the same paper in which he stated:

[The very] goal of the history of development as the science [i.e., the very goal of embryology] which deals with the multitude of changing forms, must exactly establish the general affinity between different animals and the search for the plan of their organization. (1, *AC*, p. 256)

But the problem of identification of the embryonic layers was an important one in Metchnikoff's research precisely because he (as all others) saw in it the attempt to establish the most general and basic structures in embryonic development. Therefore, in respect to Metchnikoff's devising the goals of comparative embryology, the conclusion that formation of the layers was different in various animals and that their identification was hardly possible by a histological criterion must have been a pessimistic conclusion.

Metchnikoff's Early Opinion of Recapitulation

The Darwinians

The goal of embryology, from Metchnikoff's point of view, was to establish a general affinity of different animals and to discover the plan of their organization. Attempts to solve questions related to this goal determined the essence of embryology's modern period (the 1860s).

> However, beside this strictly comparative-embryologic direction yet another one appears at the present time—a more applied direction having in view *application of the facts submitted by the history of development* [i.e., embryology] *for reinforcement and spreading of the teaching about transformation of species.* (1, *AC,* p. 256)

In this regard, applied direction was offered (according to Metchnikoff) by Fritz Mueller (9), Ernst Haeckel (40), and Carl Semper (41).

Fritz Mueller's research originated in Darwin's belief that individual development of an animal must preserve some features of its ancestor's organization. He studied larval forms of some crustaceans, searching for the simplest and, at the same time, the most common of various representatives of the class. He chose Nauplius, which in the eighteenth century had been described by the Czech, Otto Mueller. Nauplius is a six-legged larva of one of the lower crustaceans; its basic structure is shared by larvae of other lower crustaceans. These larvae were so similar in form and organization that they became the test for membership in Crustacea; thus certain parasitic animals previously considered as belonging to mollusks and worms were firmly enrolled in this class after discovery of their Nauplius-like larvae. Fritz Mueller concluded that Nauplius had preserved, in the most complete fashion, features common to its crustacean ancestor. In order to prove the hypothesis, he attempted to find Nauplius-like larvae in the higher crustaceans, whose known larvae embraced a more complex organization. He presupposed that the features of the common ancestor of the class had been completely effaced when he unexpectedly found a Nauplius-like larva of one South American crustacean of the highest order *(Penaeus).* He considered this discovery as the main argument "for Darwin," although it is obvious that the argument does not support in any way the idea of natural selection. If the discovery could be considered as a support for Darwinism, it should be taken only as a general idea of a successive transformation of organic forms. It is worth mentioning that Metchnikoff understood the inflated influence of *Origin of Species* on morphology in this period:

> Appearance of the treatise *Origin of Species* also influenced morphology, i.e., the science about constitutions and affinity of organic forms. However, the influence was conditioned not by the establishment of natural selection's theory but by the restoration and reinforcement of the theory of the successive descent of species. (42, p. 216, 1950)

This observation was written in 1876, but in the period 1865–1870, as we will discuss further, Metchnikoff's position in this respect was essentially the same. Fritz Mueller was convinced by the results of his research that individual development repeated, in an abbreviated way, the entire history of its species.

In a short period, several weeks or months, changing forms of fetuses and larvae represent a more or less complete and true picture of the transitions of the species through immeasurable millennia. (9)

Starting from this idea and his discovery of the Nauplius-like larvae of the higher crustaceans, F. Mueller reduced the lower and the higher crustaceans to a basic form. He decided that all particular differences and variations of the basic form could easily be explained as results of adaptation to the external environment. His work may be considered both as having a powerful intellectual impact, shifting the current biological thought in favor of the evolutionary idea, and, at the same time, as a manifestation of that shift.

Metchnikoff cautiously viewed Fritz Mueller's principle that development of a single animal repeats the whole history of its species. First, he questioned Mueller's criteria:

Which of the different modes of development at present occurring in a class of animals may claim to be that approaching most nearly to the original one is easy to judge. . . . *The primitive history of a species will be reserved in its developmental history the more perfectly, the longer the series of young states through which it passes by uniform steps; and the more truly, the less the mode of life of the young departs from that of the adults, and the less the peculiarities of the individual young states can be conceived as transferred back from later ones in previous periods of life, or as independently acquired.* (9, pp. 120–121, 1869)

Metchnikoff believed that these rules could not be accepted unconditionally. Although in conformity with the data obtained from studies on crustaceans, application of the rules with other reconstructed genealogies was more problematic. For instance, Metchnikoff noted that the jellyfish, *Aurelia,* has a long succession of transformations. By analogy with crustaceans and according to F. Mueller's rules, the hypothesis predicts that this case might accurately reflect the genealogy of the species and its closest relatives. But such is not the case, for *Pelagia noctiluca,* closely related to *Aurelia,* develops in a totally different manner; *Pelagia*'s ciliated larva quickly metamorphosizes into a form similar to the adult. Again, the parasitic worm, *Aspidogaster* hatches from the egg in a form similar to the adult, without demonstrating its genealogy. But closely related *Distoma* demonstrates one of the most intricate genealogies: a complex reproductive cycle in which two asexual generations alternate with a sexual form (1, *AC,* p. 258).

Of course, these discrepancies were easily explained by *the Darwinians* (Metchnikoff's term for those who saw the goal of comparative embryology in reconstruction of genealogical relations) by merely arguing that in some cases *reduction of development* had taken place (i.e., some stages may be reduced in time or effaced completely). After all, F. Mueller conditioned the accuracy of recapitulations by the additional principle that "the less the mode of life of the young departs from that of the adults," the more truly the primitive history of a species will be reserved in its developmental history. But, in many cases, this additional principle is not explanatory. Metchnikoff gives an example (1, *AC,* pp. 260–261): the larvae of many turbellarians have a similar life pattern to that of their adult forms. The larvae so closely resemble the highest ciliated infusorians that some researchers suggested a close affinity between these two groups. The Darwinians, using these suggestive embryological data, were eager to link all worms to the ciliated infusorians. But beside these turbellarians (flatworms) there are others (i.e., the order Nemertina [roundworms]) whose development is mediated by another larva *(Pilidium)* that is markedly dissimilar to the infusorians. The development of those turbellarians presents a more complicated succession. If the latter form of development is viewed as the authentic presentation of turbellarian history, then the development through the infusorian-like larva should be recognized as a result of reduction. But why then should the similarity between the infusorian-like larva and infusorians be ignored?

The idea of a parallelism between individual development and development of its corresponding species (as Metchnikoff often noted) is not necessarily connected with a Darwinian understanding of evolution, but it reflects a widespread idea of old *naturphilosophie* (e.g., correspondence with von Baer's opinions on the nature of individual development, see later discussion). Therefore, dealing with the Darwinists' approach, two different questions must be posed: (a) What kind of boundaries are defined by the actual facts of comparative embryology as applied to F. Mueller's principle? (b) Does Darwinism provide the principle with a new explanatory power? Metchnikoff wrote:

> Detailed knowledge about the history of animal development in no way can unconditionally support the opinion that in a history of an individual development a history of its species is repeated with just some small limitations. Applying the principle in practice we meet in the majority of cases the difficulties which in no way can be avoided. And if we consider history of development as solely the origin of knowledge about descent of species, then we will be forced, as may others, to add fantasy to facts. (1, *AC,* p. 260)

The first among the "others" was Haeckel.

> Looking in this exclusive way at embryology, Haeckel in his systematic survey of organisms derives conclusions without any limits and in any respect does not feel uneasy proposing the most paradoxical and premature hypothesis. Of course he is forced to contradict his own principle, even though this does not rescue him from mistakes. (1, *AC,* pp. 258–259)

These objections do not mean that Metchnikoff rejected F. Mueller's principle as such, but Metchnikoff identified problems in the very application of F. Mueller's hypothesis. Because Darwinians took recapitulation for granted, their concern was not to prove various cases, provide evidence for the mechanism, nor vigorously examine anomalies to their presumptions, but rather to explain deviations from the clear and strict parallelism between (speaking in Haeckel's terms) ontogeny and phylogeny. From Metchnikoff's point of view, to reconstruct phylogeny (43) through ontogeny, then, by the very virtue of the task, already assumes as one possible solution the idea of recapitulation. But then the very problem is to find cases of recapitulation and give sound reasons for belief that in any given example recapitulation, in fact, occurs. Concluding his arguments against the Darwinians Metchnikoff wrote:

All this said . . . , does not serve at all to destroy the very principle of F. Mueller and his followers. I only point at the difficulties which are met at every step and which render it impossible to apply this principle on a large scale. I consider it as very sound to look upon history of development of different individuals as the abbreviated genealogy of the species, but only in those few cases where the development does not represent permanent leaps. But I do not think it is legitimate to construct hypotheses pulling in every way between different species the genealogical relations which are impossible to prove by means of the data presented by science. (1, *AC,* p. 258)

The message contains something more than just a warning of possible frequent exceptions to the drawn parallelisms. Metchnikoff argued that the principle could be applied "only in those few cases where the development does not represent permanent leaps." But what did he mean when he referred to "leaps?" Is circular reasoning being applied? Perhaps, in a given case, Metchnikoff asserts that there are no leaps simply by applying F. Mueller's principle? We can surmise Metchnikoff's meaning by turning to his explanation of F. Mueller's sound results in research on crustaceans.

Peering attentively into the essence of the crustacean transformations, we notice that they can be reduced mainly to a gradual formation of the joints and extremities which is performed by highly regular and continuous formation. No matter how diverse the metamorphoses are, nevertheless they are not connected with the presence of a large amount of temporal (provisional) organs and this is highly important for finding a common plan in the development of a whole class. But on the other hand, we can assert quite soundly that in the whole realm of animals there is no other class that develops so regularly and gradually as the class of crustaceans, and because of this, it is impossible to generally apply such hasty, and at the same time, broad conclusions as are suggested by the case of crustaceans. (1, *AC,* p. 257)

Thus, individual development is a result (an end) of a corresponding species development; the order of individual development is elaborated in the history of the corresponding species. But there is no reason why the latter history should necessarily be submitted to the same order that has elaborated itself. If it occurs that the history of a species is considered as a reproduction of the same "logic" at different stages of that history (as seen in the case of the crustaceans) and to that degree in which this kind of reproduction is maintained in the history of the species, continuity of development may be accepted (i.e., parallelism between individual and species development). But in that case in which the history has been more innovative, the parallelism is not so obvious. Thus, we noted Metchnikoff's example in which he discussed two types of turbellarian development: (a) a truncated cycle where the larva resembled higher infusorians and (b) a cycle that expressed more stages of transformations but in which the larva was dissimilar to infusorians. Recall, according to F. Mueller's principle, individual development preserving more stages of transformation presents the history of the animal group more completely, whereas the other path of individual development (in this case, beginning with the infusorian-like larva) should be considered as an abbreviation of the authentic history. But after all, it is possible to use F. Mueller's idea of parallelism by observing and ultimately judging that a given stage ("image") of development is similar to another infantile or adult form found in animals of other groups. Only appealing to such an "obviousness" (i.e., to something that is immediately revealed by intuition) permits the additional criterion of length of development. In the case of dual turbellarian maturation, the "obviousness" testifies to the genealogical relation with the highest infusorians. The second pattern does not propose such an obvious solution of the genealogical question, but being subjected to the criterion of the length and complexity of individual development, this second path testifies that the first is but an abbreviation.

Why then should visual criteria alone not be acceptable if the entire theory is built on resemblance? From Metchnikoff's point of view, this difficulty arose from the presupposition that the group history is submitted to certain rules whose elaboration it cannot control. In this case, an assumption is made that one course of development is closer to the authentic group genealogy and the others represent different degrees of deviation from the authentic pathway. But if the group history is not assumed as required to always repeat the same strategy, but rather assumes that the history is its own author in respect to the elaborated strategy, then there is no need to decide which of the two criteria are more convincing—the "obviousness" of a given similarity or the length and complexity of a particular individual development. Metchnikoff concluded his turbellarian example by noting:

> The given example demonstrates that very similar animals (in our case, for example, Nemertes and Tetrastoma) develop entirely differently, i.e. that *in development one end can be achieved in different ways* entirely independently from that accepted by F. Mueller's abbreviated course of development. (1, *AC*, p. 261)

Thus, Metchnikoff believed that the validity of F. Mueller's principle (named later "the biogenetic law" by Haeckel) was limited to few cases: only where the group developed in an uninterrupted way and where the history did not radically change its strategy in elaborating new forms. Ignoring these limitations, the Darwinians put themselves in a situation in which they were forced to *ad hoc* hypotheses because they believed in a strong parallelism (excepted only by certain insignificant restrictions) between individual development and the development of the species. This belief did not allow them to notice that history had elaborated different strategies in the creation of new forms (this was especially true of Haeckel). Correspondingly, instead of true attempts to prove that a given case provided recapitulated features, they would rather accept a hypothetical parallelism and then attempt to explain by other *ad hoc* hypotheses why concrete facts would not fit their assumed constructions. And here we come to Metchnikoff's second general question concerning the relation of comparative embryology to the attempt of reconstructing genealogical relations.

Does Darwinism (as represented by F. Mueller and his followers) truly provide a new explanatory power whose application to comparative embryology would effectively reconstruct evolutionary relations? The fact that certain taxonomic relations between adult organisms were also reflected in their embryonic stages was not a Darwinian discovery. Neither was the idea of species transformation a Darwinian innovation. The true novelty of Darwin's theory was the attempt to introduce a new explanatory principle underlying transformation—natural selection. It is now broadly appreciated that true Darwinism was not broadly accepted in the nineteenth century, and the concept of natural selection had little influence on the theories of F. Mueller and his followers. Further, even in the twentieth century, Darwinism has had a restricted impact on theories of individual development and ontogenesis (see app. A). Metchnikoff however was one of the first who recognized that Darwinians omitted the central principle of natural selection in the construction of their ontogenetic theories. He understood that they only asserted the parallelism without explaining how natural selection might be operative. Instead, these Darwinians invoked natural selection when they required an explanation for deviations from the constructed parallelism. It was always possible to cite natural selection as providing those deviations as secondary adaptations. Correspondingly, this theoretical position would not allow definition of different types of affinity between various groups of organisms. The statement that affinity is due to some commonality in descent does not by itself establish that affinity. Metchnikoff correctly observed:

> Though many of the most zealous admirers of the species' transformation theory believe that to speak about the systematic similarity of organisms immediately means to preach Darwinism, but in reality they are entirely erroneous. Similarity between all organisms in general, and between their different groups in particular, is (and was) broadly recognized and its existence cannot be doubted. But not everyone thought it possible to explain this similarity by *the blood kinship* between organisms, considering the explanation as too hypothetical, devoid of a firm basis and, at the same time, in no way changing the fact of similarity of forms and organism structure. (1, *AC,* p. 261)

We may now summarize Metchnikoff's conclusions about the scientific value of the approach of F. Mueller (and his followers) to comparative embryology: First, the approach may not be broadly applied and can give true results only in a comparatively narrow scope of cases. Second, the theoretical foundation of the approach is rather weak and any attempt to exploit the foundation for extension of the approach to broad generalizations ultimately leads to invention of arbitrary hypotheses that lack any scientific significance. Third, when we omit the defects of this approach, it is no more than an applied aspect of comparative embryology, which has its own goals totally independent from the applied aspect. Finally, for realization of its goals, comparative embryology does not require any speculations about historical relations of species. Metchnikoff concluded:

> Keeping this in mind, many others, entirely independently from the question about transformation of species, formulated their goal as comparative studies in development of animals exactly in the same way as comparative anatomy existed much earlier than Lamarckism and Darwinism, and in the same way as it [comparative anatomy] even now can pursue its goals apart from a theory of the common descent of the whole organic world. Comparative history of development [i.e., comparative embryology] deals with facts from which it makes immediate conclusions leaving aside discussions about ways of different species descent. (1, *AC,* p. 261)

Von Baer

It is a mistake to understand the appeal "deal with facts" as an expression of a positivistic attitude, leaving aside any attempts to develop a theoretical approach. We suggest that any experienced researcher in a field of typology possesses an intuitive vision of the respective typologized forms. The vision may be acquired only through

experience of working with the "facts" rather than a preconceived theoretical interpretation. The experience and the intuitive vision cannot be replaced by a theoretical
construction, but it still requires that reflection to establish the research goals and
definition of its field of investigation. We saw that Metchnikoff formulated the goal
of comparative embryology as establishing a general affinity between different animals and finding their plan of organization. Working tirelessly with vast amounts of
zoological data and searching for derivative "facts" that hinted at the underlying
"plans" and species "affinities," he concurrently felt the need of a central concept to
comprehensively organize the material, orient the research, and explain the phenomena. That central concept (in those years) he hoped would be assigned to Remak's
theory of embryonic layers, which, in turn, had been developed from von Baer's
model. Metchnikoff was then a direct descendent of von Baer's goals and understanding of the nature of comparative embryology. Besides von Baer's influence in embryology of the time, the personal relations between young Metchnikoff and his famous
fellow countryman (who greeted Metchnikoff's results with favor and apparently
patronized the young scientist [44]), we note von Baer's direct influence on Metchnikoff's writing of this period. We cited earlier Metchnikoff's 1886 work that criti-
cally reviewed the situation of the 1860s when German embryologists saw in stages
of individual development an "expression of a general plan [that] was appreciated in
an ideal manner" (21, p. 419, 1950). But what does Metchnikoff's own concept of
"a general plan" mean, if not von Baer's *Bauplan?*

Metchnikoff characterized himself in 1869 not as an adversary of the idea of transformation of species but as the adversary of the theory of "the *limitless* transformation of species" (1, *AC,* p. 261). What are these limits? Perhaps we hear an echo of
von Baer's idea of limited physical evolution that does not influence the "ideal plan."
Von Baer established four great *Bauplans* for the animal realm that corresponded
closely to Cuvier's four types. Cuvier's system was a result of descriptive morphology
of adult organisms, whereas von Baer understood type as a mode of individual development (45). As in Cuvier's arguments against naturphilosophical transformism, von
Baer in his skeptical attitude toward Darwinism did not allow any transformations
of one type into another, but he admitted the possibility of physical transformations
(which did not change the general "ideal plan") within each type (46). We can hardly
doubt that these ideas were the basis of Metchnikoff's skepticism toward limitless
transformations.

In some sense, the very interest in defining the types of embryonic layer formation
(i.e., formation of the earliest structures of development) and their future role must
be considered as due to von Baer's influence. He argued that the earliest stages of
individual development possessed the clearest phyletic information and the most
authentic characteristic of their respective type *(Bauplan).* Later stages, although
reflecting phylogeny, were less reliable as evidence of the true phylogenetic course.
But if Metchnikoff's general theoretical position of that time was von Baerian, his
practical results and the conclusions obtained from them hardly can be considered
as strongly supporting that position. Von Baer was a strong opponent of the recapitulation concept if it was a repetition in embryonic developmental stages of its lower
ancestor adult forms. According to von Baer, the *Bauplan* was already established in

the very beginning of embryogenesis, initiating and controlling development. Different species within a given type were then formed by individualization of this general plan. Development proceeded from the general to the individual, from a more homogeneous state to a more heterogeneous one. This common tendency created the illusion of recapitulation to the degree in which two different species proceed in their development through similar embryonic stages. So, the similarity that created the opportunity to refer to recapitulation was explained not through repetition (in embryonic stages) of lower adult organisms (or their features), but as a similarity between embryonic stages of different animal groups.

Comparing, on the one hand, von Baer's interpretation of similarity in embryonic stages and, on the other hand, the recapitulationist idea, Stephen J. Gould contrasted their two attitudes to Darwinian evolutionary theory:

> There existed in 1859, two major interpretations for the significance of embryonic stages. Each had been formulated under creationists tenets, but each could be easily restructured in evolutionary guise. These were, of course, von Baer's principle that development proceeds inexorably from the general to the special and the recapitulationists claim that embryonic stages represent adult forms of "lower" creatures. Both were quickly given their evolutionary meaning: Darwin accepted von Baer's principle but stood the original explanation on its head. F. Mueller, Haeckel, [Edward] Cope and [Alpheus] Hyatt independently recognized the irresistible promise of recapitulation as a key to the reconstruction of phylogeny. (47, pp. 69–70)

Is it really important to decide whether embryonic structures are similar to ancestral embryonic or adult forms? "If the goal of evolutionary theory is only to set up a series of pragmatic guidelines for the reconstruction of evolutionary trees, then it makes no difference" (47, p. 73). But the stakes are established when the other aspect of the question is considered: In what way can the phyletic information be reproduced in individual development? And which principles or mechanisms provide the preservation of phyletic information?

> If related animals merely repeat their ancestral embryonic stages without alteration, we have a simple case of evolutionary conservatism. If, on the other hand, the tiny human fetus with gill slits is (in essence) an adult fish, then we must seek an active mechanism to "push" the adult shapes of ancestors into early embryonic stages of descendents. The search for a mechanism of recapitulation dominated the theoretical side of late nineteenth-century comparative embryology and provoked a major debate within evolutionary theory. (47, pp. 73–74)

We would add that before the problem took the form of a theoretical question about the mechanism of recapitulation (from 1880 to 1895), it had already appeared in the 1860s as a practical issue of comparative embryology. If similarity between embryonic stages of different groups of animals (or between embryonic stages of one of them and adult forms of another) may be considered as strong evidence for their particular relationship, is the opposite true? If a definite type of a systematic relationship is established between two animal groups and there is information about the embryonic development of one of them, how then (and in what degree of accuracy) can the embryology of the other group be related to the first? In preferring von Baer's interpretation of the meaning of the embryonic stages, there is no reason why both extrapolations (the conclusion based on embryonic data and extended to systematic relations and vice versa) should not be of similar reliability. But if a "pushing" mechanism is at work in individual development (i.e., the mechanism changing in some aspect the order of phylogeny), the situation changes: presence of similar embryonic stages may testify to some systematic relations, but not necessarily vice versa. Thus the difficulties that are connected with attempts (based on systematic relations) to comprehend a plan—a general pattern of embryonic development for different animal groups—may be considered as indirect evidence in favor of the recapitulationist idea.

The difference between von Baer's antirecapitulationist position and the position of the Darwinian recapitulists actually reflects (in an implicit way) two different understandings of organismic integrity—its wholeness. From von Baer's point of view, the embryo of an animal at every stage does not coincide with any adult form of another animal, that is, it is, at every embryonic stage just an undeveloped representative of its type. Only with the end of embryogenesis will the type reach its final form and, thus, its perfection. The last stage of individual development (the adult form) is the stage that reveals the primordial plan of this species. Each of the embryonic stages is but a step toward that realization. The recapitulists assumed, implicitly, the same supposition: the adult form was the realization of the design that has been provided by the history of the species. After all, they studied embryology of a particular organism, that is, its history leading to *this* final stage. But at the same time, they assumed that in the course of individual development the organism runs through other adult forms, that is, through other final realizations of different primordial designs. It follows that individual development is not so much a short record of the corresponding history of species, but rather a rewriting of that history, and it leads to another basic plan, to another basic mode of development. Thus Metchnikoff embraced the concept of viewing developmental history of "different individuals as the abbreviated genealogy of the species, but only in those few cases where the development does not represent permanent leaps" (1, p. 258). Then the integrity of an organism was provided not by a single (predicted) plan, whose realization was the adult individual, but by some activity (mechanism) that was responsible for reconstruction of the intermediate designs and their adaptation within the final stage. In cases where a systematic relation has been defined, through comparison of the adult forms, the relation might be proven or refuted by comparative embryological data. The classical example is the barnacle, whose plan in no way relates to the arthropods; since Cuvier these organisms were classified with the mollusca, but further study established close similarity of their larvae to the larvae of arthropods, a fact that allowed their reclassification among the latter. But the opposite is not true. Exactly because the idea of recapitulation is accepted, no judgment of individual development is offered that originates from an opinion about the systematic relatedness of some form (i.e., if the systematic relation was established by similarity of adult forms). Reliance on the relation is not possible because integrity of an organism is provided not by some final realization of its plan, but rather by an activity that integrates recapitulations of a particular development type. Mentioned earlier, Metchnikoff offered the example of two closely related groups of turbellarians (in regard to their adult form) that developed in radically different ways.

Summary

Based on the formulation described, Metchnikoff's position in those years (the 1860s and early 1870s) is quite clear:

(a) Comparative embryology is a tool in establishing systematic relations which, mainly owing to Darwin's influence, were regarded as the resultant representation of evolution. But this role is only an applied function of comparative embryology, having its own tasks independent from that of reconstructing the evolutionary tree.

(b) The independence of comparative embryology from reconstructing genealogies is clearly seen in cases of apparent disruption of the parallelism between systematic relations and orders of individual development. In those cases, it is apparent that the history of a species is not only an element that should be reduced to the systematic, but the history must be understood as a creative process acting "within" individual development.

(c) The disruption in the parallelism between comparative embryology and taxonomy is rather an argument in favor of the recapitulationist reality and against von Baer's understanding of embryological stages. When the Darwinians (first of all, F. Mueller and Haeckel) insisted that the parallelism had but few and insignificant exceptions for each particular case, they had not fully realized the implications of the recapitulation idea. They did not see that the recapitulation idea actually *contradicts* the idea of a strict parallelism between genealogy and individual development. That is why Darwinism offered little to the understanding of F. Mueller (and his followers). In their interpretation, recapitulation appeared in the guise of the old naturphilosophical idea of parallelism; in their practice, the Darwinians were forced to invent *ad hoc* hypotheses, unsupported by embryological facts.

(d) Although many facts speak in favor of the recapitulationist position (i.e., against von Baer's position), von Baer was correct in determining the reality of a "type" as a mode, or plan, of individual development; and, the "plan" rather than a systematic position represented the integrity of the organism. But if the *Bauplan* is to be understood simply as a succession of morphological structures, the limits of von Baer's understanding of individual development have not been overcome yet. To comprehend the basic plan an activity (or more activities?) running through individual development must be found for integration, otherwise no plan will be discovered and the approach to defining the integrity of organisms will be lost. Metchnikoff concluded that his own attempts (as well as those of others) to comprehend the embryonic layers using only morphological and histological criteria as the basic structures in invertebrate development had failed. But why was he certain that this activity was indeed real? Why did he not assume that organisms lacked integrity and that individual development is but a superposition of a mosaic of uncorrelated and unintegrated forms? We will see that in his future scientific development, Metchnikoff assumed (although during different periods) both of these positions.

CHAPTER 3

Metchnikoff's Embryological Studies after 1872

Genealogical Questions

After 1872, Metchnikoff radically changed his intellectual goals and methods of his embryological studies. Correspondingly, he altered the range of his scientific objectives. If in the previous period he regarded any problems of phylogenetic reconstruction as, at best, an application that added little in the pursuit of comparative embryology's proper goals, he now considered metazoan phylogeny (especially the problem of multicellular origin) as the decisive aspect of comparative embryological studies. In this period, he viewed the approach to embryology through phylogeny not only as a morphological problem, but also as having physiological significance. Earlier, Metchnikoff had studied a broad variety of animal groups, now (in accordance with the central problem—the origin of metazoans) he concentrated primarily on the lowest organisms—medusae and sponges. However, this shift in Metchnikoff's general attitude toward comparative embryology might be expected as a logical development of his scientific studies from the earlier period.

Prior to 1872, Metchnikoff considered the task of genealogical reconstruction as external and only applicable to the primary theoretical goal. If there was, indeed, a strong parallelism between phylogeny and ontogeny (either explained by von Baer's theory or by that of the recapitulists), what could it contribute to embryological studies? After all, any phylogenetic process, as related to a given ontogeny, has occurred in the distant past, and its current basis is the ontogeny itself. Therefore, to incorporate the parallelism particular individual development must be understood; of course, the latter assumes a subject of its own. If the theory of recapitulation is correct, then not only parallelism between the history of species and the corresponding individual development is expected, but some discrepancies between them are also predicted. If, on the one hand, a recapitulation provides a repetition of a feature of adult ancestors in the individual development of their descendants, then, on the other hand, this very fact means that an old "plan" of individual development has been inscribed in the new ontogeny. The very process of such a "rewriting" must mean that a given individual development realizes a new "plan," which could not be reduced to genealogical relationships between the preceding phylogenetic stages. Thus the discrepancies between genealogical relationships (as they are represented in a resulting form of the systematical relationships) and the types of individual development are not of secondary significance. Discrepancies do not necessarily allege cenogenic adaptation of the embryo to a specific environment, but rather testify to radical developmental leaps, typical phenomena in elaboration of new ontogenetic forms. Indirectly then, the discrepancies testify to the recapitulation theory.

Thus the history of species, as it is represented in systematic relationships (if only we assume that the latter, indeed, represent the history), cannot provide a true support to those most difficult cases where comparative embryological research requires such a structure. Firmly established facts of recapitulations may significantly contribute to establishing such systematic relationships. But to conclude conversely, from a given systematic relationship to an expected type or particularity (types or particularities) of recapitulation does not necessarily follow. Is the history of the species then relevant for elucidation of a corresponding individual development? Being pushed out the door, history appears through the window. If in an individual development, old "plans" (presented by recapitulations) are "rewritten" in a new context, then the recapitulated structures (features) carry two separate "meanings": (a) the role of the structure in the old context (in the developmental type of the ancestors) and (b) the role of the structure in the new context of a given individual development. In other words, at each stage where individual development proceeds from a recapitulation, it is, in fact, a process that transforms recapitulated functions. From this point of view, individual development realized a *physiological* transformation of morphologically conservative structures. Thus for Metchnikoff, homological structures possessing some physiological commonality, namely, the basic functions that are determined by their "meaning" in the recapitulated integrity, will be adopted in a new functional context as development proceeds.

As early as 1871, Metchnikoff argued against the generally accepted definition of homological organs as those that, having common origin and similar morphology, are different in relation to their functions.

> Considering an organ physiologically, it is possible to keep in view not only the final goal of its performance but the very processes realized during [the performance]. From this point of view it will appear that many organs considered in textbooks as analogical, actually also differ in regard to physiology; at the same time homological organs have very many physiological similarities. (1, *AC*, p. 194)

Thus, in order to understand how an embryological stage proceeds from a recapitulated structure, its primary functional "meaning" inscribed in a future functional context of the subsequent embryonic stages must be established. But the comprehension of the primary functional "meaning" is only its reconstruction in a supposedly ancestral adult form. The logic demanded Metchnikoff's return to the genealogy problem. His career began in advocating those goals and methods of comparative embryology that were fully independent of any themes of reconstructing phylogeny. In the position of the recapitulists, who argued for a strong parallelism between history of species and corresponding individual development, he saw an immediate challenge to that independence. Paradoxically, Metchnikoff's critique of those who prized comparative embryology, first for its assistance in the cause of phylogenetic (*genealogic* in Metchnikoff's terms) reconstructions, led him to later cross the line that would force him to conclude that reconstruction of phylogeny is not simply an applied aspect of comparative embryology, but a powerful and inevitable aspect of comparative embryological research itself.

Ultimately, Metchnikoff so concluded. But the factual history of his intellectual development shows that this radical shift in Metchnikoff's theoretical position was not exclusively due to pure speculation. Rather, his meditation prepared the semantic space within which he finally came to integrate both his old results and the new scientific realities. In this respect, Metchnikoff's most important conclusion from his research was pessimism concerning the possibility of establishing a morphological and histological identity for the primary embryonic layers. This pessimism marked the first failure to identify objective principles that would provide a general orientation for comparative embryological studies, and thus, at least in this case, sovereignty of comparative embryology failed its desirable objective confirmation. As a result, Metchnikoff's groping was the first factor that prepared his general theoretical shift.

The second factor in determining Metchnikoff's altered theoretical position was the recognition of alternative patterns as forming the second embryonic layer (i.e., not invagination, but delamination or introgression). Henceforth, his future interest was directed to the problem of mesoderm separation from the entoderm as well as a major preoccupation with the development and role of mesodermic cells.

The third factor contributing to Metchnikoff's mature theory was Haeckel's *gastraea* theory, which appeared in the second volume of *Die Kalkschwaemme* in 1872. In the famous polemic launched against that hypothesis, Metchnikoff elaborated a new vision of the relationship between embryological and genealogical research. He moved from an implicit intellectual possibility to an explicitly argued theoretical position.

In 1872, Metchnikoff prepared publication of his work on the development of medusae and siphonophores (published two years later) (2). Careful observation of the living jelly fish larva, *Geronia hastata,* revealed the splitting of the blastoderm cells by a growing jellylike mass. He thus discovered a new pattern of entoderm formation, delamination. This paper is noteworthy for the clear expression of the importance of genealogical relationships to support Metchnikoff's embryological conclusions. Thus he argued that siphonophores were descended from medusae through the polymorphism of organs.

In 1869, Haeckel had published an extensive work on siphonophores (3), which Metchnikoff called an essential contribution (2, pp. 36–37); but at the same time, he began in the "Studies" (4) his complex criticism of it. His initial volley was directed at Haeckel's belief that the pneumatophore (or gas sac) of animals was ultimately derived from the entoderm; Metchnikoff demonstrated that, in fact, pneumatophore development was independent of the entoderm, for he believed that it was the primordial medusa that had changed its function. From 1873 to 1878, Metchnikoff published a series of papers on sponges. In these, he elaborated his general opposition to Haeckel's "philosophical scientific method," developed the criticism toward the *gastraea* theory, shifted his own attention to the origin and the functions of the mesodermic cells, turned to the problem of intracellular digestion, formulated his physiological approach to the task of genealogical reconstruction, and proposed his famous *parenchymella* hypothesis. Another series of studies devoted to the development of the planarians (started in 1877 and continued through the middle of the 1880s) was subjected to the same goals and to the same scientific logic.

Because our purpose is to trace Metchnikoff's scientific evolution as the prehistory of the phagocytosis hypothesis, we should remember that all major steps leading to his major insight, including formulation of the *parenchymella* hypothesis, had been made five years prior (around 1878) to his presentation of the phagocytosis hypothesis (1883). During this period the polemic with Haeckel played an exceedingly important role, at times appearing as if the argument was the very source of Metchnikoff's theoretical inspiration. Earlier, as we noted, Metchnikoff expressed his skepticism in regard to Fritz Mueller and Haeckel's belief in a clear ontogenetic-phylogenetic parallelism; he considered the very task of phylogenetic reconstructions as no more than an application of comparative embryology from which limited immediate support for his embryological research was expected. With little at stake, their intersection was tangential. Metchnikoff appreciated certain limitations regarding the nature of individual development as contributing to phylogenetic reconstructions, but he was not sensitive as to how this undertaking might restrict studies in individual development. Thus, it is not surprising that before 1873 Metchnikoff's general attitude toward Haeckel's ideas was quite respectful; he translated and published *The Teaching About Organic Forms Based upon the Theory of the Transformation of Species* (5)—the abbreviated exposition of Haeckel's *Generelle Morphologie der Organismen.* Although Metchnikoff stressed various points of disagreement, he clearly expressed solidarity with the general spirit of the work (6). In his previous arguments with Haeckel on certain specific and restricted issues (e.g., the development of siphonophores), he only reproached him for inconsistency, "It is truly surprising to meet this inconsistency precisely in Haeckel who usually is not afraid of being consistent to the very end." Not until Metchnikoff began to establish his own genealogical approach to studies of comparative embryology did his defense become the central and competitive issue. Once a new position was assumed, his argument against Haeckel breathed zealously with a taint of animosity.

Gastraea Versus *Parenchymella*

The immediate impetus for Metchnikoff's critical attitude toward Haeckel's scientific style and strategy was occasioned by a concrete controversy related to a discrepancy between their respective descriptions of larval development in the calcareous sponges (7, pp. 34, 216). Metchnikoff observed that the larva differentiated into two parts: the cephalad hemisphere, containing a small cavity, was formed by narrow cells with cilia; the caudal portion was formed by large round cells without cilia. The ciliated cells invaginated into the round cells, forming the gastrula, followed by the round cells blending into a syncytium. Skeletal needles soon appeared in the syncytium, and the ciliated cells, which formed the entoderm, apparently lost their cilia in the process. Haeckel's description of the metamorphosis was radically different. He related that the layer forming the skeleton, which he called the exoderm (8), arose not from the nonciliated cells (as Metchnikoff observed), but from the ciliated ones—

and to complete the contradiction, he claimed that the entoderm was produced by the round cells. Metchnikoff commented on Haeckel's presentation:

> It is easy to see the reason why these opinions are so radically different from my observations if we carefully look through the chapter concerning the history of development of the calcareous sponges [in Haeckel's corresponding paper, pp. 328–338, see n. 7]. It turns out that Haeckel actually never observed the postembryonic development of sponges, but only surmised it a priori. Thus his words are quite remarkable: "The transformation of the swimming gastrula in the earliest and most simple state of attachment which we call *Ascula,* apparently arises very quickly [after becoming a swimming gastrula] *and has not been observed yet. However about the transformations which take place here* [*during this process*] *it is possible to conclude on the basis of comparing the Ascula with gastrula*" [emphasis added]. (9, *AC,* p. 33)

Apparently, Metchnikoff continued, Haeckel incautiously compared the swimming larva with the young, developed sponge: the conclusion, however, was erroneous. Surprisingly, Haeckel often cited this transformation, which he proudly established only by inference and treated as an established fact, not as a supposition—as it truly was derived. For instance, Haeckel wrote, "I call the syncytium of the calcareous sponges the entire mass of tissue arising from the blending of larval ectodermic cells, covered with cilia" (7, p. 160). Or further, "Each of the entoderm cells release one long oscillating outgrowth" (7, p. 216), and so on.

Metchnikoff noted:

> He forgets completely that he himself never saw either the blending or the release of the cilia. Is it the vaunted philosophical "scientific method" of Haeckel's research in whose neglect he condemns the embryologists (the "ontogenists") so harshly? (9, *AC,* p. 34)

Metchnikoff's conclusion is severe:

> Haeckel just concocted the metamorphosis of the calcareous sponges (and concocted it unsuccessfully), taking as the starting point the similarity with the hydroides instead of having come to this only at the end of the research. (9, *AC,* p. 36)

However, Metchnikoff does not admit that he also used analogy for support. Thus in the same paper (cited earlier), he asserted that the sponge layer that produced the skeletal needles was identified as mesoderm; this assertion is made by analogy with the skeletogenic layers of echinoderms—thus he used inference by analogy as proof for his opinion. But the right to use analogy is exactly the issue in question because the homology of the sponge layer is the very problem of both his paper and the corresponding aspect of Haeckel's work.

Haeckel's steadfast prestige as a theoretician had been shaken. In loosening Haeckel's authority, the articulated argument helped Metchnikoff recognize and formulate his own theoretical position, which prior to the controversy was more an implicit assumption than a well-defined program of research. In his paper of 1876 on the same topic of sponge development and morphology, Metchnikoff broadened his critique of Haeckel from simply citing certain factual mistakes to explicitly rejecting what he called Haeckel's naturphilosophical method, which opposed the results "acquired in the positive direction" (10) [positive direction refers to an empirically oriented science in contrast to a speculatively based hypothesis]. The polemics with

Haeckel's *gastraea*-theory became the theoretical axis of Metchnikoff's further embryological work. The task to reconstruct the hypothetical common metazoan ancestor could be viewed from our modern perspective as a romantic undertaking, inspired by new Darwinian sentiment to establish the final genealogical unity of Metazoa. But left unexplained are the emotions and labor spent in the arguments surrounding the hypotheses, which appeared in publications devoted to concrete and specific comparative embryological research. The popularity of the issue was based on its practical implications rather than a grandiose goal pertaining to a Weltanschauung. To picture a hypothetical ancestor was intended to provide researchers with support in identifying the embryological structures with which they were dealing. Thus, referring to the controversy of the *gastraea*-theory, Metchnikoff asserted:

> Modern researchers more and more undermine the basis of the theory, whose rapid expansion (and acceptance at least by many of the young scientists) can be explained in an essential degree by the longing thirst of the morphologists to gain a foothold for the ordering of the huge mass of the accumulated material. (11, *AC*, p. 259)

Cuvier and von Baer were the ardent propagators of the physiological (functional) approach to studies in morphology. As we have discussed, the idea of recapitulation implied a new meaning for a physiological approach. It actually required differentiation between a functional activity of the structure in question within the context of the given organism's integrity and a function of the same structure within the context of the recapitulated integrity. From this point of view, individual development appeared as an adaptation of basic functions provided by the ancestor's history in the development of a given species. Thus the genealogical reconstruction (similar to Haeckel's) played the role of models that provided the starting point for establishing the basic functions of embryological structures, and thus the very possibility to identify those structures.

The *gastraea*-hypothesis assumes cavital digestion as the primordial method of metazoan nourishment and, correspondingly, the entoderm as a universal and specialized structure is predicted. In other words, the *gastraea*-theory is the model that permitted the identification of the inner layer, first as the entoderm and second as the primary structure in relation to the middle layer, a derived structure. In difficult cases, that is, the development of sponges, the hypothesis was used to justify the transfer of the embryonic-layer concept that had been elaborated for animals of higher groups. The publications of those embryologists who were involved in the controversy around the *gastraea*-hypothesis reveal a vision not of a desired integration of animal genealogical relationships inspired by the *gastraea*-hypothesis, but rather the concrete difficulties in identifying the morphological realities.

Here then is Metchnikoff's exposition (given in 1876) of Haeckel's *gastraea*-theory:

> Having the intention to apply the ["biogenetical"] law to the whole animal kingdom, he [Haeckel] turned to "ontogeny" and began his search for the indications of the common animal ancestor. Haeckel turned to the theme exactly at that time when certain groups of researchers, especially several Russian zoologists led by Professor Kowalevsky, devoted themselves to the formulation and elaboration of the basic questions of comparative embryology. In the very beginning of his research in this direction, which immediately yielded several brilliant results, Professor Kowalevsky

found that the developmental processes of many animals are highly similar. He found that upon forming the vesicle resulting from the cleavage of the ovule, a deepening was formed which then transformed into the digestive tube, hence the fetus (already in the very early stages of development) consisted of two concentric sacks (the external skin, and the internal digestive), and the internal sack was opened outward by a pore (the primary mouth). Professor Kowalevsky also found that while in some animals the process took place within the ovule membrane, it occurred in a larval stage in others; the double sack having its surface covered completely with cilia liberated itself from the ovule membrane and began its independent life in water. After his discovery of this larval stage in lower representatives of the vertebrate animals (so-called lancelet fish, *Amphioxus*), Professor Kowalevsky came to the conclusion that the stage "represents the basic plan of (at least) very many forms." He even thought it was likely that this manner of development would be universal for the entire animal kingdom. But he did not dare to assert this because comparative embryology was still at the beginning of its formation and it is impossible to propose such basic conclusions without a sufficient number of positive data. At first he doubted the validity of alternative primary developmental processes which had been described by other authors. But later he was convinced in their accuracy, which confirmed his cautious attitude to the problem. But, as frequently occurs, a large generalization that has not been proposed by a cautious scientist, restricted by the demands of the positive method, may be made by a less cautious dilettante. In this way, universal and even elegant theories may be born, which however, lack only one thing—durability. In the given case, this role of the dilettante has been performed by Haeckel in his so-called *Gastraea* theory. Everything positive and fruitful in the theory belongs not to him, but has been done by others, mainly by Professor Kowalevsky. The only thing which belongs to Haeckel is the extension of that developmental process, discovered by a Russian scientist, upon the entire animal world (except Protozoa [Metchnikoff uses the word *infusoria*]) and establishing long terminology (sometimes appropriate, sometimes—absolutely useless) and classification with a completely scholastic tint. . . . Haeckel divides the animal kingdom as a whole into two large groups: (1) the Protozoa, monocellular, and (2) the "intestinal animals," whose body consists of tissues and which always have an intestinal tube. These animals of the second group *(Metazoa),* to whom belong all vertebrates, mollusks, arthropods, echinoderms, worms, and zoophytes, are descended from the common ancestor whom Haeckel calls the "gastraea." In the epoch of primordial life on earth . . . the sea was inhabited by different kinds of *gastraea,* of which no immediate trace remains, but who appear now during development of very different animals, as the larval form discovered by Professor Kowalevsky and called by Haeckel, "the gastrula." This gastrula is that double sack which I described above. Its structure is very simple. It has the appearance of a microscopic oval larva swimming by ciliated lashes and consisting of an upper (skin) layer and an internal (intestinal) layer. The last is opened outward by a mouthpore (Haeckel's "primeval mouth"). The primeval *gastraea* is different from the gastrula "only in one essential feature—it likely possessed already separated organs of reproduction." The *gastraea* had been descended from another (even more primitive) form, which Haeckel calls "plannea" and which had the appearance of a vesicle formed by one layer of small cells and which had neither a mouth nor any other organ. Some of the *gastraea* of the primordial sea were swimming on the surface and as a result, developed radiant organization. Meanwhile others inhabited the ocean floor and in crawling, developed bi-symmetrical organization. . . . The *gastraea* of the first kind gave origin to the radiant zoophytes; the symmetrical *gastraea* gave origin to the primary representatives of worms and other taxa of intestinal animals. Among currently living organisms (besides, of course, the larval form of the gastrula), the hydras and some of the simplest sponges (i.e., the representatives of the zoophytes) are most closely related to the *gastraea.* That is in short the theory of the *gastraea*. Haeckel sees its scientific basis in the similarity of all gastrulae in all studied animals, and in the fact that the two layers, which form it, are completely identical (homological) in all intestinal animals. (*SBW*, pp. 230–233)

As Metchnikoff noticed:

> Haeckel speaks himself that "the *gastraea*-theory cannot exist without proof of the true homology of two primary embryonic layers in all intestinal animals. (*SBW*, p. 233)

Haeckel believed that the homology had been fully proved. In contrast, identification of the embryonic layers was for Metchnikoff a most difficult problem. For him, proof of the homology was not a means for a reconstruction of the hypothetical metazoan ancestor, but he viewed such a reconstruction as support in his main task of identification of developmental structures. Hence, his criticism against the *gastraea*-theory was oriented, first of all, against Haeckel's assurance that the homology of the layers in different animals had been proved. Being unconvinced that different gastrulas were homological, Metchnikoff did not see any reason to accept Haeckel's assumption that the difference in organization and formation of the gastrulas are results of secondary adaptation and transformation of a single ancestral *gastraea*.

From Metchnikoff's point of view, the hypothesis provoked (from the very beginning) at least two objections (leaving aside personal matters). The first was of a rather general nature, which appeared as having no obvious connection with embryology. Specifically, *gastraea* is a poor model for the primordial multicellular organism because it did not represent *the transition* from the monocellular to the multicellular organism. *Gastraea* was a swimming, reproductive, digestive sack. Its very structure was conditioned by the central function, cavital digestion. But any model of the primordial multicellular organism (as soon as it is concerned with the pattern of nourishment) must model the transition from intracellular to extracellular digestion. In any case, the embryological connotation of the genealogical argument is quite clear. In Haeckel's model, the second layer was destined from the very beginning to serve the function of extracellular digestion. The model did not provide for the difference between the original function of a recapitulated structure and the new function of the same structure within the new integrity. The model had been developed on an organism whose second primary embryonic layer was organized in accordance with the central function—extracellular digestion. As the structure responsible for that function, it entered nomenclature as the entoderm. Then the model demanded that every secondary mass (postblastoderm) of cells should be considered endoderm. Correspondingly, the model did not differentiate between extracellular digestion and the original, recapitulated function of the second layer. The second layer cannot be anything but a structure adopted to the performance of extracellular digestion. This general objection raised several questions closely related to the issue of the true homology of the embryonic layers. Does the entoderm (if the name designates the covering membrane of the digestive cavity) always appear as the primary structure following the blastoderm and preceding the mass of cells usually referred to as mesoderm? Is differentiation between these two structures always possible? Is extracellular digestion the universal function of all multicellular organisms? Is the invaginated gastrula the true pattern of forming the second layer, and is any other pattern (e.g., delamination—discovered by Metchnikoff) only a cenogenic aberration? These questions determined the directions of Metchnikoff's research and, correspondingly, the second type of objections (born from observations and experiments) to the *gastraea-theory.*

In 1874, Metchnikoff studied the sponges, *Halisarca dujardinii* and *H. pontica* (12). The outer layer of the larvae was formed out of narrow cylindrical cells. The segmentation cavity was gradually filled with migrated cells from the outer layer. In this paper, Metchnikoff called these cells mesoderm. Within the mesoderm, these cells further developed canals covered with cells, which he called entoderm. As Metchnikoff wrote, "I have found no trace of invagination or any other similar way of formation of the inner cells" (12, p. 354). The issue of identifying these cells becomes the question of defining their function as different from extracellular digestion. It is natural that Metchnikoff's attention turned to the phenomenon, described twenty years earlier by Johann N. Lieberkuehn (13) (and then almost forgotten), which initiated a series of remarkable studies of *Spongilla* capturing carmine, colored granules and other solid particles. As Metchnikoff noticed (in 1878), no essential attention had been paid to Lieberkuehn's results. Before Metchnikoff, Haeckel in his book on sponges touched on the topic in connection with the question concerning capture and processing of food. Haeckel wrote:

> The flagellated cells of the entoderm seems to be the only organ of digestion, capturing, assimilating, and absorbing food. It seems to me very doubtful and unlikely that beside this [layer] the syncytium of the exoderm can accept food. (7, p. 372)

And he repeated more explicitly:

> The syncytium of the exoderm apparently is excluded from any participation in digestion and assimilation of food stuff; it [the syncytium] receives its nourishing material through the flagellated cells only in an already assimilated form. Of course, in the experiments with feeding pigmented granules, the latter can penetrate also in the sarcode of the syncytium from the dermal or gastral surface, as well as from the surface of the canals. Anyway, these foreign bodies apparently are mainly pushed in the syncytium by an external mechanical force. (7, p. 377)

What Haeckel called the syncytium of the exoderm, Metchnikoff considered mesoderm. It is obvious that Haeckel's conclusions did not directly follow from either Lieberkuehn's or his own observations, but rather from his model of how the two primary embryonic layers were formed.

Metchnikoff began his studies with *Halisarca,* but the calcareous and siliceous sponges gave similar results. He stated that in all of his previous observations he found foreign bodies within entodermal and mesodermal cells. He experimentally proved the absorption process by adding to water carmine or indigo particles and then observing among the mesodermal cells varying amounts of the dye. The cells of the entoderm also contained many granules. Metchnikoff had difficulty observing how the particles penetrated the mesodermal cells, "But it seems to me very likely that at least some of the cells with granules of carmine came from the cells of the entoderm" (12, p. 372). He observed that many of the entodermic cells that had protoplasmic outgrowths traveled into the canals. In some cases, all the canals of

Halisarca pontica disappeared; thus the entire body of the sponge as well as the ecto-dermal cover appeared like a mass of amoeboid cells containing carmine.

> The facts which prove at least a close connection between the cells of the mesoderm and the entoderm, would be possible at first glance to interpret as evidence of descent of all mesodermic transparent cells from the tubes of the canals. However, the history of development teaches us this is not the case, because the mesodermic cells are formed earlier than the system of canals, and the latter arises immediately from the mesoderm. (12, pp. 372–373)

The transformation of *Halisarca* canal cells to mesodermic cells, followed by the complete disintegration of the canals, presented Metchnikoff proof of a close kinship between the two sponge layers. But further, beyond mutual dependence and trans-formation, he suspected that the mesodermic structures were primary in relation to the entoderm. Lieberkuehn had already observed (14) that in freshwater sponges dur-ing winter periods there are no flagellated chambers, but only amoeboid cells. Metch-nikoff concluded:

> I can confirm the information. . . . As far as I could observe the flagellated epithelium of "the entoderm" disappeared not only with low temperature but in general under the influence of unfavorable conditions. (12, p. 375)

All these facts led Metchnikoff to deduce that

> among all parts of the sponge's body, the inner flagellated epithelium must be con-sidered as the most inconstant. . . . We can assume that the cells of this layer, trans-forming from flagellated into amoeboid, lose their characteristic properties and assume the features of the typical cells of the parenchyma. (12, p. 376)

This inconstancy and (in the sense of embryological development) secondary nature of the entoderm cells pressed him to doubt cavital digestion as the primordial func-tion of individual and phylogenetic development. From this point of view, the pres-ence of foreign particles in the mesodermal cells obtained quite a different meaning.

Metchnikoff appealed to Lieberkuehn's original observations of infusoria pene-trating the sponge's parenchyma, followed by the protozoan's disintegration and dis-appearance. Metchnikoff confirmed those findings by observing living *Oxytricha*'s destruction in *Spongilla*. In some cases, within a quarter of an hour its chlorophyll granules were found in mesodermic cells, whereas in other cases, similar processes took several hours and were not always complete. For instance, he observed a large number of *Euglena* captured by a sponge: their protoplasm dissolved, but many of the chlorophyll granules were left undigested. With these observations, Metchnikoff began his research program in intracellular digestion. But already in the "Spongio-logische Studien" Metchnikoff wrote:

> It is possible to infer the conclusion that the so-called mesoderm, the cells of which are able to capture food substances, is also able to more or less digest them. (12, p. 374)

What do all these facts offer for the identification of the embryonic layers in sponges? Metchnikoff derives the conclusion that determines his *parenchymella*-hypothesis as the alternative to Haeckel's *gastraea*-theory.

I think . . . that the sponges differ particularly by the very fact that their mesoderm appears very early, so [the mesoderm] in many representatives of the group, functions as the material for the formation of the subsequent entoderm. Then to speak of two layers in sponges, in my opinion, should be done in a completely different sense. Relying on the fact that both of the inner layers [of the sponges] are separated from each other not clearly, and both morphologically and functionally (the digestive activity) are similar, it should be possible to designate as the primary embryonic layers only the external epidermis and the neutral parenchymatic inner layer. From the latter, the definitive layers of the mesoderm and entoderm develop as the secondary formations. . . . The further differentiation of this inner layer into two distinct layers is only the first step in that direction along which follow further and more definitely the other more developed animal forms. Because an oral opening has not yet formed in the sponges, they do not have a separate organ system for capturing food. (12, pp. 377–378)

Each of these facts place the *gastraea* hypothesis in a compromised position. Comparative embryology also offered evidence against Haeckel's theory. Among the Coelenterata, the most primitive classes (the hydroides, the siphonophores, as part of the coral) have an entoderm that forms in the same parenchymatic fashion, and only the higher Coelenterata have a gastrula formed by invagination.

When Haeckel accepts the *Gastrula invaginata* as the primary larva form but considers the larva of the hydroids without an oral opening as a secondary cenogenic transformation, he leaves the assumption completely arbitrary and unfounded. . . . The facts which I have presented . . . rather speak for the gastrula as a secondary larva form. (12, pp. 381–382)

In parallel with the sponges, Metchnikoff initiated study of parenchymatic digestion in turbellaria. In 1877, he published "On the Digestive Organs of the Fresh-Water Turbellarians" (11) and "Studies in Development of the Planarians" (15). Again, he searched for parenchymatic digestion and embryological proof that the parenchyma was a primary formation in relation to the entoderm. From his observations, Metchnikoff concluded:

The facts show, first, that among the freshwater turbellarians there are those forms whose digestive systems appear either as an unbroken mass of parenchymatic cells or as an intestinal sack which is not fully formed. Second, the facts show that even turbellarian digestion, with a fully formed intestine, has the apparent features of the parenchymatic type, that is the food penetrates into the intestinal cell and undergoes digestion. . . . There are among the turbellarians, those which possess the usual way of digestion [the absorption of intestinal fluid contents by the intestinal cells]. (11, *AC,* p. 256)

Metchnikoff asks: Is it possible to recognize that for most turbellarians the parenchymatic organization of the digestive organs is a primary phenomenon? He admitted that the embryology of the turbellarians was obscured by many secondary phenomena and thus he could not provide a definitive answer. But he still concluded that although the comparative morphological approach does not provide the final solution (in this case), it suggests that parenchymatic digestion is a primary phenomenon. If the assumption was true, it presented further evidence against the *gastraea*-theory as well as another vision of the primary ancestor of metazoans, *parenchymella.*

The "gastrula" can not play the role which is attributed to it . . . that is [the *gastraea* theory] can not be recognized as the ontogenetic recapitulation of the basic primordial form of the six types of animals. . . . In the same way as the intestinal cavity has descended from the parenchyma, and the intestinal (cylindrical or ciliated) epithelium has been descended from the amoeboid, in the same way "the gastrula" had to appear as a result of transformation of "the parenchymella," i.e. as a result of secondary processes. (11, *AC*, p. 257)

Accordingly, some trace of the primordial parenchymatic status ought to be saved in the development of certain modern metazoans, especially among lower animals, rather than those species in whose development the gastrula is recapitulated. Apparently, the traces of this primordial status is found in the development of the sponges, the lower *Coelenterata*, and some of the turbellarians. If the gastrula is not the reflection of the primary stage but a result of secondary transformation, then it is clear that the gastrulae of different animals are not homological. For instance, the difference between the oral gastrula and the anal gastrula reflects not secondary transformations of a primary state of gastrula but the fact that any gastrula itself is a secondary phenomenon (in relation to *parenchymella*). Metchnikoff concludes the paper "On Digestive Organs of the Fresh-water Turbellarians" cautiously. The ideas he expressed there, he proposed to consider not as a firmly established theory, but rather as a program of future research. He similarly concluded his "Spongiologische Studien."

Thus, Metchnikoff came to the *parenchymella*-hypothesis as the alternative to Haeckel's *gastraea*. The simplest exposition of this alternative is found in Olga Metchnikoff's biography (written under her husband's supervision):

Metchnikoff, however, discovered among primitive multicellular animals, such as sponges, hydroids, and lower medusae, a stage of development still more simple than the gastrula: this stage is without a digestive cavity and only assumes the gastrula form in its ulterior evolution. He also made the remarkable discovery that, in the most primitive multicellular animals, the endoderm is formed, not by means of invagination, but by the *migration* of a number of flagellated cells from one pole of the wall of the blastula into the central cavity. These cells draw in their flagellum, become amoeboid and mobile, multiply by division, fill the cavity of the blastula, and become capable of digesting. They originate the digestive cells of the complete organism and give birth to the mesoderm, which explains how the latter comes to contain a number of devouring cells even though these do not constitute digestive organs properly so-called. Metchnikoff gave to that stage the name of *parenchymella*, for the migrating cells constitute the endoderm in the condition of a parenchyma.

The invariable presence of this stage in the simplest multicellular animals, the primitive amoeboid state of the endodermic cells, cases of ulterior transformation of the parenchymella into the gastrula form in certain animals, the absence of a differentiated digestive cavity, all that proved, according to Metchnikoff, that the parenchymella is more primitive than the gastrula, and is therefore entitled to be considered the prototype of multicellular beings.

He saw a confirmation of this in the fact that primitive adult animals also have no digestive cavity but merely an intracellular digestion (sponges, turbellaria).

He concluded that the common ancestor of multicellular beings was a being constituted by an agglomeration of cells without a digestive cavity, but endowed with intracellular digestion, like that of the "parenchymula" stage of development. He therefore gave to that hypothetical ancestor the name of *parenchymella*.

Later, in 1886 [Olga Metchnikoff is referring to Metchnikoff's *"Embryologische Studien an Medusen,"* Vienna: A. Hollder, 1886], he definitely formulated his theory of the genesis of multicellular beings, and having already stated the phagocyte theory, he substituted for the name *parenchymella* that of *phagocytella,* which indicated at the same time the primitive mode of digestion of that hypothetical ancestor.

Reduced to its simplest form, it presented, according to Metchnikoff, a certain analogy with a colony composed of unicellular beings of two kinds: the first, flagellated, forming the external layer, and the others, amoeboid, occupying the centre of the colony and capable of digesting. (16, pp. 108–110).

Let us now examine the 1886 account given by Metchnikoff:

The concept of the embryonic layers has been borrowed from the embryology of higher animals and then transferred upon the invertebrates; because of this anti-genealogical method, a set of defects have been established which have still not been eliminated. For instance, defining the embryonic layers in doubtful cases, too often [only] topographical indications have been employed. Thus we must accept, as an essential progressive step when, for the first time, Haeckel (*Biologische Studient,* vol. 2, *Studient zur Gastraea-Theorie,* Jena, 1877, p. 258) clearly formulates the opinion that the embryonic layers (at least the two main layers) must be considered as primary organs. In this way, a firm, and at the same time, purely genealogical orientation was acquired. . . . Because we do not know the origin of the multicellulars, the absence of a firm foundation was the main difficulty in the genealogical interpretation of the embryonic layers. In order to formulate that, we must begin with hypotheses which would agree with the greatest amount of factual material.

Although transitions between *Protozoa* and *Metazoa* among modern animals apparently do not exist, an attempt to compensate (to certain extent) this gap in our knowledge was made by hypothetical constructions. It is possible to assume two ways by which such a transition could be performed: either by differentiation of protoplasm around separate nuclei of some multinuclear *Protozoa,* or by unification of many individuals of a *Protozoa,* colony into a multicellular whole. A close relationship between *Ciliata* and *Turbellaria,* to wit between their larvae, was often assumed in the preceding decades, and thus it seemed natural to assume between them a genealogical kinship and to construct a hypothesis of *Metazoa*'s origin. (17, *SBW* pp. 423–424)

Then Metchnikoff analyzes phenomena that may be considered as arguments against the transition hypothesis:

We saw . . . how formation of the entoderm in medusa takes place in different ways. . . . The entoderm arises either at many points of the embryo, i.e., in a multipolar way, or only in one part of it, i.e., in an hypotropic [underturning] (concentrated) way [an illustration shows a collection of cells at the inferior pole about to embark to form the inner layer]. The multipolar method of entoderm formation is performed: (a) as the multipolar immigration of the embryonic cells from the surface into the embryo; (b) as the primary delamination through the cross division of the blastoderm's cells; (c) as the secondary delamination after preceding formation of the morula; and (d) as the mixed delamination when the entodermic cells are formed partially by cross division and partially by migration. It is impossible to differentiate between some of these ways of formation because they are connected by intermediate transitions. The hypotropic (or concentrate) formation of the entoderm is performed either by the way of immigration of the blastodermal cells of the larva *bottom* or by way of a true invagination, i.e., gastrulation. A special form of epiboly that is observed as a kind of variation after uneven cleavage, should be also related to this type. . . . It is easy to see that accepting the hypothesis of *Metazoa*'s descent from multinuclear *Protozoa* we leave without explanation such processes of embryological development as the immigration from the surface, primary delamination, invagination. . . .

It is known that the *gastraea*-theory solves many [of the problems] by reduction of different processes to primary invagination, and partially aids us to understand the complicated processes of entoderm formation, as, for instance, in the invertebrates. At the same time, it encounters serious difficulties in explanation of delamination, as it was recognized by Haeckel, yet in the first formulation of his theory. . . .

Haeckel believed it is possible to overcome this difficulty by assuming the "secondary falsification of ontogeny." In his main work [*Studient zur Gastraea-Theorie,* vol. 2, 1877, p. 267 and p. 247 fn.], he repeats frequently the assertion that delamination, only if it truly takes place in the animal world, is a cenogenetic process which "arises, as a secondary phenomenon, from the palingenetic process of invagination." In any case, Haeckel does not any more closely approach consideration of such a falsification. It baffles all the more so, because Haeckel himself acknowledged difficulties for his theory precisely in this question. For a long time, Haeckel and his school (the brothers Hertwig) had doubts about the very reality of delamination. (17, *SBW,* pp. 429–430)

The most powerful argument against the *gastraea*-theory was multipolar formation of the entoderm which, as Metchnikoff believed, in no way was to be considered as a secondary phenomenon in relation to invagination. But this was not the only target of Metchnikoff's critique:

Because [the *gastraea*-theory] was proposed in that time when cavital digestion was assumed as universal, and it was unknown that lower animals digested food intracellularly, [the theory] does not correspond any more to our modern physiological knowledge. (17, *SBW,* p. 433)

Another set of arguments against the theory was related to the difficulties (not connected immediately with the problem of entoderm formation) that arose in the attempts to prove the homology of all gastrulae and to interpret differences between them as secondary phenomena. After this critical analysis of the *gastraea*-theory, Metchnikoff proceeded with similar arguments against two other hypotheses concerning the origin of the primordial metazoan—those of Balfour (18) and Buetschli (19). Metchnikoff concluded:

If we now review the discussed theories, we see that they are unable to unite, in a general perspective, the entire sum of the known embryological material, and further they suffer from lack of a physiological explanation. Another way was thus found. In the course of my research of sponges ["Spongiologische Studien." *Z. wiss. Zool,* Vol. 22, pp. 349–387, 1879], I made certain cautious comments, which from my point of view, were in agreement with the acquired data about formation of the entoderm in the lower *Metazoa* and with the newly described phenomena pertaining to intracellular digestion. I believe that the entoderm did not arise at once, in the form of a pipe-like stomach with a terminal pore, as seen in the gastrula, but that these formations have an underlying long process of historical development that eventuates in the formation of an unbroken parenchyma digesting intracellularly. In its turn, the parenchyma was similarly not formed at once, but gradually, as cells of the blastoderm migrated into the blastocoel. Finally, the bilaminar *parenchymella* arose by reduction of the embryonic process and a progressive differentiation of the digestive apparatus, which was transformed into the gastrula. (17, *SBW,* p. 439)

Metchnikoff speculated (or [as he stated] proposed, some "a priori consider-ations") about the evolutionary processes that led to formation of *parenchymella:*

At the beginning, an inequality, that was to lead to a further differentiation, had to arise between the individuals of the colony [referring to a *Flagellata* colony as the origin of the hypothetical primary multicellular organism]: while some individuals were mainly engulfing food, others were more adapted to locomotion and attraction to food. For mobile colonies, there was a certain advantage for individuals contain-ing food particles (i.e., loaded and therefore heavier) not to remain on the periphery but to move closer to the centre. Another advantage was that feeding individuals were in conditions permitting [more perfect] accomplishment of their function. It is known that many *Flagellata* turn (from the state of the monad) into the amoeboid state when they are feeding. . . . Further, it is easy to imagine that feeding individuals reproduced more frequently; so, a certain correlation between a more intensive feed-ing and reproduction could be formed. One more reason for immigration was the impossibility for the colony to broaden its surface beyond a certain limit, a fact of particular significance among swimming colonies. Because an increase in the indi-vidual's number made it possible to increase the [general] activity [of the colony], it was doubtlessly favorable when the cells, which could not find their place on the surface, adapted to an existence within the colony. It is likely that for a long period, the individuals of the same colony differed from each other only quantitatively: the locomotive cells obtained food particles by the movement of the flagella and them-selves engulfed the smallest of the particles. Even in our time, it is possible to observe in some *Coelenterata* random engulfment of food by ectodermal cells. On the con-trary, the inner amoeboid individuals were able to engulf larger particles which could not be caught by the locomotive elements. It is likely that during the process, the amoeboid individuals almost reached the periphery and (through the multiple pores of the external layer) caught particles at the surface of the colony. . . .

Gradually, differentiation in the described direction reached increasingly higher lev-els; the locomotive cells were more or less losing their function of capturing food; the function was increasingly adopted by the amoeboid phagocytes; the finest ran-dom pores between the locomotive elements could be enlarged and turned into pores that in such great number are found on the surface of sponges. To the extent of the proceeding individualization of the colony (the individual of the second order), the surface individuals differentiated into the *ectoderm* (the kinoblast), meanwhile the amoeboid inner individuals differentiated into the phagocytoblast (the parenchyma or the mesoentoderm). The cells of the latter, in the case of their inability to engulf larger food particles, formed around them the plasmodium, similar to that as occurs now in the entoderm of siphonophores and in the mesoderm of many animals. The increase in activity of the multicellular organism (provided by the two primary organs) led to satisfaction of the requirement of food; it is likely that larger plant and animal organisms were eaten. In order to make feeding possible, one or a few entrance pores, which was to lead to a mouth formation, had to arise. . . .

I have earlier called the transitional form between the *Flagellata* and the *Metazoa,* from which the latter were descended, the *parenchymella.* Now I would like to rename it phagocytella *(Phagocytella),* because this name indicates a very character-istic peculiarity of the form. . . . *Phagocytella* possessed two primary organs—the kinoblast and the phagocytoblast which were not separated yet from each other in that distinct way in which the embryonic layers of the majority of *Metazoa* are sep-arated; it is likely that the replenishment of the phagocytoblast by the intruding cells of the kinoblast continued for a long time. In regard to developmental history, it is possible to say that the ova of *phagocytella* (it had to have sexual reproduction) underwent even cleavage, the blastomeres divided in three spatial dimensions, and the blastocoel (which was then gradually filled by individual cells and by central products of the cells' division) rose early. (17, *SBW,* pp. 447–449)

Metchnikoff then concluded the exposition of the *phagocytella*-hypothesis:

Elucidation of the question about the origin of the multicellulars is necessary for obtaining a basis for comparative morphology. In any case, as long as the anti-genealogical direction is dominant in elaborating the problem of the embryonic layers, solutions to the most important questions will be prevented by insurmountable obstacles. That is why I think that, in absence of positive data, hypothetical constructions can be considered as legitimate. (17, *SBW,* p. 455)

All theoretical reasons (including the explicitly formulated objections to Haeckel's theory) that finally led to the *parenchymella* hypothesis already had been articulated around 1876. Many of the most important observations that Metchnikoff laid as the basis of his hypothesis were already completed in the 1877–1879 period. The very term *parenchymella* appears for the first time not later than 1877.

Metchnikoff continued his studies of the turbellarians during the next decade, until the middle 1880s. Between 1881 and 1885, he published a series of works grouped under the title *Comparative Embryological Studies,* in which he continued to polish his *parenchymella* hypothesis and compiled massive new material in its support. His critique of Haeckel became even more pointed. From Metchnikoff's point of view, Haeckel's *gastraea*-theory was no more than a popularization of Kowalevsky's publications, which at the same time avoided those difficult problems that Kowalevsky himself saw quite clearly (20). Kowalevsky attempted to create a theory that encompassed a common formation for the embryonic layers in lower Chordata *(Amphioxus)* and invertebrates. He believed that the invaginated gastrula was the stage of development of all animals possessing a segmentation cavity. He thought that the blastopore (the opening of gastrula), in all gastrula, developed into the anus, but soon he found that it was true only in some cases; in other cases, the blastopore developed into the mouth, and still in other cases, the blastopore closed and the anal opening formed anew. The hypothesis of homology of all gastrulae which Kowalevsky expressed in 1866, was not again repeated. But Haeckel continued to invoke it as a firmly established fact.

In order to reconcile these contradictory facts concerning the blastopore, Otto Buetschli (21), and after him, Berthold Hatschek (22) proposed a new hypothesis: the primordial *gastraea* would have a round opening, which in further evolution developed from an oval form to a slit. This formation would allow the bifurcation of the slit into two openings by fusing together the middle parts of opposite edges. One of these openings would then develop into the orifice and the other into the anal opening. The slit shape determined bilateral symmetry. In order to check the hypothesis, Metchnikoff attempted to study gastrulae of many different animal classes. He concluded that most of his observations would not support the hypothesis, for example, both the sea urchin's anal gastrula and the annelid, *Polygordias*'s oral gastrula express radial symmetry; the sea urchin's mouth appeared too far from the blastopore. In the nemertines, although the radial gastrula was retained, the transition to bilateral symmetry was applied not to the blastopore, but to the development of the ectodermal sack, and so on. *Comparative Embryological Studies* prepared Metchnikoff for concluding his embryological work with "Embryological Studies in Medusae," which appeared in 1886. In the latter work, Metchnikoff discussed a similar circle of problems, but now having already formulated (in 1883) his phagocytosis hypothesis, his new theory presented the embryological problems with an essentially novel perspective. Here we are interested only in the development of the ideas and information that prepared for the birth of the phagocytosis hypothesis, thus neither "Embryological Studies in Medusae" nor the fourth and fifth parts of *Comparative Embryological Studies* (published in 1885) are germane.

Summary

Let us now summarize both the general theory that oriented Metchnikoff's pre-phagocytosis research and the general result of that work. Development of comparative embryology accumulated extensive factual material that required theoretical principles to order the data. The idea of recapitulation played the central role of guiding the conceptual framework of these studies. The old naturphilosophical idea of recapitulation was based on the assumption that a universal scheme underlaid any development. It was the universality of the scheme that provided for the similarities between different specimens and thereby also provided the very fact of recapiculation. The authority of this naturphilosophical idea was shaken in the 1860s, in part by virtue of the new Darwinian spirit and in part by new-found discrepancies between systematically presented evolutionary relations and comparative embryological data. In this newly created atmosphere, recapitulation no longer appeared as a manifestation of a general scheme directing a developmental process. On the contrary, recapitulation demanded that a structure must be adopted in a new context of development, and the recapitulated function of that structure must be reconciled within the new context. From this point of view, individual development is a process ordered by a vector, the starting point of which is the recapitulated structure as the carrier of its ancient function, and the end point is the structure as functioning in the new context. Thus, identification of embryological stages was recognized as essentially dependent on genealogical reconstructions. This intellectual disposition explains why so much attention was paid by experimental embryologists to such theories as Haeckel's *gastraea.*

Why was Metchnikoff so critical of the *gastraea*-hypothesis? From his point of view, although presumptively modern, it was disguised old *naturphilosophie.* Specifically, Metchnikoff argued that it is was not modern gastrulae that recapitulated the ancient *gastraea,* but the hypothetical model recapitulated the actual gastrula. The hypothesis did not demonstrate what kind of ancient recapitulated structure was adopted in processes that lead to formation of the second layer as the entoderm, but it ascribed to the primordial ancestor—the completely formed entoderm and its corresponding function—cavital digestion. Thus recapitulation appeared in this case as a repetition of a universal scheme of organization, similar to von Baer's *Bauplan.*

Metchnikoff's *parenchymella* hypothesis attempted to compensate for the defect of Haeckel's argument. But was it too radical? Metchnikoff proposed a hypothetical transitory organism, linking Protozoa and Metazoa, where intracellular digestion was the recapitulated ancient function, which in further development gave place to a new function—extracellular digestion. But what about the fate of the ancient function itself? We said that according to the new idea of recapitulation, the function was supposedly "inscribed" in a new context. But the metaphor of "inscribing" should not mislead; because there is no guaranteed general scheme of development, expectation that the ancient function will be harmoniously adapted in the context of a given individual development is not assured. The recapitulated structure may yield its "biological meaning" to a new structure, but at the same time, this does not mean that it ceases to perform its ancient function. If it abandoned that original function, the recapitulated structure would now contradict the very definition of recapitulation.

Thus mesodermic cells yielded their basic function of the organism's nourishment to the newly developed structure—in this case, the entoderm of the digestive cavity without stopping to perform intracellular digestion, as such. Thus, the organism appears as a set of heterochronic (in respect to the order of evolutionary origins) structures, each of which performs its function in accordance with its own "biological meaning," not concerned with any harmonic integration with other structures.

Thus, Metchnikoff came to the idea of disharmony as the basic characteristic of every organism. The idea played a fateful existential role in his personal life, and was crucial in his scientific and metaphysical research. His research after 1872, as compared with the previous period, added to this idea of disharmony two particular features. First, he realized that establishing the fact of recapitulation required a special geneaological approach to comparative embryological studies. Second, his studies in recapitulation and genealogy took a specific "mesodermic orientation." These additional genealogical and mesodermic dimensions of his research resulted in formulation of the *parenchymella* hypothesis.

CHAPTER 4

The Problem of Evolution in Metchnikoff's Works

Introduction

Whenever Metchnikoff reflected on the history of the phagocytosis theory, he always stressed that it had originated in his early studies of invertebrate comparative embryology. That research had focused on the question concerning the phylogenetic fate and ontogenetic role of amoeboid mesodermic cells as well as on a related phenomenon—intracellular digestion. However, there is no self-evident link between the phenomenon of intracellular digestion and the concept of a specialized protective system. In fact, the very idea of a special defensive activity in a host was novel and not easily compatible within the traditional view of ontogeny as the self-revelation of an organism's "nature" (i.e., the expression of the organism's underlying plan). In this perspective, the healing forces of an organism were regarded not as the expression of a special protective mechanism, but as the immediate manifestation of the organism's integrity (its "nature"), whose very essence was thought of as a self-establishing and self-supporting wholeness. The organism as a whole was viewed as this self-protecting "device"; correspondingly, the phenomenon of acquired immunity generated not so much consideration of how, or even whether, the organism protected itself, but rather of the nature of the etiological factors that failed to recur. The logic of Metchnikoff's studies in comparative embryology formed his nontraditional approach: he saw ontogeny not as a revelation (through individual variations or specific expressions) of a single integrity, but as a disharmonious interplay of different centers of activity pertaining to different phylogenetic stages and, correspondingly, presenting different designs of integrity. If, under this premise, it was possible to consider one of these conflicting centers as a harmonizing force in its continuous "disharmonious" relations with other constituents, then the idea of a special self-supporting and self-protecting subsystem was ready to emerge. In this context, we must carefully analyze Metchnikoff's work specifically as relating to Darwinism, whose impact was surely the most important influence on his scientific and metaphysical development.

The profound impact on Metchnikoff of Darwin's *Origin of Species,* read in 1863, cannot be overemphasized. Olga Metchnikoff wrote relative to that experience, "The theory of evolution deeply struck the boy's mind and his thoughts immediately turned in that direction (1, p. 41)." The review Metchnikoff (then eighteen years old) wrote immediately after that first encounter was largely unfavorable and his relationship to Darwinism, until late in his career, remained critical. But after the mid-1880s, Metchnikoff's intellectual posture grew more closely akin to the natural selection theory, and his retrospective musings on his earlier negative relationship to Darwinism was glossed over to present the past as more consistent with the current state of affairs (2). We must understand why, in Metchnikoff's retrospective reassessment of Darwinism, this interesting chronological peculiarity occurs (previously noted by Daniel P. Todes [3]). Between the 1860s and early 1880s, that is, during the time of the highest success of Darwinism in Russia and Germany (in the two countries with which his scientific activity of that time was most closely associated), Metchnikoff remained very critical of Darwin's interpretation of evolution. But during the later period of Darwinism's eclipse, Metchnikoff professed himself to be an ardent supporter. Thus Olga Metchnikoff's biography, written in France in the last years of her husband's life and according to her own evidence (1, pp. xxi–xxiii) composed under his immediate supervision, depicted him as "a true Darwinian," from his very entry into science.

It is difficult to identify a worse environment for Darwinism than France of the early twentieth century. The general status of natural selection had fallen on hard times, as Peter J. Bowler notes:

From the high point of the 1870s and 1880s when Darwinism had become virtually synonymous with evolution itself, the selection theory had slipped in popularity to such an extent that by 1900 its opponents were convinced it would never recover. Evolution itself remained unquestioned, but an increasing number of biologists preferred mechanisms other than selection to explain *how* it occurred. (4)

Of the status of Darwinism in France in particular, Robert E. Stebbins writes:

Even in the mid-twentieth century Darwin was not prominent in French schoolbooks. . . .

By 1900, the transformist position was clearly predominant in France, as it was in most countries. . . .

The French still receive Darwin as one who offered one, but not the only, explanation for the idea of transformism, of which they more than the English were the originators. With a different sense of proportion than the Anglo-Saxons, they still perceive less sense of high drama in Darwin and Darwinism than do their foreign counterparts.

There was no "Darwinian Revolution" in France, just as there was no political revolution in England in 1789, 1830, 1848, and 1871. (5, pp. 162–163)

There is the opinion that Metchnikoff's conversion to Darwinism reflected his wish to defend the phagocytosis theory, providing general biological support for it (6). However true that opinion might be, it leaves us without an explanation concerning the terms by which Metchnikoff came to agree with Darwinism, which for Metchnikoff was not an ideology (at least not *only* an ideology), but a scientific theory. For many years he was concerned with the problems that the theory could pose in his own field—comparative embryology of invertebrates. Metchnikoff actively dealt with the possible applications and explanatory power of the theory—and likewise with the limits of such application. If he forgot the principal problems of his original argument with Darwinism, it only reflects that Metchnikoff for the sake of his own theory neglected the constellation of problems out of which his theory had been born. But after formulating the phagocytosis theory, he always stressed its general biological background, remarking that the theory had originated in his comparative embryological studies of the mesoderm—and the contradiction in his position relative to Darwinism must reflect other issues.

It is true that arguments around Darwinism always provoked extratheoretical passions—religious, cultural, national, ideological. For many people, acceptance or rejection of Darwinism was a matter of personal (i.e., unobjectivized, extratheoretical) taste. It is also true that these nonscientific motives could affect even the most objective and careful scientific critique of Darwinism. But in this last case, these arguments could exercise their influence only by being embedded in a corresponding conceptual framework. Whatever the extratheoretical sources of Metchnikoff's criticism (first against Darwin, then followed by reconciliation), Metchnikoff explicitly formulated what he viewed at that time as the inner inconsistencies of Darwinism's conceptual apparatus as well as the alleged discrepancies between Darwin's ideas and many empirically observed phenomena. If his conversion into the Darwinian faith was not associated with a conclusion that reconciled those inconsistencies and discrepancies, why would he deceive himself in the attempt to provide support of his hypothesis with a theory that, as he believed, was false? If Metchnikoff's conversion to Darwinism was a marriage of convenience, then he was converted not because of a newly acquired hope to solve the difficulties of his previous relations with Darwin's teaching, but because he hoped that in others' eyes, the conversion would make his own theory more appealing. Suspecting Metchnikoff with such tactical cunning, we deprive him of any prudence. Being one of the most informed and broadly erudite biologists of his time, spending enormous efforts for scientific defence and popular propaganda of the phagocytosis theory, he could not be unaware that his conversion had taken place in those embattled times when the popularity of Darwinism had begun to wither. Although his own attitude toward Darwin's ideas was growing increasingly friendly, Darwinism, for most biologists, was rapidly dying. Of course, Metchnikoff might have sincerely deceived himself, forsaking his principal disagreements with Darwinism for the sake of defending his own position. We doubt that this motive is applicable in Metchnikoff's case. Darwin's idea was not so popular as to be evoked as an effective defense for a potentially related, but essentially different, cause. Darwinism could only provide for itself.

We will deal in detail in chapter 6 with the assault made by various German scientists on Metchnikoff's theory. But here we must note that one of the most cumbersome problems was Paul Baumgarten's accusation that the phagocytosis theory was teleological (7). Metchnikoff first argued that the theory had nothing in common with teleology but had been completely built "upon the principles of evolutionary theory" (8). In his next critical paper (9), Baumgarten responded ironically to this argument: because of Darwinism's spell, everything that refers itself to that teaching obtains meaning solely because of that reference. Recall Bowler's observation that in the 1870s and 1880s Darwinism became "virtually synonymous with evolution itself." So, it is not strange that Baumgarten (in 1889) understood Metchnikoff's reference (of 1887) to "the principles of the evolutionary theory" as exploitation of Darwinism's spell. The understanding was all the more natural because Metchnikoff spoke about the phenomenom of phagocytosis in Darwinian terms, that is, the struggle between organisms. But exactly during the greatest popularity of Darwinism, Metchnikoff never identified (at least explicitly) the theoretical foundation of the phagocytosis theory with Darwin's approach to evolution. Thus, "the principles of the evolutionary theory" in no way should be understood here as another expression for Darwin's principles. So, there is no reason to regard Metchnikoff's self-proclaimed conversion to Darwinism as either self-deception or as conscious tactical mimicry. We will argue that the phagocytosis theory could be considered by its author as an answer (or its starting point, at least) to the questions that earlier alienated him from Darwinism. We will argue further that accepting, after 1883, the idea of adaptive evolution and natural selection as the basic power of evolution, he maintained his own interpretation. For a man who (already in the 1860s and 1870s) had carefully distinguished between the respective ideas of adaptive evolution and Darwinian natural selection, it was but natural for Metchnikoff to maintain independence from Darwin's teaching during its greatest popularity; it was just as natural for him to posture and proclaim himself a Darwinist when the very idea of selection seemed endangered. We believe that the evolution of Metchnikoff's attitude toward Darwinism after 1883 reflected not self-aggrandizement, but the innermost logic of the mutual dependence between Metchnikoff's phagocytosis theory and his version of Darwinism.

The Early Critique

As we noted earlier, Metchnikoff wrote, in 1863, a critique of *Origin of Species* (10). At that time, he was a student at Kharkov University and was to start his original research in comparative invertebrate embryology only several years later. So, we cannot expect at this point a general theoretical reflection, one that was only elaborated later as a result of original research. But the less this essay reflects Metchnikoff's original scientific contribution, the more it presents his personal temperament and general intellectual orientation. The youthful critical aggressiveness and ambitiously emphasized independence of judgment were to pervade his scientific posturing throughout his life. The general intellectual horizon of the essay apparently reflects both the influence of the conceptual framework exploited by the idea of transformism as such and some peculiarities of the Russian intellectual climate in the 1860s. As Alexander Vucinich writes:

> Darwin's theory could not have come to Russia at a more propitious time. After the Crimean defeat, the country was in the midst of a national awakening that called for a critical reassessment of dominant values and engendered a strong sentiment in favor of fundamental reforms. (11, p. 226)

The secularization of thought was one of the most powerful determinants of the time. Many years later, Metchnikoff wrote of the factors determining the secular orientation of the Russian intellectual generation coming to age in the 1850s and 1860s:

> In this relation, an important role was played not only by popular articles in Russian general journals but also by foreign popular books and brochures. There were first of all those works in natural sciences which outlined generally current opinions on nature and life. The main place among them was occupied by [Ludwig] Buechner's *Kraft und Stoft*, which circulated in the 1850s not only among university students, but also in the upper grades of the high schools. Many started to study German in order to read the works of Buechner, Vogt, Moleschott in the original. However, some of the books appeared soon in hectographed Russian translations and promoted further the spread of the positivists and materialistic Weltanschauung which seemed to be able to answer all the questions asked by young people. (12, *AC,* pp. 9–10)

Actually, Metchnikoff recalls here his own conversion to secularism and materialism during his years at the lycée. As Olga Metchnikoff wrote, her husband began to read books and publications forbidden by the Russian censors (including Alekesandr Herzen's newspapers, *Polar Star* and *The Bell*).

> Little by little he lost the faith which he had held when under his mother's influence. Atheism, however, was to him more interesting than disappointing: it incited in him a state of general criticism. Ardently passionate in this as in all things, he preached atheism to others and received the nickname of "God is not." (1, p. 29)

In these years, he was surrounded by a group of friends who were devoted to science and an intellectual culture. Olga Metchnikoff continued:

> He studied German so as to read in the original the classical materialistic writers Vogt, Feuerbach, Buechner, Moleschott, etc. (1, p. 31)

In this respect, Metchnikoff's early development reflected a common experience resulting in political radicalism. Despite this intellectual background and the strong impression made by the close personal acquaintance with such pillars of the Russian movement as Mikhail Bakunin and Herzen, Metchnikoff never sympathized with any political form of radicalism. He always expected science, not a political revolution, to improve human society. But in his adherence to science, he remained a typical Russian nihilist of the nineteenth century, drawing his highly idealistic inspirations from a rejection of traditional idealistic values. Any assertion of life's present form as historically independent was rejected by this radical mentality. From this perspective, Darwinism (as any evolutionary theory) represented an antitraditionalist kindred spirit. Even many years later, arguing how Darwinism in Russia had been so readily accepted, this nihilism was inclined to view the absence of a firmly established theoretical tradition as a special advantage of the Russian spiritual atmosphere. A. O. Kowalevsky wrote:

> Darwin's theory was received in Russia with profound sympathy. While in Western Europe it met firmly established old traditions which it had first to overcome, in Russia its appearance coincided with the awakening of our society after the Crimean War and here it immediately received the status of full citizenship and ever since has enjoyed widespread popularity. (11, pp. 229–230)

It is highly remarkable that Metchnikoff himself, in his 1902 essay devoted to this very Kowalevsky, explicitly refers to Russian nihilism as the source of their respective spiritual development. In describing the frame of mind with which they began their scientific careers, Metchnikoff cited Evgeni Bazarov—the hero of Ivan Turgenev's *Fathers and Sons* who is the most paradigmatic image of mid-nineteenth-century nihilism in Russian literature (12). And immediately following a quotation where Bazarov favored Buechner's *Kraft und Stoft* in contrast to Aleksandr Pushkin, Metchnikoff reflected:

> Appearance of Darwin's *Origin of Species* at the end of the 1850s gave a very signif-
> icant new impetus in the same direction. Joining man with the animal world by the
> commonality of origin, Darwin strengthened thereby the hope to solve the problem
> of man's Being by means of studying the laws ruling living things. (12, *AC*, pp. 10–
> 11)

These words are the more remarkable as they inadvertently convey the paradoxical essence of nihilism, that is, the intention to solve a metaphysical problem ("the problem of man's Being") by means of "physics" ("studying the laws ruling living things"). Thus, inspiration was drawn from metaphysics, but the formulation and realization of the goal was placed in the physical world. This train of thought reflects nothing other than the *metaphysical* configuration of this mentality, whose influence is still tangible in Metchnikoff's explanation (written in 1913) of Darwinism's successful reception in Russia. His point of view coincides with Kowalevsky's opinion, namely, the principal reasons why Darwinism was so welcomed in Russia was the absence of a theoretical tradition. Metchnikoff wrote:

> The guiding thought of the majority of the biological works which have been pro-
> duced in Russia during the last half-century, was Darwin's teaching about transfor-
> mation of species. While in Europe it ran into numerous prejudices and quite often
> met persistent resistance, it took root at once on Russian unplowed fields and formed
> the basis of many special studies. All questions about structure and development of
> organisms were elucidated precisely from this point of view. (13, *AC*, p. 52)

It is true that the Russian nihilistic mentality fondly received Darwinism. But the same attitude was self-deceptive when it failed to recognize its own dependence on certain theoretical traditions. Russia of the 1850s was not that theoretical virgin soil depicted many years later by Kowalevsky and Metchnikoff. In the same essay, "On the History of Biology in Russia," Metchnikoff recognized that in the beginning of the 1860s there were in Russia such "stars of the first magnitude in pure and applied biology, although already outdated ones [as] the great naturalist Carl Ernst von Baer and Doctor [Nikolai] Pirogov" (13, *AC*, p. 50). Certainly, von Baer's preeminent position in pre-Darwinian evolutionary discussions is well known (14). Aside from his promotion of limited evolution, there continued in Russia a strong tradition of Lamarckism. We have already mentioned how in his early works Metchnikoff attributed the popularity of Darwinism not to the convincing power of the natural selection idea as such, but to the renovation and enforcement of the old Lamarckian (even pre-Lamarckian) idea of transformism. In the 1860s and 1870s, Metchnikoff offered this explanation of Darwinism's popularity in both Russia and Germany. Rather than the absence of a theoretical evolutionary tradition, the presence of a strong

Lamarckian history conditioned the success of Darwinism in Russia during the early 1860s. Francesco Scude and Michele Acanfora write:

> It seems that Russian biologists reacted in a unique way to Darwin's work mainly because Russia was the only major country in which evolution, justified mostly by theories with a strong Lamarckian bent, was already rather well established among professional zoologists some time before Darwin and Wallace entered the scene, that is by the 1840s. As a result, in Russia the *Origin* immediately started a technical debate concerned almost solely with mechanisms, particularly on the ways in which natural selection would be an essential complement to the already accepted ones. (15, p. 732)

It is noteworthy that even in 1913, Metchnikoff asserted that the guiding role of Russian biology had been played by "Darwin's teaching about transformation of species" (13, *AC,* p. 52), he did not say—"Darwin's teaching about natural selection."

It is true that many Russian scientists (among them Metchnikoff's friend Kowalevsky) accepted Darwinism on the appearance of *Origin of Species.* It is equally true that Darwin's popularity increased continuously with each publication (16). (It is another question as to what degree this popularity reflected a true appreciation of Darwin's theoretical novelty.) But it is not true that Metchnikoff accepted Darwinism with the same readiness. It was not only in Western Europe of the 1860s and 1870s that Darwinism had "met persistent resistance" (as Metchnikoff stated), for there was at the same time a certain hesitancy in Russia as well. And one of the most intelligent critics of Darwin's ideas was Metchnikoff. Although in his work of 1863 Metchnikoff did not approach Darwinism from the perspective of original research, he had already outlined the main points restricting unconditional acceptance of Darwin's ideas:

(a) To assess the degree of theoretical value and novelty of Darwin's teaching it is necessary to keep in mind the difference between the idea of natural selection as the main force of transformation and the very idea of transformism.

(b) The idea of natural selection, as presented by Darwin, is quite unclear itself, and Darwin's reliance on Malthusian principles makes the idea even more vague and vulnerable.

(c) In any case, natural selection as the explanatory principle is insufficient to formulate the cause of species diversity.

(d) It is impossible to formulate in terms of natural selection the evolutionary tendency to perfection or, if there is no such a trend, simply to establish a biological concept of perfection that would be relevant to the intuitively obvious differences in levels of organization.

The main idea (or in Metchnikoff's language, the main formula) of Darwin's *Origin,* as the young reviewer saw it, was:

> All species of the animal and plant realms have been formed as the result of permanent slow changes of one or a few original species and their descendants during geological periods and are still going on before our eyes. This hypothesis is not a new one: it was ardently defended by [Lorenz] Oken and [Jean-Baptiste] Lamarck; Étienne Geoffroy Saint-Hilaire (although very cautiously) defended it. But Cuvier and after him almost all the other paleontologists revolted against it. (10, *SBW,* pp. 656–657)

Darwin's merit is not in the invention of the transformism idea, but its defense. We should also credit him for his intention

> to find the laws according to which the transformations of species (from one into another, from less complex to perfected) are carried out. (10, *SBW*, p. 657)

It is well known that Darwin believed both in the reality of the general evolutionary tendency (although not absolutely dominant) to develop toward perfection and in the sufficiency of the natural selection idea to explain that tendency. The reality of attaining perfection is self-evident for young Metchnikoff. Darwin made an attempt to discover the principles of species transformation, that is, to find the principles driving the perfecting process. Although in this early review, the idea of progressive development displayed itself with the power of a common prejudice, invulnerable to scientific self-reflection, this theme was to turn into a significant scientific problem for Metchnikoff (17). But already, completely accepting the idea of adaptive evolution, Metchnikoff here believed that Darwin had too hastily equated adaptation with perfection. After quoting Darwin's position that according to the theory of natural selection new forms are more perfect than their predecessors (i.e., every new species developed through the struggle for existence acquired new advantages in relation to its close competitors), Metchnikoff concluded:

> This opinion about activity of natural selection can be refuted by many factors. Its main defect consists in the equation of the concepts: advantage and perfection of organization, while the concepts must be strictly distinguished. (10, *SBW*, p. 669)

Darwin's primary mistake, as Metchnikoff argued in this review, was "a false generalization of Malthusian theory" (10, *SBW*, p. 668). Metchnikoff did not assert the Malthusian principle was wrong: "Not daring to prove the validity or fallaciousness of Malthusian law" (10, *SBW*, p. 666), Metchnikoff simply observed that "Darwin is very mistaken in applying Malthusian law upon the animal and plant realms"(10, *SBW*, p. 667). First of all, Metchnikoff argued, Malthus, who borrowed his data from the statistics of North America, asserted that humankind developed according to geometrical progression. Darwin, in his turn, never observed such speed of reproduction, but he suggested a *tendency* to reproduce with this frequency. Metchnikoff, in turn, postulated that the struggle for existence explained why such population growth cannot be fully realized. What is even more important is the difference between Malthus and Darwin in interpreting the question concerning the rate of increased food production.

> Malthus believes that agricultural products, which of course consist of organisms, increases according to arithmetical progression; Darwin, on the contrary, assuming in all organic creatures the same striving for rapid reproduction, views thereby food as striving for an increase in accordance with the same geometrical progression. (10, *SBW*, p. 667)

These arguments do not mean that young Metchnikoff denied the evolutionary importance of the struggle for existence. Quite the opposite, he wrote of the struggle as if it were self-evident and broadly recognized; there is not even the slightest trace of doubt. Rather, Metchnikoff focused on the causes of the struggle for existence and other related phenomena for which the struggle might be causative. As the legion of Darwin's critics before and after him, Metchnikoff in his review of the *Origin* asserted,

> The striving to rapid reproduction is an effect of the struggle for existence but not the cause of it, as [Darwin] . . . believes. (10, *SBW,* p. 667)

The ease with which Metchnikoff accepted Darwin's major concept reflected his affinity to the established tradition of transformation. And this same posture reveals a misunderstanding of Darwin's originality. As many others, Metchnikoff regarded the struggle concept not as a way to avoid the otherwise unavoidable discussion of evolution in terms of feelings, desires, and motivations, but exactly as one more way to deal with living phenomena in these terms. Thus, he objected to Darwin's contention that the most intensive struggle takes place between individuals of the same species. He disagreed with Darwin on this point because the idea was a result of a quasi-Malthusian approach, and

> beside this [i.e., the unfounded extention of Malthusian principle], the opinion is wrong because, as everyone knows (!), common dangers and obstacles do not excite struggle between individuals subjected to these disasters, but on the contrary, force them to unite together in one society in order to fight back the current obstacles by united, more reliable efforts. (10, *SBW, p.* 668)

The general conclusion is categorical. He viewed the main defects of the *Origin* as

> the wrong generalization of the Malthusian law and attributing a special significance to the principles of natural selection and extinction. (10, *SBW,* p. 672)

Darwin's vision of evolution, as mediated first and foremost by the relations between organisms, is criticized as neglecting the more traditional (and self-evident) vision of evolution immediately influenced by reactions to the external environment. Metchnikoff wrote:

> All of these defects [in *Origin*] are rooted in a too superficial view on the influences of external environments upon organisms, which influences are, of course [*sic!*], the main factor of organization and life. (10, *SBW,* p. 672)

He concluded:

> Thus, having considered Darwin's treatise, although in a very superficial way, we must, however, recognize the fallacy of his theory in its most important, essential theses. . . . But rejecting Darwin's theory, we do not mean by this to throw a stone at the very idea of transformation of species; on the contrary, we admit for the theory a great future and, although we do not have convincing facts in favor of its absolute truth, we, however, with a deep faith in it, can boldly and without hesitation join its most zealous advocates. (10, *SBW,* p. 672)

The Middle Period

In 1869, six years later, Metchnikoff published in Russian *(The Teaching About Organic Forms Based upon the Theory of the Transformation of Species)* (18) his abbreviated exposition of Haeckel's *Generelle Morphologie* (19). Here Metchnikoff is more favorably oriented to Darwin. In the preface he wrote:

The activity which was excited in science by Darwin's teaching on the origin of species is the best proof that his ideas about organic life of nature appeared, in its proper time. (18, *AC,* p. 23)

If we recall that in the same year Metchnikoff published "The Current Situation in Science Concerning Development of Animals" (20) (discussed at length in chap. 3) in which he clearly stated a negative assessment of the approach realized in morphology by the Darwinians, in general, and by Haeckel, in particular, we would not anticipate the almost ecstatic tone in which he referred to Darwin and Haeckel:

On the other hand, the French academicians led by the old man [Marie-Jean-Pierre] Flourens and all the conservatives of the museum rubbish still try now to stop the tide of the ideas which are hostile for them, but on the other hand, the majority of the best German and English zoologists and botanists ([Franz] Leydig, [Carl] Siebold, [T. H.] Huxley, [Édouard] Claparède [the naturalist], [Karl] Naegeli, and very many others) have expressed themselves in favor of the [Darwinian] teaching. Still others, applying Darwin's opinions to special studies, have reached already remarkable results and continue to develop in different fields of natural science the most essential part of his theory.

Finally, Ernst Haeckel, a professor of Jena University, was the first, who undertook to rebuild the whole science of natural organic forms according to the new teaching about the origin and development of the forms. (18, *AC,* p. 23)

In this work, Metchnikoff does not doubt the importance and essential success of Haeckel's undertaking. So, why is there such a striking difference between two works published in the same years ("The Current Situation in Science . . ." and the comments to the *General Morphology*) in the assessment of Darwin and Haeckel? In the first paper ("The Current Situation in Science . . ."), Metchnikoff complained that until the beginning of the 1860s, although extensive data in invertebrate embryology had been accumulated, neither principles of organization nor a general theoretical goal for these studies had been provided. He made the same complaint about morphology in general, by noting of Haeckel's *General Morphology:*

Until now morphology is nothing else but a collection of factual data (although very rich but too heterogenous). . . . The more material accumulated (and its stock [has] increased since Cuvier's time and continues to increase with remarkable speed), the more is felt the lack of a carefully considered plan which would give an opportunity to reduce this multiplicity of uncoordinated facts to a unity, not to an abstraction, but one which would coincide as closely as possible with living reality. That is what Haeckel has undertaken. (18, *AC,* pp. 23–24)

From this point of view, the attempts of the Darwinians to bring order into the chaotic data was welcomed by Metchnikoff. But in "The Current Situation in Science . . ." essay, Metchnikoff revolted against the tendency to see in comparative embryology only a means for reconstructing phylogeny. On the contrary, he saw in the reconstruction only an application of comparative embryological studies that had their own problems and goals. Comparative embryology is a powerful tool in establishing genealogical relations, but the newly evolved practice of the Darwinians to totally reduce studies in individual development (the problems of production, diversity, similarity, and affinity of forms) solely to establishing genealogical relations leads necessarily to a tendency to create arbitrary phylogenetic hypotheses and to substitute true embryological studies with speculations. Metchnikoff did not doubt that

Haeckel was the champion of this trend. Thus the purpose of criticizing Haeckel in "The Current Situation in Science . . ." essay reflected Metchnikoff's understanding of the relationship between phylogeny and ontogeny (i.e., the understanding that he considered as decisive in his own formulation of the goals and methods of comparative embryological studies). On the other hand, his edition of Haeckel's *General Morphology* was addressed (as Metchnikoff stated) to nonspecialists (18, *AC*, p. 24). What he cherished in the book was not an elaboration of any essentially new approach to studies in his own professional field, but a universal evolutionary vision as the most powerful expression of the *Zeitgeist*.

Metchnikoff's attitude to Haeckel's *General Morphology* is not a matter of scientific research, it is a matter of science as ideology, science as Weltanschauung. Metchnikoff wrote:

> We consider as one of the most important of Haeckel's contributions, his intention to explain the organic world by the same mechanical laws which govern the phenomena of non-organic nature. . . . Leaving aside some unimportant blunders and gaps, which are always unavoidable in any first attempt, we mainly attempted to present, with all possible clarity and completeness, the development of Haeckel's basic thought—"the thought (as he himself defines it on the last page of his introduction) about the unity of organic and non-organic nature, the thought about a universal dependance of all (without exception) natural phenomena on mechanical causes, the thought that the generation and development of organic forms are the necessary results of the eternal natural laws which do not allow any exception." (18, *AC*, pp. 23–24)

Reproducing Haeckel's formulations of "struggle for existence," "the law of divergency," "the law of natural progress," Metchnikoff (unlike in his other works) does not argue in any way with the concepts. Instead he states:

> The theory of transformation of organic forms proposes the opportunity to reduce to universal forces of the world those mysterious sources which produce organized living beings. Correspondingly, we have the right to say with Haeckel that this theory is the only scientific basis for both history of development and morphology in general, which are placed by the theory under the command of the cause-effect law. (18, *AC*, p. 76)

It is not surprising that under the spell of this universal mechanical-evolutionary vision, peculiarities of Darwin's evolutionary doctrine are minimized. Darwin is prized only as presenting the most convincing evidence in favor of the great idea of transformism, not the most compelling explanation. The true value of Darwinism is conditioned only by its participation in the great tradition of transformism. And Metchnikoff sympathetically expounds Haeckel's point of view:

> The theory of the species' transformation cannot be exclusively attributed to any of those famous naturalists whose names are now connected with it—to Lamarck, Geoffroy, Goethe, Darwin or Wallace. It is possible to say about it the same thing which can be said about all great discoveries and inventions, that is, the theory is much more a product of its time than of a personal genius of one or another scientist.
>
> Actually, the same views (!) on organic life were proclaimed already in the beginning of our century by Baer, [Matthias] Schleiden, V[ictor] Carus, and by others, and even earlier by the mystical naturphilosopher Lorenz Oken and the poet Goethe. (18, *AC*, p. 76)

The triumph of Darwinism in the nineteenth century was conditioned mainly by those for whom the *Origin* had appeared as the powerful stimulus to renovate and establish as dominating the old idea of transformism. Thus, in Britain, as Bowler writes,

> [T. H.] Huxley . . . had little real interest in natural selection or the geographical evidence. Huxley was, in fact, a typical pseudo-Darwinian; he acknowledged the *Origin* as a key stimulus in the conversion to evolutionism, but he used the idea in a manner significantly different from that advocated by Darwin. The situation was equally complex in other countries. In America, the botanist Asa Gray supported Darwin with arguments drawn from biogeography, while the paleontologist O. C. Marsh adopted Huxley's version of pseudo-Darwinism. In Germany, the most prominent Darwinian was Ernst Haeckel, whose adherence to Darwinian principles was even looser than Huxley's. It was Haeckel who created the popular vision of progressionist evolutionism that was Darwinian in name alone. French biologists largely ignored the *Origin* and were only converted to evolutionism in later decades through a revival of interest in Lamarckism. (21, p. 72)

From the very beginning, that is, from the 1860s, the evolutionary idea overshadowed for the majority of Darwinians the real message of the *Origin*. It is not surprising that by the late nineteenth century, the term *Darwinism* "was used as little more than a synonym for evolutionism by writers who had no real interest in what Darwin actually said" (21, p. 73). Metchnikoff's position in his comments on Haeckel's *General Morphology* appears to coincide with the similar orientation of the other Darwinians of the time. However (as we noted), there was another aspect in his approach to Darwinism. On the one hand, Darwinism was a powerful manifestation of new scientific thinking, proposing confirmation of Metchnikoff's mechano-evolutionary Weltanschauung (i.e., those principles that constituted his intellectual horizon). And there was nothing in Darwinism that Metchnikoff could consider as contradicting or menacing his deepest beliefs. On the other hand, Darwinism as the source of his metaphysical inspiration did not overshadow those questions that arose in applying those themes to his own morphological studies. And in this peculiarity of Darwinism, the idea of evolutionary *mechanism* was the most important issue that again and again provoked Metchnikoff's criticism. This ambiguous attitude reflects, although in a special way, the general ambiguity of Darwin's reception in the nineteenth century. As David Hull argues (22), the term *Darwinism* did not reflect any coherent set of ideas pertaining to the mechanism of evolution, but rather the camp of Darwinism was formed by those who proclaimed their loyalty to Darwin as the leading figure in establishing the general idea of evolutionism. In these circumstances, it is very difficult to define any difference between the Darwinians and the anti-Darwinians in their broad scientific beliefs. Thus, Hull writes about Saint G. J. Mivart whose works (starting in 1871 with *On the Genesis of Species* [23]), remained paradigmatic for anti-Darwinian criticism during the nineteenth century:

> Mivart could easily have become a Darwinian. His views about evolution differed in no important respect from several key Darwinians. Like Huxley, he thought evolution was more saltative than Darwin did. Like Gray, he thought it was directed. And like so many Darwinians, he did not think natural selection could do all that Darwin claimed of it. Yet he soon became one of the Darwinians most effective critics. (22, p. 797)

This similarity between the Darwinians and their opponents signifies more Darwin's failure than his success. After all, both his opponents and his proponents had refuted (the first explicitly, the second implicitly) either the entire or partial Darwinian formulation of evolution's principal mechanism.

> The similarities that can be discerned between pseudo- and anti-Darwinism lie in the fact that both were largely expressions of the morphological approach to biology and the developmental view of the history of life. Both movements tended to picture evolution as the unfolding of orderly trends, without the element of haphazard divergence, introduced by Darwin's concern for the accidents of migration. . . . For every anatomist such as Huxley who looked for patterns of evolution that at least did not violate Darwinian principles, there was another like Mivart who constructed orderly patterns based on the old idea of linear development. (21, p. 74)

There is no doubt that starting with 1869, Metchnikoff's arguments against Darwinism originated as the criticisms of a morphologist; however, his vision is unique compared to his colleagues of the period. How well the morphologists debated the issue is another question. Bowler has extensively discussed how the morphologists neglected the perspective offered from studies of organisms living in the wild and in the process failed to appreciate the Darwinian message (21, p. 74; also see app. A herein for a more current view of the debate between morphologists and Darwinians). In light of this observation, Metchnikoff's critique assumes particular interest in its novelty. Further, Metchnikoff's later conversion to Darwinism (proclaimed explictly in the 1890s) in no way had been motivated by field naturalists' studies, but only by the logic of his development as a morphologist. So, how did the developmental descriptive approach motivate his criticism and his ultimate reconciliation with Darwinism?

The most expressive manifestation of the morphologists' developmental approach to evolution was presented by the idea of a parallelism between evolution and individual development: the degree individual development could be viewed as an adequate model of evolution determined the extent that a vision of evolution was shaped by the model. We remember that as early as 1869, Metchnikoff voiced strong opposition; in "The Current Situation in Science . . . ," he admits this parallelism rather as an exception than a rule (20). Nothing similar to Mivart's intention to construct "orderly patterns based on the old idea of linear development" (21, p. 74) could be found in Metchnikoff's anti-Darwinian criticism. On the contrary, in the strict parallelism of the "biogenetic law," he saw the inherited vice of the linear-development pattern as embedded in the new divergent evolution of such Darwinians as Fritz Mueller and Haeckel (24). We have discussed Metchnikoff's "antilinear" position of 1869, to which he returned in his 1871 paper, "The Goals of Modern Biology" (25), which was devoted to a critique of Herbert Spencer's *Principles of Biology* (1864).

> Due to the activity of some (mainly German) scientists, the theory of species transformations, or so-called Darwin's theory, quickly became the key dogma of science. Considering the principles of the theory as the only basis for all phenomena of organic life, Darwin's followers have brought the theory to the extremes which they proudly call "the inevitable postulates" of the theory. However, there have gradually accumulated such facts in science, which in no way can be brought in accordance

with the now dominating teaching about the origin of species. . . . Careful studies demonstrate that frequently very similar animals, living in the same circumstances and going through a long series of transformations [26], develop in very different ways. (25, *AC,* pp. 124–125)

And Metchnikoff concludes:

Of course, all these facts cannot prove that there is no transformation of species in nature, but nevertheless they hinder the explanation of the commonly accepted theory about the general pattern of transformation. (25, *AC,* p. 125)

Metchnikoff's anti-Darwinian position *was* the position of a morphologist. But it hardly fits to that morphologist paradigm as presented by Bowler. And we can understand why Bowler writes:

Darwin failed to complete a truly Darwinian revolution in biology because he was unable to wean the morphologists away from their fascination with abstract patterns expressing the underlying unity of living forms. (21, p. 74)

Can it truly be said that Metchnikoff the morphologist was fascinated with the vision of the descent of species as *evolution* (in the sense of expression or self-revelation) of abstract patterns (27)? If so, it would mean that Metchnikoff took the underlying unity of living forms as a self-evident and guaranteed reality. The idea of individual development as a revelation or manifestation of an underlying unity (but not as the only process that provides the unity of living things) dominated morphology at least since Aristotle's interpretation of the concept morphe. Discernible in Metchnikoff's early writings is an implicit acknowledgment to that traditional morphological orientation. It is enough to recall how Metchnikoff formulated in 1869 the goal of embryology:

The goal of the history of development as the science which deals with a multitude of changing forms, has to be precisely the establishment of a general affinity between separate animals and the search for the plan of their organization. (20, *AC,* p. 256)

The evolutionary approach of Fritz Mueller and Haeckel assumed a strong parallelism between genealogy and individual development and could be considered as typical examples of a morphological approach to biology and the developmental view of the history of life. But Metchnikoff's early criticism in regard to both of them could be viewed as a reflection of a much more radical morphological position. In this early period, he considered the role that studies play in individual development in reconstruction of genealogical relations as an exclusively applied function of comparative embryology. These genealogical (phylogenetic) reconstructions, from his point of view, could not offer much to comparative embryology.

Though many of the most zealous admirers of the species' transformation theory believed that to speak about the systematic similarity of organisms immediately means to preach Darwinism, but in reality they are entirely erroneous. Similarity between all organisms in general, and between their different groups in particular, is (and was) broadly recognized and its existence cannot be doubted. But not everyone thought it possible to explain this similarity by the *blood kinship* between organisms, considering the explanation as too hypothetical, devoid of a firm basis and, at the same time, in no way changing the fact of similarity of forms and organism structure. (20, *AC,* p. 261)

That is why Metchnikoff was in full agreement with those who

> entirely independently from the question about transformation of species, formulated their goal, as comparative studies in development of animals exactly in the same way as comparative anatomy existed much earlier than Lamarckism and Darwinism, and in the same way as [comparative anatomy] even now can pursue its goals apart from a theory of the common descent of the whole organic world. (20, *AC*, p. 261)

Metchnikoff always believed in the decisive importance of comparative embryological data for reconstruction of genealogical relations. At the same time, he minimized the role of such reconstruction in comparative embryological studies. Is this then not an example of morphologist maximalism (20)?

For Metchnikoff as the embryologist of the van Baerian era, identification of an organic form meant, first of all, identification of a type (a form) of development. At this point, he agreed completely with Haeckel, "The definition of species, which would be tentatively true theoretically and useful practically, is possible only on the basis of history of development (18, *AC*, p. 98). However, identification of a developmental type (form) became not just a task of empirical observation and description. We saw that in his studies of invertebrate embryology, Metchnikoff hoped to find the possibility for such identification in studies of the primary embryonic layers. The technical difficulties of the descriptive morphological identification provoked the general questions about legitimacy in applying Remak's concept of the primary embryonic layers (elaborated for the vertebrates) to the embryonic laminated structure in invertebrates. Or, more generally, the difficulties provoked questions about the principles of comparison and equation of those morphological (histological) realities that had different developmental fates. It is but natural in these circumstances to search for those features in the developmental structures that had been acquired *before* those structures took part in the given type of development, that is, *before* they accepted the burden of a particular developmental fate. Thus, the theme of homologies naturally entered Metchnikoff's deliberations.

However, if homological structures are defined as having a common phylogenetic origin, but at present perform different functions, then to establish their unity again is a matter of phylogenetic speculation. It is possible to avoid this approach only in cases where a particular form (i.e., the structures themselves) carry evidence that they are the same structures of the ancestor. To describe a structure as an organ is, first, to describe functions of the structure as pertaining to the organism as a whole. Consequently, the presentation of an ancestral organism in its descendant means that in a given ontogeny the primary, ancient function of the structure is discernible from the functions adopted in the descendant's development. Thus, discovering homologies relies on establishing two different functional contexts of the same structure. Actually, for Metchnikoff, the term *recapitulation* means coexistence of two heterochronic (in the sense of relating to different phylogenic stages) functional contexts. Although this position was explictly expressed by Metchnikoff only in the 1870s, even by the mid-1860s (as discussed earlier) adhering rather to the recapitulationist position than that of von Baer, he rejected recapitulation as a confirmation of parallelism between phylogeny and ontogeny. Quite the opposite, Metchnikoff consistently argued that many systematically related animals exhibiting apparent close genealogy at the same time often portray strikingly different types of individual development. Thus, there is no reason to expect uniformity for inscribing phylogeny into a given type of ontogeny. In like manner, there is no reason to consider the order of phylogeny as a provision of ontogenetic unity. Finally, why assert that ontogenetic unity itself has been provided? Recapitulation means coexistence of two heterochronic functional contexts of the same structure, but it does not mean that any form of reconciliation, coordination, or mutual "translation" of the contexts is guaranteed. Correspondingly, recapitulations provide disharmonies that might be harmonized in some cases, but not necessarily. The concept of individuality did not confer harmonized wholeness, that is, where every component manifesting an underlying unity perfectly fitted to a design. The issue then became how inherently disharmonious elements became harmonized, and a new dynamics was introduced. From 1868, the opposition harmony/disharmony became the central theme of Metchnikoff's general biological and philosophical meditations.

It is obvious from this intellectual perspective that the concept of individual development does not imply the concept of a unity underlying development. The progressionist's view of individual development was rooted in the assumption that the process in question is a *revelation* of (real or ideal) unity that preceded and actually directed development. But it is obvious that Metchnikoff's position excludes that assumption. Thus, at least in this case, the morphologist position is not the position of the progressionist.

In 1863, in his early review of the *Origin*, Metchnikoff wrote of progress in evolution as a self-evident tendency whose universal domination was beyond doubt. He did not question its universality and dominance. He only critiqued Darwin's ability to provide a sufficient scientific explanation. In 1869, having already conducted original morphological research, Metchnikoff in discussing Herbert Spencer's *Principles of Biology* questioned the very reality of progress as the dominant tendency of evolution. Spencer asserted that his "law of progress" was based on von Baer's teaching about the development of animals as proceeding from homogeneity to heterogeneity. The assertion provoked Metchnikoff's criticism:

> Is it true that there is in the nature of the organisms the law of progressive development according to which all biological phenomena form the successive processes of separation (differentiation) and unification (integration)? (25, *AC*, p. 117)

Actually, Metchnikoff asks here (as it becomes evident from his further discussion) not one, but at least four questions:

(a) Is progress formulated in accordance with the criteria of differentiation and integration, indeed, a universal tendency of individual development?

(b) Does our intuition of developmental levels satisfy these criteria?

(c) Are those processes that satisfy our intuition of progress, indeed, universal and dominant evolutionary phenomena?

(d) Could a theory of adaptive evolution (including, of course, Darwinism) provide a conceptual means for describing developmental levels (levels of perfection) and, in addition, for drawing distinctions between directions of evolution (progressive, regressive, or stable in respect to a level of organization)?

First, Metchnikoff argued against von Baer's belief that the dominant tendency of individual development is differentiation (i.e., the processes leading to transition from homogeneity to heterogeneity). He argued that in too many cases development does not proceed through differentiation. On the contrary, very often a radical shift in development may be performed through the disappearance of already existing specialized structures and, likewise, through a simplification of organization. On the other hand, there are no less (maybe even more) examples that contradict Spencer's second criterion of progress: "Integration is even a less necessary attribute of development than differentiation" (25, *AC,* p. 119). There are many examples that seemingly confirm Spencer's "law of progress," but these cannot prove universality or dominance. Metchnikoff wrote that Spencer's theories "may be applied to some cases but they do not correspond to phenomena forming whole series and which therefore cannot be considered as exceptions" (25, *AC,* p. 122). Metchnikoff supported his argument with extensive examples: there are many cases when a simplification of organization corresponds to our intuition of a regression. These cases could be seemingly explained as degenerative exceptions (e.g., the transition of the sponge's mobile larvae into the immobile adult form, with corresponding simplification of organization). But for every example of this kind, there can be found another example where transition to an active stage is followed not by further differentiation, but by simplification of organization.

It is obvious that the intuition of progress is related for Metchnikoff (if not for all his contemporaries) not to the morphologically defined succession of developmental stages, but to intuitively classified levels of activity. Some of his remarks leave us to define the intellectual structure that supports this intuitive classification. Thus, referring to a parasitic crustacean, as an example of regressive ontogenetic development (the type of development that was actually ignored in Spencer's defence of the "law of progress"), Metchnikoff noticed:

> It cannot be generally said that in this kind of development the sum of organs is diminishing but, what is important, the organs of so-called animal life (legs, eyes) are replaced in this case by the organs of vegetative life (the organs of reproduction) and exactly this serves as the typical sign of true regressive development. (25, *AC,.* p. 120)

We discern that the intuitive gradation of life's activity that supports these judgments about progressive and regressive developmental directions appeals to the traditional opposition of "the vegetative life" and "the animal life," which, in turn, may be traced to Aristotelian metaphysics and the cosmic hierarchy of entities ordered in accordance with degrees of liberation from their "natural places." We doubt that this historical-metaphysical dimension of thought consciously existed for Metchnikoff. He could turn to the history of a problem (and often did) in order to observe what had been done, what data had been obtained, and what approaches had been successful. In other words, he could turn to history as to an object. But we believe his positivistic ideology would never allow him to turn to history as a reality that actually functioned in his own mentality to form his own conceptual apparatus. This would explain why we do not encounter in Metchnikoff's writings any conceptual explication of the ordering intuition that conditioned his vision of progress as progress in life's activity. He could not ask how to express conceptually the reality whose criteria (presented as features of an object) he was seeking. He could not ask, because concept would mean, in this case, a set of objectively presented criteria. However, it is obvious that the intuitive paradigm of progress (and regression) was not presented for him merely by the fact of individual development. Individual development *could* present progressive (or regressive) features if the development went through a shift in the degrees of activity that, in its turn, could be comprehended actually only through specific intuition. (How is this intuitive position possible without an appeal to Aristotelian metaphysics to explain why the shift toward "the organs of animal life" must signify progressive development?) But neither a positivistic orientation toward objects nor a nihilistic habit of solving metaphysical problems by "physical" means allowed Metchnikoff to deal explicitly with intuition. He simply disallowed Spenser's criteria of differentiation and integration because they failed to satisfy his own intuition.

Metchnikoff did not question the reality of biological progress, but he criticized Spencer's specific notions. But what is more important, Metchnikoff questioned the *universality* of biological progress, no matter how the criteria were defined (either in accordance with Spencer's differentiations and integrations or with his own criterion of the shift from "the organs of vegetative life" to "the organs of animal life"). Even according to Metchnikoff's own criteria, progress is not universal and there were many cases when apparently progressive and regressive paths of development alternate during life of the same animal or even in the development of the same organ (25).

Any concept of universal progress implies that the unity of the process in question is provided. The problem of individual development, as formulated by Metchnikoff, the morphologist, excluded any assumption of an underlying unity of development. In like manner, the concept of development could not coincide with the concept of progress. "Development appears to be a much more general phenomenon than progress" (25, *AC*, p. 121). This is a natural conclusion because, "as we saw, development may be progressive, regressive, and substitutive (i.e., formed by shifts of parts)" (25, *AC*, p. 122). Progress is the revelation or the establishment of unity. The concept of unity is intuitively (in this case) correlated with the concept of activity. Lack or decrease of activity reflects, similarly, absence of progress or regress and, at the same time, absence or destruction of unity (Metchnikoff's concept of disharmony). Even in Metchnikoff's late writings on the disharmonies of human nature and the prolongation of life, we observe this opposition of "vegetative" and "animal life's organs" is still at work as an essential component in structuring his vision of harmonies and disharmonies, that is, in structuring his approach to the problem of unity in individual development. For instance, Metchnikoff formulated as one of the basic disharmonies the conflict between the mesodermic phagocytes, representing in the organism the ancient "vegetative" function of intracellular digestion, and the noble and progressive nerve cells that represent the functions of "animal life" (28, 29). The same can be said of another favorite topic, the disharmony between early maturated reproductive organs ("vegetative" life) and the relatively retarded development of the nervous and muscular system (30, 31).

It was commonplace in nineteenth-century philosophy to view freedom not merely as an attribute of political and social life, but foremost as life itself, in its innermost essence, in its autonomy, and in its self-responsiveness. This vision of freedom was the most essential element in the nineteenth-century concept of progress. In its turn, the intuition of progress as an increase in levels of freedom was equally characteristic of German idealism, naturphilosophical biology, and Spencer's philosophy. The vegetative–animal organ opposition was also broadly used by Metchnikoff to structure the levels of freedom, thus designating the direction of progress (32). In this respect, there was nothing original in Metchnikoff's understanding of progress. The true originality rests in his restriction in accepting *universality* of progress. The reasons (as already expounded) were rooted in his vision of the basic problem of invertebrate embryology, that is, in his refusal to accept as self-evident that individual development must be a revelation of an underlying unity provided by preceding evolution.

Thus Metchnikoff's argument with Darwinism cannot be explained merely by discounting Darwinian evolution to satisfy his morphological intuition of linear progressive development. He was not enamored with the typical morphologist position; at the same time, his criticism of Darwinism was from the vantage point of morphology. Any evolutionary teaching must provide a language for an evolutionary interpretation of ontogenetic development. But from Metchnikoff's point of view, such a provision does not imply that evolution necessarily provides a unity of individual development. Yet because any theory of evolution attempts to explain those processes that finally lead to the formation of organic forms, it follows that any evolutionary teaching must present its own explanation of how these processes are mediated by ontogenetic development. Metchnikoff's true problem was not to describe evolution in accordance with the pattern of individual development, but rather to understand that development as mediating evolution. Actually, this issue remains a critical question for modern evolutionary theory (see app. A), as Leo Buss writes:

> The synthetic theory of evolution, with its emphasis on the individual as the unit of evolutionary modification, is frequently, and justly, criticized as a "theory of adults"—one which has failed to address the diversity of ontogeny. Evolutionists, even today, seek to understand how development will illuminate patterns in evolution, not how evolution will illuminate the details of the developmental process. (33, p. 65)

We described how Metchnikoff (in his earliest essay) reproached Darwin for underestimating the role of the external environment, placing a false emphasis on interindividual relations (i.e., to mediate environmental influence by competition between organisms), which was deemed too internalistic. Then, in 1869 and 1871, with his own experience in morphological research and with his own formulation, Metchnikoff recast Darwinism as an externalistic doctrine. He observed (1871) that "the too 'consistent' supporters of Darwin's teaching" had too readily accepted all the peculiarities of organisms as arising by adaptation to the external environment or by deviation of inherited transmission. Of course, although there are many examples of these types of adaptations and deviations,

> if a theory does not offer an explanation of some significant phenomena, though it is not sufficient for its direct refutation, it is necessary, anyway, to be aware of its too broad generalization. (25, *AC,* p. 125)

And there are too many phenomena that could not be explained as resulting from adaptations and deviations:

Modern science demonstrates to us now and then examples of organisms, which, being perfectly similar by most of their features and living in very similar conditions, may be different only in a single, but most important, aspect. (25, *AC,* p. 122)

In these cases, the similarity of external conditions does not allow for the explanation of the differences as a result of divergence of adaptations. On the other hand, because the feature missing in a particular group of animals plays a crucial role in the life of other closely related groups, it is impossible to understand the presence of that feature in these groups as inheritance that, owing to its adaptive insignificance, has not been exposed to the pressure of negative selection (34).

All this does not mean that Metchnikoff refuted the idea of adaptive evolution, for he stressed that the very similarity between close groups testified to the similarity of their environments (24). His argument rests upon two tenets:

(a) To insist on the adaptive character of a given feature does not offer an evolutionary explanation because there are different forms of adaptation to the same environment. Correspondingly, we have to explain processes leading to the divergence of adaptations, otherwise the evolutionary explanation is a tautology. That is, we believe that a given feature has arisen from evolution because this particular feature seems to be an adaptive one, and evolution, by definition (for the Darwinians) is the production of adaptations.

(b) On the other hand, Metchnikoff doubts that all (or even all of the most essential) peculiarities and diversities in developmental form can be explained by adaptation.

In other words, Metchnikoff questioned not the legitimacy of adaptation as an explanatory principle. First, he challenged the application of the principle independently from considering developmental processes (i.e., he could not accept adaptation as a phenomenon that is not mediated by development), and second, he refuted the universality of the principle.

In this 1871 essay, Metchnikoff is mainly concerned with the very idea of adaptive evolution, and he almost ignores the struggle-for-existence issue as the mechanism that selects variations according to their adaptive capacity. Metchnikoff touched on this problem only once (and then not directly) in referring to Spencer's attempt to refute Malthus (i.e., the proposition that an increase of organization is always followed by decrease of reproduction and, because evolution tends to increase the perfection of organization, there is no danger of overpopulation). Only in respect to this argument did Metchnikoff allude to the Malthusian principle as the explanatory basis of evolution. Metchnikoff argued that Spencer's assertion is but another reflection of general evolutionary progress and final reconciliation of all contradictions. Facts testify rather in favor of the opposite view: an increase in organization is followed in most cases by an increase of reproduction. But concluding the argument, Metchnikoff does not mean to turn to an analysis of the Malthusian principle or any other that would lay claim to explaining the mechanism of natural selection. He used the argument as a vehicle in approaching the main topic of his essay: there is no evidence of a unity underlying evolutionary processes nor, indeed, is there evidence of programmed progress.

Having been convinced that productivity and, correspondingly, increase of population in no way follow any laws of purposeful progress leading to the good of mankind, we should naturally ask ourselves: Is it true that there is in the nature of organisms the law of progressive development? (25, *AC,* p. 117)

Rejecting adaptation as the universal explanatory principle of evolution, did Metchnikoff keep in mind any alternative theory? Definitely not. In this respect, he formulated his opinion quite clearly:

[Pierre-Simon] Laplace's cosmogonic theory, which is completely rejected, is the best demonstration of how carefully we must deal with all-embracing theories. This theory explained the formation of all cosmic bodies from the common cosmic matter so simply and demonstratively that human mind was unintentionally inclined toward it. . . . Despite all, the theory lived less than a century. Step-by-step, both astronomy and geology found many facts which positively demonstrated that, no matter how brilliant Laplace's theory was, it however was not correct. Science preferred to admit its own ignorance in respect to the origin of the earth and the other celestial bodies but not to follow the wrong path. (25, *AC,* p. 127)

The Mature Position: Origin of Metchnikoff's Disharmony Concept

In 1876, Metchnikoff published his definitive work on the problem of transformist theories: "Essay on the Question About the Origin of Species" (35). He concludes the essay with these remarkable words:

Almost every time I expounded a particular question, I could not avoid mentioning the incompleteness of our knowledge, which is especially painful in such basic subjects as, for instance, the struggle for existence, natural selection, and variability. . . . One of the main goals of this essay was to precisely point at such questions and thereby to make their scientific elaboration more accessible and to ease the serious studies of "transformism." (35, *SBW,* p. 238)

But this is only one of his goals, and it pertains to the future success of the transformist idea. What about other objectives? How are they related to Metchnikoff's own embryological research questions?

It could not have been accidental that exactly at this time Metchnikoff decided to elucidate for himself the basic problems of current evolutionary teachings. As described, Metchnikoff's embryological studies of this period (after 1872) witnessed a change in his view of the role in which the genealogical perspective might play in comparative embryological studies. Previously, he regarded the task of phylogenetic reconstruction as no more than an application of comparative embryology, which could not be particularly helpful in the pursuit of its proper goals. He explicitly expressed this opinion in 1869 ("The Current Situation in Science . . ."). Although more sympathetic with the task of phylogenetic reconstructions in his comments on Haeckel's *General Morphology* (1869), his attitude was addressed not to the way in which Haeckel conducted experimental research in morphology, but rather to the German's Weltanschauung. The same can be said about his essay on Spencer's *Principles of Biology* (1871). Here he was sympathetic with Spencer's task of philosophical generalization, but he warned against drawing too broad conclusions that ignored the true diversity of morphological data. While discussing the importance of comparative embryological data for formulation of evolutionary theories, Metchnikoff did not describe in what respects these theories might affect embryological research. After 1872, he became increasingly interested in the problem of metazoan origins, this, in turn, was provoked by his attempt to provide a genealogical approach to identifying the primary embryonic layers. As discussed, he was not satisfied with the morphological and histological criteria for identification of the layers, but rather by physiological criteria that by his interpretation of the recapitulationist idea demanded the genealogical reconstruction of the ancient function of the structure in question. Unlike his previous essays, in the work of 1876 Metchnikoff directly refers to the importance of genealogy for morphological studies, "Morphology is designated, first of all, by establishing the natural system, i.e., the genealogy of the organic world" (35, *SBW,* p. 236). The change of position in regards to 1869 is striking. Earlier he also believed that a morphological similarity *might* be a result of a genealogical unity. But he refused to see that a genealogical approach could in any way be helpful for establishing morphological affinities or, more generally, he refused at that time to admit that the evolutionary vision had anything to do with establishing the subject matter of morphology. By 1876, Metchnikoff claimed that his view of morphology was, in principle, evolutionary and that morphology was designated by genealogy.

Thus this essay reflects a radical change in Metchnikoff's vision of the role the genealogical perspective was to play in morphological research. The changes were, of course, provoked by his studies in comparative embryology, but the last section of the essay explicitly demonstrates that he undertook the investigation of evolutionary thought for the sake of his own central research problem, namely, the identification of the primary layers in general, and of the mesoderm, specifically. The last section is appropriately devoted to discussions of Fritz Mueller and Haeckel, for the theme of transformism and morphology was the fitting culmination to the design of the entire essay, whose focus was Metchnikoff's argument against Haeckel's *gastraea* theory. (As we have discussed, the same argument was prominent in Metchnikoff's comparative embryology publications, which repeated again that morphological criteria of the homology of the primary layers—either the similarity in their formation or the organs that develop from the layers—are insufficient [35, *SBW,* p. 233].) Haeckel's genealogical reconstruction (the *gastraea* theory) exploits for its own foundation the same morphological criteria; it does not prove the alleged homology of the primary layers, but presupposes an unproved homology (35, *SBW,* pp. 233–236). Thus, Haeckel's evolutionary approach to morphology becomes exclusively a morphological approach to evolution.

Haeckel was not concerned with the question of how that residue of an evolutionary idea, which was not reducible to morphological observations, could possibly be helpful. In fact, he considered only the opposite side of the relationship: How could morphological data aid in establishing the general evolutionary vision. Several years earlier, Metchnikoff had viewed the relationship in the same fashion and had asserted the applied significance of genealogical studies. In those years, his criticism of Haeckel's hypothesis (or Spencer's) warned against too hasty a generalization unsupported by observed facts. Some dose of this criticism can be found in the essay of 1876, but his argument against the *gastraea* theory reveals a more complex interaction between morphology and evolutionary theory. From this perspective, it is clear that Haeckel's theory appeared as a poorly constructed generalization because it *started* with the assumption of homology that had been defined in accordance with morphological criteria instead of providing genealogically directed morphological research that could possibly prove or refute homology. Thus, this concluding criticism of the *gastraea* theory reveals the mutual dependence of Metchnikoff's theoretical criticism and the concrete problems of his comparative embryological studies.

There is no doubt that Darwin powerfully influenced morphology:

> The appearance of *Origin of Species* influenced morphology, i.e., the science about structure and affinity of organic forms. However, this influence was determined not by the theory of natural selection, but by restoring and reinforcing the theory of the successive descent of species. (35, *SBW,* p. 216)

For Metchnikoff, the leading Darwinians (Haeckel and Spencer) represented eclectic mixtures of Darwinian elements with old ideas of *naturphilosophie,* Lamarckian, and even pre-Lamarckian theories. Metchnikoff was also confused as to what degree Darwin's own ideas were novel and free from earlier influences. He therefore devoted a significant effort on expounding the history and the different versions of the general evolutionary idea, discussing quite thoroughly the opinions of Charles Bonnet, Carolus Linnaeus, Georges-Louis Buffon, Peter Simon Pallas, Bernard-Germain Lacépède, Immanuel Kant, Jean-Baptiste Lamarck, Étienne Geoffroy Saint-Hiliare, Johann Wolfgang von Goethe, Karl Ernst von Baer, Georges Cuvier, Johannes Peter Mueller, Artur Schopenhauer, Ludwig Buechner and many others (35, *SBW,* pp. 9–87). He saw the belief that the idea of natural selection was sufficient to explain the evolutionary tendency toward perfection as the principal peculiarity of Darwinism. Metchnikoff clearly expounded Darwin's caution of invoking the exclusiveness of natural selection as an evolutionary force, but he criticized Darwin's seeming belief that natural selection was the only factor conditioning an increase in levels of organization. As already noted, Metchnikoff's concern with the problem of evolutionary increase in levels of organization reflected not his fascination with the pattern of individual growth, but, on the contrary, his belief that progressive development could not be considered as a general law of individual growth; this skepticism in regards to the universality of progressive individual development formed a parallel to Metchnikoff's rejection of considering individual development as revealing a provided, underlying unity. Thus, it is quite understandable that the true semantic axis of the essay is the problem of the relationship between the idea of natural selection and the possibility of interpreting levels of organization in that context. In this respect, Metchnikoff's approach appeared similar to the typical progressivist critique of Darwinism. In some sense, it *was* similar. But Metchnikoff was no less critical of the progressivist theories than those of Darwinism. Having discussed the ideas of Askenasy, Koelliker, Naegeli, and Weissman, Metchnikoff offered, in conclusion, a general appraisal of anti-Darwinian teachings in Germany. (Metchnikoff also applied his critique to the British Darwinian critic, St. George Jackson Mivart.) In Germany, the entire school of transformists, although admitting some role for natural selection, considered the inner striving for development, which they understood as *progressive* development, as the most important evolutionary factor. From their point of view, the morphological features, which are most important for systematic organization, are formed by this striving to perfection; but natural selection, in its turn, affects only the *physiological* features that are most important in the struggle for existence.

> The school has done much more in critical aspects than in the positive establishment of a new principle. At least, it has proposed as a hypothesis, but without proof, that natural selection affects the physiological side, i.e. the only significant side in the struggle for existence, but it [natural selection] almost escapes [influencing] the forms. Furthermore, it drew attention to the nature of variability and proved that neglect of this side of the problem led to an essential misunderstanding. . . . The school established only that the variations could not occur in all possible directions; it did not go beyond it: it failed to prove that there were only few ways of variability, all the more it failed to prove that it [variability] occured in one progressive direction. (35, *SBW,* pp. 118–119)

Adaptation of a given structure to the external environment means that this structure (being transformed or not) performs a new function(s). So, the assertion that selection (resulting from the struggle for existence) first affects physiology is quite a natural conclusion. But such a picture of evolution cannot satisfy how evolution (in this case, the process of adaptive changes in the physiology of a structure) will illuminate the details of the developmental process (in this case, the developmental process that forms the structure in question).

Metchnikoff shared this dissatisfaction with other morphologists of his time. But he in no way shared the belief (so popular among them) in a general progressive tendency of developmental and evolutionary processes. In his own analysis of Darwin and Wallace's use of natural selection as an explanatory principle, Metchnikoff came to the conclusion similar to those of other anti-Darwinian morphologists. He wrote:

> We do not find in Darwin (with the exception of his treatise *The Descent of Man*) any attempt to demonstrate in a direct way, i.e., by immediate examination of facts, the possibility of applying natural selection to a given systematic group and the degree of its effectiveness [in regard to such a group]. (35, *SBW,* pp. 169–170)

Metchnikoff finds such an attempt in Alfred Wallace's interpretation of natural selection's activity in the case of the Malayan *Papilionide* (*Contributions to the Theory of Natural Selection.* London: Macmillan, 1870), with whose conclusions he disagreed. Metchnikoff believed that more critical evaluation of the facts utilized by Darwin and Wallace to support the natural selection theory demonstrated:

> First, in those cases where an effect of the factor is most obvious and undoubted, a durable heredity (as in the case of the protective coloration) appeared in assistance; second, natural selection rather affects more hidden characteristics than those which constitute the morphological peculiarities of races and species; and, third, exactly these latter peculiarities cannot always be reduced to the activity of natural selection. (35, *SBW,* p. 171)

And further, he stated even more categorically:

> Major facts of organic nature's real life do not accord with the basic principles of the selection theory. (35, *SBW,* p. 177)

Metchnikoff noted that Darwin himself admitted that in some cases, features that are indifferent in regard to adaptation can be preserved not because of selection, but becuse of "the nature of the organism or to the nature of the external environment."

> The only difference in the opinions is that Darwin considers these cases as exceptions from the general rule, and because of this he pays very little attention to them, meanwhile they actually form a widespread and major phenomenon. (35, *SBW*, p. 182)

It is clear that this skeptical attitude toward the central role allegedly played by selection of adaptive characteristics conditioned Metchnikoff's corresponding attitude to Darwinian interpretation of the material that selection operates on (i.e., variability) and the corresponding selective mechanism (i.e., the struggle for existence). Like most of his fellow morphologists—who in their discussion of evolution were interested not in adaptive variations of given structures, but rather in the evolutionary realization of the processes that led to formation of the structures—Metchnikoff's vision of variability was much more saltatorial than that of Darwin (35, *SBW*, pp. 137–142). Metchnikoff believed that even the facts gathered by Darwin contradicted the conclusions regarding the abolition of abrupt species change (35, *SBW*, p. 139). Darwin had argued that crossbreeding eliminates abrupt variations; naturally, Metchnikoff returned the argument, asserting that precisely "such [abrupt] variations have more chance for durable existence than small individual peculiarities" (35, *SBW*, p. 141). Similarly, he supported Fleeming Jenkin's argument in favor of collective variations (36). Having noticed (35, *SBW*, p. 182) that Jenkin's paper actually changed Darwin's basic belief in the leading role of individual variations, Metchnikoff wrote:

> *In order to be able to start to act, it is not sufficient for natural selection to have mere individual deviations; it is necessary to have a certain sum of individuals which have changed in advance in a similar way, or, in other words, a certain race must be formed before the beginning of the selection's activity and independently from the latter.* (35, *SBW*, p. 183)

Correspondingly, his unwillingness to accept the leading role of individual variations as the main arena for operation of natural selection led to Metchnikoff's refusal to accept the competition between individuals of the same species as the most creative evolutionary factor.

Metchnikoff believed that there were several forms of the struggle:

> (1) The competition between individuals of the same species; (2) the competition between individuals of different species; (3) the struggle between individuals of different species (for example, a struggle of a beast of prey with a herbivore); and (4) the struggle between living creatures and the elements (the struggle against hunger, drought and so on). (35, *SBW*, p. 146)

Thus, the "real" struggle takes place between individuals of different species, either as they compete for sustenance or in their respective encounters with abiotic environments. In this last case, the individual also represents its group in the opposition to the "living world" and the "dead world." Individuals, inasmuch as they represent themselves but not their corresponding groups, do not reach a higher degree of conflict than competition. For instance, the relation of struggle between predator and its prey is constitutive in relation to the very essence of corresponding species: at least one of them cannot exist without this struggle. But such a relation as competition of plants for light or water does not necessarily mean that at least one of the competitive species cannot live outside of this relationship; so, this kind of struggle for existence is a detail of individual life, it is something that might happen under certain circumstances, but it does not comprise the essence of the species' nature, thus falling under the rubric of *competition,* but not *struggle.* The same can be said about the struggle for existence that takes place between individuals of the same species. This relationship, according to this logic, should also be called *competition,* as distinct from *struggle.* Thus, variations within a species can lead only to competition (i.e., not the crucial role that leads to struggle). Likewise, the Malthusian principle cannot be accepted as the main explanatory principle of the driving evolutionary force and

> intensive reproduction is very far from having such an important significance in the generation of the struggle as it has been assumed by Darwin: . . . in this respect, competition and struggle between heterogenous forms undoubtedly play a much more important role. (35, *SBW,* p. 152)

This "collectivistic" opposition to Darwinian "individualism" is in no way something original or unusual for biological thought of the nineteenth century (37). After all, the old naturphilosophical idea of evolution, which assumes an underlying common scheme of evolution and individual development, excluded a consideration of individual variations as the only (or even the main) source of evolutionary creativity. Under various disguises, the idea was still at work in different versions of the morphologist's criticism or reinterpretations of Darwinism. Thus, it is not surprising that in such anti-Darwinian or pseudo-Darwinian expositions, evolution appeared more altruistic than in the original Darwinian interpretation. Metchnikoff sympathetically discussed Naegeli's evolutionary ideas, which were supported by his rich direct botanical observations. Hans Naegeli believed that the ouster of a weaker competitor by the stronger seemed a self-evident phenomenon only superficially and could exist only as an exception. The idea seemed to be self-evident and was only tested against hypothetical forms (38). From his point of view, not the intraspecific struggle of individuals and ouster of variations, but coexistence of different forms and socially organized life, favors formation of new species (39).

Bowler argues (21) that Darwin's "individualistic" approach to evolution was of such radical novelty that it was not easily recognized by his contemporaries. This "collectivistic" approach even dominated the opinion of the cofounder of the selection theory, Wallace. In this connection, Bowler writes about Wallace's initial position:

> The title of the 1858 paper was "On the Tendency of Varieties to Depart Indefinitely from the Original Type." . . . It generally has been assumed that it contains the essence of the theory already worked out by Darwin, although there are actually considerable differences between the ways in which the two naturalists presented the idea. . . . Wallace had been impressed with Lyell's discussion of the "war of nature" between species and understood struggle for existence at this level. Like Darwin, he read Malthus because he too was interested in the problem of human evolution. But the 1858 paper uses the idea of population pressure to drive home the severity of competition between varieties already established within a species, that is, between distinct populations *not* between individuals. Darwin always had thought of struggle

as an individual level and made this the basis of his theory. Wallace instead presented selection acting between varieties, eliminating those least fitted to cope with the overall conditions of the species' range. (2, p. 174)

The formulation and popularity of the collectivistic version of evolution did not require a specific Russian cultural and social context. It was implied by the dominating tradition of evolutionary thought. What was unique in the Russian reaction to Darwinism was not a theoretical peculiarity of the collectivistic alternative, but the very fact that so many Russian intellectuals identified with an alternative vision opposed to British (or Western, in general) analytical rationalism and individualistic historical being. The unique Russian feature of the reaction was the recognition in this old collectivistic version of the evolutionary idea something more congenial to Russian mentality than the new individualistic alternative as it was represented by Darwin. We noted earlier that this generally formulated opposition to the analytically self-dissecting and self-atomizing West, being extended to its logical limit, turned paradoxically into acceptance of Western thought as the real soul of Russian culture (37).

Similar paradoxical results can be found in the formulation of collectivistic alternatives to Darwin's ideas. For instance, from Todes's point of view (3, 40), Metchnikoff is a typical representative of those Russians, who comparing the importance of evolutionary factors, paid much more attention to the interspecies struggle than to the struggle between individuals of the same species. Although completely true, this interpretation is incomplete. What prize did Metchnikoff pay to support this specific attitude? In his final reconciliation with Darwin's teaching, Metchnikoff reserved his collectivistic objections against Darwin's version of the struggle for existence. On the other hand, as we will discuss further, he was finally able to accept the idea of the struggle as the leading force of evolution because he began to consider individual development as a process resulting from the struggle between different parts of the same organism and different cell lineages. Thus, he dipped the interspecies struggle into the individual organism itself and actually considered, as most important, the struggle between parts of the same organism. Arguing for primacy of the interspecies struggle, Metchnikoff created of it the very soul of individuality. To establish peace among individuals of one species he proclaimed a war between parts of each individual organism, *the war of the individual against itself.*

Thus Metchnikoff (in the 1870s) did not reject the idea of evolution through selection, but he believed that selection could not be considered as the primary evolutionary force. From his point of view, selection could affect rather some functional changes than those essential morphological transformations that led to a new systematic group. Selection can operate only to facilitate the establishment of those variations that, having been formed independently from selection, represent at once an essential transformation toward a new systematic group. Correspondingly, what matters, from Metchnikoff's point of view, is not random individual variations, but the variations that are directional and essentially general, not small changes but radical shifts in organization. Accordingly, the real struggle (as the principle of selection) takes place not between individuals who, belonging to the same group, manifest slight variations of the same features, but rather between different groups (or individuals as representatives of different groups) and with inanimate elements of nature.

There is nothing original in these objections to Darwinism. Like the majority of the morphologists of his time, Metchnikoff could not accept the idea of adaptive evolution, considering adaptive transformations as real but secondary phenomena. But unlike the majority, he expressed himself in this 1876 essay against the idea of linear evolution. Although this originality is not of a unique nature, and Metchnikoff was not the only one of that time who expressed skepticism concerning the universality of the "law of progress," his argument against the progressive vision of evolution reflected (as we have said) his professional concern with the problem of identification in comparative embryological studies. Actually, the central issue of the essay concerns the possibilities of interpreting morphological transformations in terms of adaptive evolution. As noted, the problem of identification of developmental structure became the problem of genealogical reconstruction: establishing the given structure's function in relation to the integrity of an ancestral organism. It is natural from this perspective that Metchnikoff estimated any evolutionary theory, first of all, by its abilty to propose an objectively founded scale or principle for comparison of evolutionary defined integrities. Correspondingly, the problem of perfection and progress remains crucial. Metchnikoff discusses the problem here even more carefully than in his previous works. He noted that Darwin (after von Baer) considered labor's differentiation as the main criterion of progress. Metchnikoff noticed that von Baer clearly saw the faults of his own principle: insects or Cephalopoda are (contrary to broad scientific belief) more "perfect" (or more highly developed) than fish, whereas the fish cranium is more perfect than the crania of birds, mammals, and humans. Then Metchnikoff analyzed Heinrich Bronn's criteria of perfection, which (similar to those of Spencer) included, beside differentiation, concentration and blending of parts (41). As in his essay on Spencer, Metchnikoff easily demonstrated that there are many cases where application of such criteria were nonsensical. The entire argument reflected the ageless biological conflict:

> Yet when we make generalizations about trends among animals and plants . . . it is almost automatic to point out the exceptions and throw out the baby with the bath. This is not a question of fuzzy logic or sloppy thought; it is merely a question whether the rule or the deviations from the rule are of significance in the particular discussion. (42, p. 15)

However, something new appears in comparison with the essay of 1871 (on Spencer). Metchnikoff explicitly attempts to fight the metaphysical context of this conjecture about levels of perfection (although as usual without revealing the metaphysical origin and meaning of the concepts). Metchnikoff quoted Bronn:

> Because we accept the human organism as the highest type of the animal realm, and because we see that it is able to reach its highest perfection only by means of the brain and the nervous system which are prevailing over other systems, and also by means of harmonious development of all other subordinated systems, . . . we discover immediately that the class of mammals is closer to such a perfection than birds. (41, pp. 110–111)

He betrayed two implicit ideas broadly accepted among naturalists: man represents the highest perfection and all organs develop harmoniously (35, *SBW*, p. 192). At least since 1868, Metchnikoff was occupied increasingly with the idea of the organism as a basically disharmonious entity. He rejected Bronn's criterion because it could not be applied to many living forms:

> But beside this it [the criterion] is affected by subjectivity to such a degree which could not leave a naturalist unshocked [Metchnikoff, of course, glorifies here his own intuition of the naturalist and his determination to oppose "subjectivity" with the prevalent view of man as harmonious and perfected]. From the objective point of view, man does not appear as the summit of harmonious development of all his parts. (35, *SBW,* p. 193)

Metchnikoff well understood that the idea of harmony was supported by the naturphilosophical idea of a provided developmental scheme. He opposed the idea in both its forms: first, as the theory proclaimed the parallelism between phylogeny and ontogeny, and then in the form of the von Baerian interpretation of the general developmental tendency. But Metchnikoff stated (35, *SBW,* p. 65) that he followed von Baer in considering the idea of parallelism, not as belonging to a single author, but as reflecting an entire stage in the development of natural sciences, that is, the *naturphilosophie* stage. This idea of parallelism not only asserted a provided scheme of development, but it ordered development and evolution in a linear and progressive fashion. In opposing the idea, Metchnikoff considered von Baer as his ally:

> In truth, Man is only in respect of his nervous system, and of that which is connected with it, the highest form of animal. . . . One must be completely prejudiced, in fact, not to see that the stomach of the Ruminant, which changes grass into chyle, is more perfect than the stomach of Man. (43, p. 242, 1828; trans. p. 231, 1853)

On the other hand, Metchnikoff considered von Baer's idea of development, which proceeds from the general undifferentiated stage toward a more and more heterogeneous and differentiated pattern, as "a further step of the naturphilosophers' theory, a more positive and definite step" (35, *SBW,* p. 67). Von Baer's radial evolution proceeding from a common center can be opposed to the linear evolution of the progressionists. But the idea of differentiation as the main developmental tendency actually presented in another form the old idea of harmonious development (i.e., the idea of development as the realization of an underlying unity). Both von Baer and Bronn's criteria of progress presupposed the vector of increased activity, which in its most general form was designated by the opposition of vegetative–animal life, and morphologically presented opposition of the organs—organs of the vegetative life and organs of the animal life. If in his earlier essays, Metchnikoff shared with others the use of the opposition as something self-evident, in this essay he was already much more sensitive to its naturphilosophical implications:

> Accentuating the organs of the animal life, we inevitably come to the conclusion that algae and fungi are much higher than all the other plants, because only among them we meet an animal-like state (zoospore). . . . The flowering plants do not present anything similar to that. (35, *SBW,* p. 193)

Of course, it is possible to object to Metchnikoff's argument by the very design of the concepts of "vegetative life" and "animal life" forming two extremes of progress; animals could have vegetative organs as residues of a lower developmental stage; however, by the very structure of the opposition, it is mistaken to seek in plants organs of animal life. But Metchnikoff committed more than just a formal error. As typical of Metchnikoff's writings, he struggled with concepts elaborated in a metaphysical context, but neither intended to refute them nor to elucidate their metaphysical origin and meaning; he sought to clarify the intuitively perceived metaphysics, not by explication of content and structure, but by finding in the "physical world" something analogical to his intuition. If, dealing with the opposition, he had not left the old metaphysical context, he would have recognized that inside that context, the zoospore more appropriately fitted a definition of the vegetative organ. As we mentioned, the opposition was elaborated in accordance with the Aristotelian scale of the hierarchy of living beings, which expresses an understanding of perfection's levels as the degrees of "liberation from the natural place." According to this scale, the zoospore manifests dependence of reproduction from the water element as the "natural place" for algae and fungi, but the flowering plants could be considered as the summit that had been achieved by vegetative life in its striving to liberate the reproductive processes from the water element. Rejecting that there were any objective data that could possibly allow Metchnikoff to base the criteria of progress on the opposition of the animal life's organs and the organs of the vegetative life, he still tenaciously clung to these very concepts. Similarly, admitting that both von Baer and Bronn's criteria of progress failed to establish a reliable correlation between the intuition of progressive development and corresponding objective data, Metchnikoff did not mean to reject the very idea of progress. Being faithful to the tasks and concepts born within this metaphysical tradition, he never attempted to explore their philosophical meaning. At the same time, failing to reformulate them in "physical" terms, he never rejected them.

Thus his thought moved within a certain circle: struggling to replace the metaphysical content of concepts with a "physical" reality, he was forced again and again to confirm that metaphysical horizon within which his task was defined and whose metaphysical nature he was to deny. In this essay (unlike his earlier composition 1871), he rejected definitions invoking levels of organization that compared the organs of the vegetative life with the organs of the animal life. But despite all this, from hereon until his death, Metchnikoff continued to define his basic concepts of "harmony" and "disharmony" in accordance with this opposition. The same can be said about his attitude toward the anthropocentric nature of biological progress. Thus, he rejected, as we saw, Bronn's criterion of progress because "it is affected by subjectivity to such a degree that could not leave a naturalist unshocked." Speaking here about subjectivity, Metchnikoff meant that Bronn's criteria reflected an essentially anthropocentric intuition of progress that assumed that Man is the highest creature (44). But several pages later, arguing that progress in organic nature is an *objective* (although not universal) phenomenon, well established by scientific data, Metchnikoff explicitly affirmed this very anthropocentric meaning of the concept "progress" and here he does not seem shocked by its subjectivity; he sees as mistaken only the early theories of linear progress.

> Since then, science demonstrated that it is impossible to speak about unilinear development. . . . But the general features of the law of organic progress are inviolable. (35, *SBW* p. 202)

Metchnikoff continued, writing that geology demonstrated the earliest organisms were the simplest:

But *the highest creature, man* [emphasis added], is, at the same time, the latest one. It [geology] demonstrated further that the lowest representative had appeared at first among plants and vertebrates, and after them appeared more and more complicated and perfect forms. (35, *SBW,* pp. 202–203)

Metchnikoff noted that because of the difficulties in elaborating objective criteria of progress, certain naturalists totally rejected any principle of perfection other than as reflected for the immediate benefit of the organism. In this connection, he mentioned Hermann Mueller, who wrote of the perfection of flowers only from the vantage of their adaptation to reproduction (45). From Metchnikoff's point of view, this approach did not solve the problem, only ignored it. From what we have already discussed, it is clear that the problem of the progress criterion, or the problem of the perfection levels, could not be solved from Metchnikoff's point of view in terms of adaptation, for adaptation pertains to the physiological transformations, not to those of organization. It is also clear that the problem could not be solved in terms of natural selection, which operates on the field of variations having different adaptive values:

Even in the hypothetical examples that have been proposed by Darwin, in order to clarify the activity of natural selection, it is impossible to find any immediate relation to progress. . . . Generally speaking, because the selection [as Darwin believed] affects individuals and races of the same species, it often appears that to draw a distinction in the degree of perfection between the winner and the loser is an unsolvable task. How is it possible, after all, to find a different degree of parts' separation [von Baer's criterion of progress, which was accepted by Darwin] among so closely related organisms, if it is impossible to sometimes make such a distinction in relation to whole orders. (35, *SBW,* p. 195)

Metchnikoff concludes:

Between perfection of organization and selection, there does not exist that essential connection which was presupposed by Darwin. (35, *SBW,* p. 196).

Selection may favor either an increase or decrease in organization, sometimes it acts without affecting those characteristics that determine the *systematic* level of the organisms (35, *SBW,* p. 200). The latter situation is the most usual ("The facts demonstrate that the most broadly widespread natural phenomena have a clear conservative character" [35, *SBW,* p. 208]). An increase in perfection is something radically different from the ability to adapt to a changing environment and selection could favor it only under steady external conditions (35, *SBW,* pp. 200–201). If selection affected a shift in the levels of organization during long evolutionary periods, corresponding to changing environments, it would be rather a regressive shift than a progressive one. ("The examples of regress agree better, in general, with the activity of natural selection than many examples of progressive development" [35, *SBW,* p. 208]). It is quite clear that it was exactly this interest to regress as the alternative direction of evolution that determined Metchnikoff's approach (in the 1870s) to parasitology (see chap. 5).

Conclusion

Metchnikoff was not searching for another illustration of the interspecies struggle concept when applying Darwinism to the consideration of such a phenomenon as parasitism. He sought to check to what degree (if at all) it was possible to describe developmental processes in Darwinian terms. Darwinians held that natural selection was a sufficient explanation of the progressive tendency. We have described how Metchnikoff doubted that hypothesis. Maybe, Metchnikoff asks, "The law of progress of the organic world, being dependent on natural selection only partially, is, on the other side, a result of an organism's inner striving to perfection?" (35, *SBW*, p. 202). He does not offer a decisive answer to the question. But it is clear that his arguments are designed to prove that changes in the level of organization cannot be described in terms of selection. Metchnikoff does not attack Darwinism because of its inability to present progress as a universal evolutionary tendency, but because of its inability to elaborate proper terms for describing the difference between progress and regress, a description he deemed impossible in terms of adaptive evolution and natural selection. Those terms (as Metchnikoff believed at the time) could describe the external fate of results that had been elaborated in individual development, but they did not fit the processes themselves. Ontogeny did not play any role in the Darwinian explanation of evolution through natural selection. In this respect, Lamarckian explanation of evolution, where an organism's activity plays a much more important evolutionary role, is from Metchnikoff's point of view closer to the goals of morphology (35, *SBW*, pp. 236–237). (This does not exclude Metchnikoff's highly critical attitude toward Lamarck [46].)

Two years later, in 1878, Metchnikoff published "The Struggle for Existence in a Broad Sense" (47). His principle position remained unchanged. In 1879–1880, he published several papers on parasitism; again no change in his approach to his evolutionary ideas, in general, and to Darwinism, in particular, is found. Then, until 1892, when he published his essay "The Struggle for Existence Between the Parts of Animal Organisms," wherein he explicitly proclaimed that the phagocytosis theory had been built upon the Darwinian theory of natural selection, there was a gap in his publications on general evolutionary problems. In his essay of 1876, the discussion of Darwin's influence on morphological research was culminated with the polemic against Haeckel's *gastraea* theory, which attack he continued in his special publications on comparative embryology. During this period (1876–1877), Metchnikoff elaborated his own alternative to Haeckel's *gastraea*—the *parenchymella* theory. Thus, it is clear that the *parenchymella–gastraea* controversy became the ultimate concretization of Metchnikoff's general evolutionary studies—the true center of evolutionary theoretical controversies. The *parenchymella* hypothesis required the identification of the mesoderm by its primordial function, which was seen by Metchnikoff as intracellular digestion. At the same time, the hypothesis asserted a basic disharmony in animals with cavitary digestion: the ancient aggressive and destructive function of amoeboid mesodermic cells was recapitulated in those organisms, which did not use that function for nourishment. In the light of the hypothesis, the organism appears as a basically disintegrated entity. In its turn, the phagocytosis idea in this regard was a proposal of how this potential disintegration might have been harmonized by an evolutionary mechanism.

To anticipate the later detailed discussion, the phagocytosis hypothesis presented immunity as a particular case of inflammation (the *diffusive* inflammation [immunity as a general, nonlocalized inflammatory reaction]). It is useful to briefly trace the developments of Metchnikoff's notion of immunity as part of the harmony/disharmony construct: At its basis, the evolutionary problematic of harmony/dishar-mony resides. On this foundation, Metchnikoff viewed physiological inflammation as an ontogenetic solution that would be applied to both physiological and poten-tially pathological conditions. It is in this latter case that immunity is a subset of pathological inflammation, where the response is generalized as opposed to site-spe-cific reactions. To reiterate, immunity is a specific case of pathological inflammation that, in turn, is a specific case of physiological inflammation that arises as a specific form of the harmony/disharmony conflict. Thus, disharmony was transformed into a specific form of the struggle for existence—now the struggle between cell lineages. The struggle of this particular case led to the establishment of organismic integrity. The concepts "struggle" and "selection" then became appropriate descriptions of developmental processes. It is clear from this point of view that the period between 1880 and 1892 represented no gap in Metchnikoff's concern with concepts of evo-lution, but rather comprises his final maturation that realized the elaboration of the conceptual framework of the *parenchymella* hypothesis and the theory of inflam-mation; the general problem of struggle for existence and natural selection was trans-formed into the concrete and specific question of the nature of inflammation. Of course, the struggle between cell lineages as the process that determines structural evolutionary transformations, is not the same as the Darwinian struggle between individuals as evolutionary units (48). Thus it is not surprising that the Metchnikoff of the 1880s did not consider himself a Darwinian, nor that he later proclaimed him-self a faithful Darwinian when the majority of the scientific community rejected the very idea of selective evolution, regardless of any concrete interpretation of the selec-tion concept. We are now prepared to consider the development of Metchnikoff's thought as a pathologist.

CHAPTER 5

Metchnikoff's Emerging Concept of Inflammation

The Status of Germs in 1880

Three broad avenues of scientific inquiry merged in Metchnikoff's phagocytosis theory: (a) the embryological definition of mesodermal origin, structure, and function, (b) an intellectual infrastructure of evolutionary dynamics applied to the organism, and (c) the emerging concepts of parasite–host interactions on a pathological level. We have considered the first two problems; now we must turn to the third problem, specifically the inflammatory reaction to microbial pathogens, whose investigation became Metchnikoff's primary arena of study (1).

In the same year that Darwin published *Origin of Species,* Félix-Archimède Pouchet presented *Hétérogénie ou traité de la génération spontanée,* an elaborate work that claimed to demonstrate that life might arise anew from inanimate solutions. Spontaneous generation had a long antecedent history and represented a problem Pasteur was advised to avoid, but he became embroiled in the issue as he perceived it was central to his notions of the central function of microbes in the economy of nature and causation of disease (2). In a series of famous experiments, Pasteur showed that sterilized fluids would not sustain bacterial growth, which might arise only on introduction of contaminated air. The academy had established the Alhumbert Prize in 1860 to help resolve the confusion; Pasteur won the prize in a dramatic public exhibition in 1862. The controversy in retrospect may be viewed primarily as a problem in methodology: Pouchet had not been able to sterilize resistant organisms or eliminate contaminating dust. But more broadly, the polemic drove the nascent field of microbiology to more vigorous experimental caution. With Henry Charlton Bastion's new assertion of spontaneous generation in 1872 (3)—after the war had seemingly been won—instigated John Tyndall's 1876–1877 demonstrations of heat resistant bacterial spores (4). More rigorous sterilization techniques were developed (higher temperatures under increased pressure); consequently, the debate had served to promote research for a firm methodological base. Neither Pasteur nor Tyndall could prove that spontaneous generation does not occur, but the controversy established techniques required to examine the question of contagion as a microbiological problem.

Although the germ theory appeared to have successes, these were, in fact, indecisive blows to spontaneous generation, which did not eliminate broad sentiment for the alternative theory. Perhaps the most dramatic incident is the case of Claude Bernard's unfinished musings on the subject, found in his desk after his death in 1877. Stunningly, he asserted that fermentation could occur independently of living processes and implied that yeast might, in fact, arise from fermentation, not cause it. Pasteur robustly defended the germ theory in oratory, repeated various experiments, and essentially quieted the nascent palace revolt, but the incident suggests the strong current of unsettled dispute regarding the nature of microbial processes in regards to host–bacterial interactions. In this context, the etiology of contagious diseases was very much in debate during the 1870s.

The triumph of the germ theory arose in the controversy of competing theories, of which the most critical was the contagion/anticontagion debate, which was essentially resolved by the 1870s (5). Of the various contagious theories, each suggested an unidentified, hypothesized particle as etiologic in some fashion (6). The zymosan theory, likening diseases to fermentation, was popularized in its nineteenth-century form by Justus von Leibig. Following the proposal by Charles Cagniard de Latour, Friedrich Kuetzing, and Theodor Schwann that fermentation was due to yeast, Liebig proposed that infectious diseases consisted of two stages: decomposition in the blood followed by multiplication of the ferment. As J. K. Crellin notes, the far-reaching feature of the theory was the importance attached to self-reproducing particles (ferments) of organic matter (6). William Farr, in fact, coined the term *zymosis* and emphasized that multiplying particles were specific for each disease. Benjamin W. Richardson, in 1859, proposed an alternative "glandular theory," based on the inability to identify the replicating particle. He offered, instead, a chemical theory (7). Richardson argued that secreted organic poisons, which were ultimately derived from normal albumen, were catalyzed by (again) an undefined particle, and it was the chemicals that gave rise to disease symptoms. The characteristic feature of this hypothesis is in the contrast to Lionel S. Beale's disease germs, which were living particles of degraded normal bioplasm. These particles were not microorganisms, but were like Farr's theory, specific for each disease—and contagious—but they differed from previous hypotheses in supposing that the particle was biological (8). According to this account, the bioplasm was not microbiological, but derived from normal living protoplasm of the body and gave rise to disease when corrupted by some alteration in its vital processes. Beale's term *disease germs* not only added confusion to the terminology, but because of its vitalistic overtones, was resisted by aspiring reductionists; experimental support seemed to be obtained by 1870, with John Burdon Sanderson's demonstration of disease induced by transfer of infected lymph (9). Finally, the graft theory, first proposed by James Ross (10) and then modified by John Drysdale (11) is primarily of interest in that it reflected Darwin's influence. The theory conjectured that detachments from a living body might become particles of contagion (in preference to living germs) causing disease by descending with successive variations "from a disease which was different from both, but which presented characters intermediate between them" (10, p. 267). To Drysdale disease was due to transplanted particles of living, detached matter (bioplasm or degraded protoplasm) grafted onto a new body (6) (Drysdale's evolutionary chart is also reproduced in Richmond's article.) None of these theories forthrightly denied spontaneous generation, and they allowed for it in some form or another. The problem could not be resolved until the practical methodology to study bacteria was developed in the second half of the 1870s, and it still lingered on with Bastian's nagging persistence (3).

Robert Koch's 1876 characterization that anthrax is caused by *Bacillus anthracis* (12)—a finding that was widely acclaimed, closely preceded Metchnikoff's phagocytosis hypothesis and led to the rapid identification of other bacterial pathogens: *Staphylococcus* (Koch, 1873), *Neisseria gonorrhoeae* (Albert Neisser, 1879), *Salmonella typhi* (Karl Joseph Eberth, 1880), *Streptococcus* (Alexander Ogston, 1882), and *Mycobacterium tuberculosis* (Koch, 1882). The identification of the etiological agent of tuberculosis (13) was heralded as of particular importance. The *New York Times* proclaimed, "It is one of the great scientific discoveries of the age." Koch's technical virtuosity, first demonstrated with his studies of anthrax and then followed with the plate technique (14), firmly established the science of bacteriology, but his observations seemed satisfied with studying the pathogenic etiology of disease, not the basis of the host response. Herein lay a basic conflict with the descriptive cellularists, who viewed the dynamic between organism and host as paramount. The later polemic between Metchnikoff and his German detractors may be viewed in large measure as a struggle with a newly emerging reductionism, where a positivistic attitude was rigidly invoked. We will see in chapter 6 how these different postures were expressed as Metchnikoff defended his phagocytosis theory.

Although by the late 1860s, Pasteur's demonstration of microbial fermentation and putrefaction were widely known and Joseph Lister's antiseptic techniques in surgery led practical credence to the bacterial origins of disease, the role of how specific microbes served as etiologic agents of contagious disease was not clearly established and led to controversy concerning the nature of the bacterial–host relationship (2, 15). In the late 1870s, the parasitic nature of the contagious diseases was still in dispute with conservative opposition led by Virchow, Bernard, and Theodor Billroth advising cautious restraint.

The case of Virchow is of particular interest because he later proved a staunch supporter of Metchnikoff's phagocytosis theory, giving the latter early encouragement and publishing his first phagocytosis papers (1884) (Metchnikoff's scientific relationship with Virchow is extensively discussed hereafter). Even by 1880, Virchow still confirmed that his sympathies lay with the catalytic theories of epidemic diseases promoted by Justus Liebig—as opposed to *contagium vivum* (16). According to E. H. Ackerknecht, this attitude probably resided in the dual intellectual leanings of the young Virchow: (a) his mechanistic interest in "pathological chemistry," which first won him recognition and (b) his antiontological bias: specific diseases were an anathema. Most germane, however, is the likely primary role of cellular pathology, which Virchow authored; in his construction, cellular pathology would view infectious agents only as secondary to primary constitutional or structural factors. In any case, between 1846 and 1860, Virchow published on fungi (coining the term *mycoses*), on several animal parasites (most notably *trichinae*), and he continued to publish micro-biological research of other researchers in his *Archives.* He was, thus, well versed in the field and understood the dynamics of contagious disease. His leadership in defin-ing the social parameters of epidemic diseases is an important part of his scientific heritage. Although as early as 1854, he had coined the expression *infectious diseases,* this actually comprised all forms of general toxic disease, and Virchow was reluctant to assign all contagious diseases to a microbial origin. As early as 1871, he noted that toxins, from bacteria or *other sources,* might be the causal agent of certain contagious diseases.

During the late 1870s and early 1880s, Virchow's opposition, in fact, seems to have largely been defensive. First, Edwin Klebs, a leader of the new school of bacteriology, vehemently attacked cellular pathology in 1878; by claiming that all cell processes were passive, Klebs abolished internal causes, confusing etiology of disease with dis-ease process, a point Virchow attempted to clarify (17). Klebs thus made disease depend exclusively on external factors (e.g., bacteria), and Virchow found himself then situated between that position and the position of Julius Cohnheim who argued that internal factors alone were causative (18)! (This debate is extensively discussed later.) Virchow's view was essentially that cellular pathology was not concerned with parasites per se because he made no claim for a general pathology. Cellular pathol-ogy, which he personified, only dealt with the behavior of body elements in basic forms of disease. Although the mycotic origin of a number of infectious diseases was shown, a general theory of infection—as promoted by Klebs—had not yet been pre-sented to Virchow's satisfaction. The vehemence of the debate is evident by Vir-chow's defense in 1877 of digestion as a chemical, as opposed to a bacteriological, process (16).

By the 1870s, the modern view of infectious diseases was widely accepted and Vir-chow embraced the achievements of bacteriology and lavished praise on Pasteur and Koch (16). The seminal point here, in regards to Virchow's sympathy to Metchni-koff, resides in the predominant interest in disease process: How does a pathogen cause disease? What are the dynamic factors between host and microorganism? What is the basis of immunity? In this sense, the didactic bacteriologists were positivists, ignoring the interrelationship of parasite and host and, thus, omitting the entire ques-tion that possessed Metchnikoff and drove his research, which like Virchow, revolved around the issue of disease process. By 1885, Virchow had formally embraced the phagocytosis theory; in defense of the theory of cellular pathology, he hailed Metch-nikoff's discoveries as crucial to the central issue of defining the fight of cells against parasitic microorganisms. Later, Virchow aligned himself with Metchnikoff against the humoralists, arguing that bactericidal sera were probably cell products (19). It is interesting to note how the microbiologists, at the earliest stage of their emerging reductionist position (first the bacteriologists led by Koch, later his allies who became humoral immunologists [discussed in chapter 7]), were ferociously pitted against an essentially descriptive, teleological orientation. The vehement rejection of Metchni-koff's phagocytosis theory by the German microbiologists extended to "character assassination" (20). The case offers a glimpse into the angry struggle between dispa-rate visions of biology—a recurrent theme we will have occasion to discuss more fully later.

The Status of Leukocytes in 1880

We must next briefly consider what was known concerning leukocyte function prior to Metchnikoff's phagocytosis theory. Metchnikoff's indebtedness to previous workers was detailed in his own work (21, 22) and has been reexamined many times (e.g., 23–27). Here we wish only to review the most crucial observations concerning the amoeboid white cell, which established the context of a new definition of inflammation. By the mid-nineteenth century, there was evidence that the inflammatory reaction was responsible for opposing noxious agents and expelling them, but this was not the general opinion; the role of the white cells in host defense and a novel description of the inflammatory process awaited Metchnikoff's synthesis.

The first observation that white cells might contain foreign particles was made by von Koelliker in 1847, who studied the spleen and noted cells containing particles. How this observation was related to splenic function was problematic and not pursued. Later Alexander Ecker (1847) confirmed von Koelliker's observation, but incorrectly concluded that the erythrocytes found within the macrophages were in a developmental phase as opposed to our current understanding that senescent erythrocytes are destroyed by the phagocytosing splenic reticuloendothelial system (28). In 1852, Virchow, observing the same phenomenon, added the notion that the erythrocytes resided in the larger cells, not as a result of active phagocytosis of the macrophage (a concept that had not yet been formulated), but by passive penetration owing to blood pressure (29). The ability of phagocytic cells to engulf particles is dependent on their mobile properties and elastic membrane. Wharton Jones is credited with first observing the similarities of leukocytes and amoebae in their contractile movements (30)—a finding confirmed by several later investigators. These observations inspired Haeckel to conduct similar investigations, from which he first concluded that elastic membranes of the cells followed, in a passive way, the content of the cells. But he later concluded that invertebrate leukocytes (and maybe those of vertebrates) did not have any membrane (31). The absence of a membrane from Haeckel's point of view, explained how these cells could passively accept particles of a solid substance. The issue then of foreign substances in mesodermal cells was first appreciated as an extension of their innate pliability and ultimate passiveness. A seminal observation was made by Haeckel in 1862 while studying the vessel system of *Thetis fimbia* (a seal mollusk); he injected indigo in water and a few hours later observed that the small vessels contained leukocytes filled with the dye particles. Repeating the experiment, he was able to watch the penetration process (32), but this research was not pursued further by Haeckel. What he misunderstood as a passive process was, in fact, active phagocytosis, which required recognition of the foreign substance and its containment. The leukocyte was first observed to undergo shape change and form projections, later called pseudopodia by Friedrich von Recklinghausen, in 1863 (33). When injecting noxious silver nitrate in the frog's peritoneal cavity, a massive inflammatory reaction resulted, and von Recklinghausen correctly described the elicited cells as particles of pus. With this background, Wilhelm Preyer in 1864, proposed that Virchow's observation (erythrocytes contained within splenic cells) was not, therefore, a passive occurence, but resulted from an active process, that is, splenic cells captured the particle (34).

By the middle of the 1860s, it was already broadly accepted by histologists that some cells of the body (both human and lower animals) have the capability of capturing foreign particles. This opinion was presented in texts by Heinrich Frey (35) and by Solomon Stricker (36), who used the term *fressen (devour)* to designate the process of capturing foreign particles by leukocytes. At last, in 1873, Alexander Kusnezoff succeeded in observing rabbit spleen leukocytes engulfing erythrocytes (37), formulating the first modern concept of erythrocyte senescence. Recall that von Koelliker (1867) considered the process as pathologic; what neither Kusnezoff nor von Koelliker recognized was that phagocytosis might represent a general property to deal with either senescent or abnormal host cells or to protect the host against invading microorganisms. Most investigators did not connect the observations with the notion of a defensive function of leukocytes. Klebs considered leukocytes as offering transportation of bacteria to the lymphatic tissue (38). Koch observed a large number of the bacilli in leukocytes of frogs that had been inoculated with anthrax bacilli, but he considered the pathophysiological role of leukocytes negatively (i.e., the cells served the bacilli as a suitable environment for multiplication and the means to disseminate to other organs (39). Thus, although histological research by the middle of the 1870s had established the capability of leukocytes to actively capture microorganisms, the general opinion did not connect leukocyte function with any defensive role against microorganisms, nor was there confidence that the process in question was truly active capture as opposed to a passive penetration of foreign particles into the cell.

Although there were a few exceptions from this general opinion, the countervailing view had negligible influence prior to Metchnikoff's seminal formulation. In 1901, Metchnikoff listed those who approximated similar views to his own (i.e., the protective functions of leukocytes) before 1883 (the year of his own discovery) and whose works became known to him only much later (22, pp. 514–519). In 1874, Peter Ludwig Panum in a paper on putrefactive poisons surmised that bacteria found in the blood are ingested by leukocytes (40); soon after, Paul Albert Grawitz noticed that mammalian leukocytes could seize fungi and thus might protect the host (41). Perhaps the fate of the hypothesis expressed by Wilhelm Roser, gives us the most impressive example of how insignificantly these notions were appreciated even by their respective authors and how little they may be considered as comparable with Metchnikoff's first immunological publications. Roser published his article in 1881, of which Metchnikoff wrote:

> It appears that not only did other biologists and medical men attach no importance to Roser's speculations, but that the author himself did not claim any great value for them. I draw this conclusion from the fact that five years after his first pamphlet he published a second on inflammation and healing in which he does not apply his theory of immunity to explain these two phenomena. (22, p. 516).

In addition to these predecessors of Metchnikoff's phagocytosis theory, there are two of whom Metchnikoff apparently was unaware. Robert Herrlinger (42) rediscovered a young German doctor, John Muellendorff, who in his doctoral dissertation "Ueber Ruckfallstyphus nach Beobachtungen im staedtischen Krankenhaus zu Dresden" (1879), had already described and correctly interpreted what Metchnikoff a few years later called phagocytosis; the dissertation was published in 1879 (43). Under the influence of observations made by Edwin Klebs, Ferdinand Cohn, Felix Victor Birch-Hirschfeld, and others, Muellendorff hypothesized that the parasites of recurrent typhus could be seized by white cells. If we are ready to reduce Metchnikoff's idea of phagocytosis to an intuitive conjecture that flashed across his mind in Messina, then it is difficult to recognize any principal difference between this guess and that of Muellendorff. But Muellendorff's hypothesis neither developed nor proposed a research program. The scientific tradition, to which he referred, had not elaborated any practical approach to investigate the functions and role of leukocytes. The only real attempts made by prior investigators concerned only one question: Do leukocytes purposefully ingest foreign particles or do the latter actively penetrate the cell? But to the extent that the question concerning the activity of leukocytes had been positively answered, the next question became self-evident: What is the significance of this activity for the host organism? In dealing with this issue none of the above-mentioned "cofounders" of the phagocytosis idea ever succeeded in presenting it as a scientific concept, that is, as a principle of organization of some research program. In sharp contrast, Metchnikoff approached the question of relevance from the perspective of studying intracellular digestion, in particular, and the role of mesodermal cells, in general. Because such a program did not exist for Metchnikoff's erstwhile competitors, their answers were by necessity limited to a speculative character. Indeed, there was disagreement as to whether leukocytes were detrimental or helpful to invading microorganisms.

The same issues arise with another competitor, an American military physician, George Miller Sternberg (24, 44). In 1881 he wrote:

> It has occurred to me that possibly the white corpuscles may have the office of picking up and digesting bacterial organisms which by any means find their way into the blood. The propensity exhibited by the leukocytes for picking up inorganic granules is well known, and that they may be able not only to pick up but to assimilate, and so dispose of, bacteria which come in their way does not seem to me very improbable in view of the fact that amoebae, which resemble them so closely, feed upon bacteria and similar organisms. (45, p. 175)

Several times Sternberg attempted to claim his scientific laurels (46). In *Immunity: Protective Inoculations in Infectious Diseases and Serum Therapy* (1895), Sternberg would remind the reader of his priority claim to the phagocytosis theory; as late as 1914, he would continue to present his case before the medical profession.

> I have no desire to detract from the credit due to Metchnikoff in connection with this theory, but in justice to myself desire to call attention to the fact that this theory was suggested by me several years before the publication of Metchnikoff's first paper on the subject. (47)

Jan Bibel concluded her comparison of Sternberg and Metchnikoff:

> As exemplified by this comparison, fame and success do not always come to those who are first. Effective communication and massive follow-up are equally significant. Even scientific ideas need to be marketed. As Sternberg himself would observe, the common use of the descriptive term phagocyte, like a trademark, focuses attention on Metchnikoff's work. (44)

We agree with Bibel that the word *phagocytosis* could play an important role in marketing Metchnikoff's theory. But we would argue that *phagocytosis* was not merely a descriptive term, but rather one that presented a highly complicated theoretical construct; the word *phagocyte* was successful not because it excited an idle curiosity, but because it reflects the origin of an idea: the problem of intracellular digestion. At the same time, it projects a new direction for immunological research. In order to realize this difference, it is enough to compare Metchnikoff's term *phagocytosis* and Muellendorff's term *Verzehrungs-prozess* (process of destruction). The latter is not a name of a real idea, but a descriptive term of an observed fact; as such, it reveals a vacancy. Metchnikoff erected an edifice of immunological theory around phagocytosis. The different intuitions that underly these two terms (*phagocytosis* and *"process of destruction"*) illustrate, perhaps in the best way, a conceptual difference between an abstract conjecture about the defensive function of leukocytes and the idea of phagocytosis. We lose the capacity to appreciate the difference only in the case of not acknowledging the theory as a developing conceptual problem, but take it as some final statement. Only in this limited sense can we say that Muellendorff or Sternberg expressed the same idea as Metchnikoff. In any case, Metchnikoff himself was reasonably modest in laying claim to priority:

> I need scarely say that in none of my publications have I laid claim to the discovery of the ingestion of solid bodies by mesodermic cells, nor have I ignored the large number of researches which have been made on this subject. . . . When [the phagocytosis theory] is once firmly established, it will be time enough to determine the exact part taken in its foundation by workers such as Panum, Gaule, Roser, etc. (21, p. 210)

Bibel concurs, "For Metchnikoff, the proof of experimentation and the progress of science would continue to outweigh the vanity of discovery of the origin of theory. He would argue for a concept rather than a claim" (44). But what does this posture reflect: simply a humane detail of Metchnikoff's personality or a radically different relation to the nature of the problem?

Metchnikoff's Biological Theory of Inflammation

The Cohnheim - Virchow Debate

Metchnikoff's lack of medical training has, in our opinion, misled even his closest associates (e.g., Alexander Besredka) to believe that his interest in pathology was a late development in his career and incidental to his zoological research.

> Until this moment [when Metchnikoff first formulated the idea of protective phagocytosis], Metchnikoff was preoccupied by questions of general biology. No pathological concept entered his mind. Suddenly, there was a complete, apparently inexplicable, reorientation.
>
> The zoologist, who so far found all his satisfaction in study of lower animals, lost all his interest in his subject and never took it up again. With his well-known passion, he turned to problems of pathology: first in animals, later in man (48, p. 9)

However, we will argue that a medical orientation was always essential to his intellectual life as well as central in forming his existential position. Olga Metchnikoff states that at age fifteen, as a student of the lycée and attending diverse lectures at Kharkov University, Metchnikoff met a young physiologist, Tschelkoff, who "consented to give him private lessons in histology." Olga continued:

> Then, fired with a passionate desire to produce something personal in medical science, and attracted by Virchow's cellular theory, [Metchnikoff] dreamt that he might create a general theory of his own in medicine. (49, p. 52)

(It is difficult to deny fate's fulfillment when we note that twenty-three years later, it was Rudolf Virchow who was among the first, by happenstance, to be in Messina and to applaud and encourage Metchnikoff's phagocytosis research (49, p. 519).) When Metchnikoff, two years later, enrolled at Kharkov University, he decided to study medicine,

> but his mother dissuaded him. "You are too sensitive", she said, "you could not bear the constant sight of human suffering." At the same time, Tschelkoff suggested the Natural Science Faculty as being more appropriate to purely scientific activity. Elie accepted his opinion and began to study physiology under his direction. (49, p. 41)

(Again, similar to the classical plot, the attempts to escape destiny led him directly to its fulfillment!) Although Metchnikoff did not become a pathologist by traditional medical training, research led him to establish a new concept of inflammation and the corresponding field of immunopathology. Escaping medicine for the sake of general biology, he was led back to pathology. Following his mother's advice, Metchnikoff avoided medicine and its encounter with human suffering, but he could not be shielded from his own melancholy, whose pessimism was applied to his theoretical musing on the fundamental biological disharmonies of human nature (i.e., his deep belief in life's imperfection and his pessimistic Weltanschauung). His suicide attempts are merely the most dramatic manifestations of these meditations. To complete the similarity with the scenerio of classic tragedy his theory of protective phagocytosis, born out of the highly emotion-laden musings on what he viewed as fundamental biological disharmonies, played the cathartic role, providing the example of self-harmonizing disharmony. As Metchnikoff himself understood, the delayed entry into medicine (pathology, then *orthobiosis*) initiated the tranquil and optimistic period of his life. This optimistic phase, of course, coincided with stabilization of his personal life, the presentation of the phagocytosis theory, and his final professional departure from Russia (50).

We have discussed in the chapters on Metchnikoff's embryological and evolutionary research, the reasons for his preoccupation with the problem of disharmony. But in medical reasoning of the nineteenth century, the opposition harmony/disharmony was much closer to the opposition health/disease than it is in the medical mentality of the twentieth century, which is reluctant to root its discussions in definitions of an organism's wholeness but prefers to speak in terms of particular normal and pathological mechanisms (51). Natural sciences of the first decades of the nineteenth century were still under the powerful influence of Romanticism, with its animation of the ancient approach to the human organism as microcosm (52). The influence of Romanticism and the idea of microcosm was explicitly tangible at least until the

1840s (53). Implicitly, for example, in the form of the human organism as evolution's highest perfection, the idea of microcosm dominated biology long after the 1840s. We saw that the idea influenced even Metchnikoff's writing on evolutionary problematics, although he rejected it explicitly. It is natural that in these assumptions, the opposition of harmony and disharmony was equated with the opposition of the healthy state and pathological processes, but not with the opposition of the norm and the pathologic. Metchnikoff's disharmony was pathologic, but it was at the same time the natural norm that in some cases might be transformed into another norm more favorable for the organism. Thus, we can say that his vision of general biology was fundamentally pathological: from Metchnikoff's point of view, there were no obvious reasons that would inevitably force evolution to provide harmonious ontogenetic development. Disharmony (hence, pathology) was for him a regular phenomenon of normal ontogeny. In this regard, it is possible to say that pathology formed the semantic horizon of his general biological thinking and structured his deepest existential experience. For many years, he was tormented by the thought that the more complex and sophisticated the creature, the more disharmonious and morbid; further, he believed that more complex organisms struggled with the more primitive (hence, more healthy) at a disadvantage.

The sudden, complete, and apparently inexplicable reorientation (which befuddled Besredka so completely) is in fact quite explicable (54). On the one hand, the phagocytosis hypothesis, which proposed a means to self-harmonizing disharmony, opened a new perspective in his vision of ontogenetic problematics and a new opportunity for solving those theoretical problems with which he was preoccupied for the preceding twenty years. On the other hand, the hope that he had found a mechanism of the organism's self-protection and self-harmonization, deprived his pessimistic Weltanschauung of what he considered as its most fundamental rational element. A new personal and intellectual optimism corresponds to the presentation of the phagocytosis theory.

Metchnikoff's transformation from zoologist to immunologist, from biologist to pathologist, is understood if we appreciate his pathological vision of general biology. But there is another reason, of a more general nature, that might contribute to our confusion. As we discussed, identification of the second primary layer as an embryological problem oriented Metchnikoff's interest to intracellular digestion; his morphological research acquired a physiological perspective, from which the phagocytosis theory was born. In this regard, we must acknowledge that physiology of the nineteenth century, to an essential degree, was still considered as a derivative of medicine. It has just begun to

> gradually emancipate itself from its intellectual and institutional roots in medicine. . . . Physiology itself was an ancient science and its students had often turned to animals (but, obviously, rarely to plants) for useful instruction in the workings of the human body. But physiology referred to the study of the functions of human body and was for the most part a matter of medical concern. (55, p. 3)

The general affinity of physiology and medicine in the nineteenth century, then is another factor in explaining Metchnikoff's conversion. However, the question remains: What did Metchnikoff know about the results and ideas of professional pathologists and, specifically, their approach to the problem of inflammation?

Our major clues to these questions rely on Metchnikoff's description in *Immunity in Infective Diseases:*

> I have never prosecuted any medical studies; but some time before my departure for Messina I listened to the reading of Cohnheim's treatise on *General Pathology,* and I was struck by his description of the facts and of his theory of inflammation. The former, especially his description of the diapedesis of the white corpuscles through the vessel wall, seemed to be of momentous interest. His theory, on the other hand, appeared to be extremely vague and nebulous. (22, p. 518)

Apparently, while in Messina, he also studied Ernst Ziegler's book.

> A perusal of Ziegler's treatise on *Pathological Anatomy* made it clear to me that in these branches of medical science there had long been accumulated a great number of observations fitted to facilitate the acception of the new hypothesis on inflammation and healing. Numerous and well-established facts on the absorption of extravasated blood, on the fate of the coloured corpuscles, etc., confirmed me in my view. (22, p. 519)

So, what facts and ideas pertaining to the phenomenon of inflammation did Metchnikoff find in Cohnheim's treatise?

Metchnikoff sojourned in Messina during 1883. Cohnheim published the first volume (containing the chapter on inflammation) of his *Lectures on General Pathology* in 1877 (56, pp. 191–306). The second edition of the *Lectures* was published in 1882 (the chapter on inflammation is in vol. 1, pp. 232–367). In regard to the issue of our concern, there are no significant differences in these two versions of Cohnheim's works. Hence, Metchnikoff's referral may be applied to either edition. Cohnheim's description of diapedesis was given in the context of discussing different anatomical transformations of vessels; it was here that he posed his central concern:

> It seems to me it would be nothing short of an insult to common sense were we to confine all possible alterations in the constitution of the vessel walls within these limits: were we, in other words, to pronounce all vessels to be healthy, normal, which are neither sclerosed nor fattily degenerated, nor in the amyloid condition. If it is impossible to judge from the appearance of an endothelial cell, or even of an entire capillary, whether it is living or dead, how, I ask, will you venture to decide from its optical characters alone whether the constitution of a vessel is normal? How can a microscopical examination exclude a possible chemical or physical, so to speak, *molecular* deviation from the normal. . . . [emphasis added] [Several examples are then discussed that Cohnheim believed demonstrated that] *the transition from intact physiological life to death is only in exceptional cases sudden, and is, as a rule, slow and gradual.* (56, p. 246, 1889)

Cohnheim concluded:

> These examples will, I think, explain the drift of my thoughts, for they show that alterations in the constitution of the vessel walls, for which the term *molecular* just now appears to be the most suitable designation, are called forth by a number of influences of the most different kinds. But if such alterations occur we are justified in asking—*what effect have they upon the circulation?* (56, p. 247, 1889)

In order to answer the question, Cohnheim conducted direct observations on veins and capillaries of the frog intestinal mesentery or on vessels of the papillary surface of the frog tongue after surgically removing the papillae. First, he observed a *dilatation,* which occured chiefly in the arteries and to a lesser extent in the veins, and least of all in the capillaries. Mesenteric dilatation was followed by a short acceleration of blood flow followed by retardation. Augmented blood flow was often absent in the tongue wound, and its retardation was associated with vessel dilatation. But the most interesting observation (according to Cohnheim) were changes seen in the veins:

> Slowly and gradually there is developed in them an extremely characteristic condition; *the originally plasmatic zone becomes filled with innumerable colourless corpuscles.* The plasmatic zone of the veins, you will remember, is always occupied by scattered colourless blood-corpuscles, which, owing to their globular form and low specific gravity, are driven into the periphery of the stream, and whose adhesiveness makes it difficult for them to escape from the wall once they have come into contact with it. (56, p. 249, 1889)

The retardation of the bloodstream apparently contributes to the accumulation of large numbers of colorless corpuscles in the peripheral zone "and here [they] become *comparatively* motionless" (56, p. 249, 1889). Although not a state of absolute rest,

> this does not lessen the striking contrast presented by the central column of red blood-corpuscles, flowing on in an uninterrupted stream of uniform velocity, and the peripheral layer of resting colourless cells; the internal surface of the vein appears paved with a single but unbroken layer of colourless corpuscles without the interposition at any time of a single red one. It is the separation of the white from the red corpuscles that gives the venous stream in these cases that characteristic appearance, anything analogous to which you will look for in vain in the other vessels. (56, p. 249, 1889)

And here Cohnheim begins that description of diapedesis that apparently so profoundly impressed Metchnikoff. After describing his findings in the capillaries and arteries (presenting many additional details) Cohnheim noted that these vessels did not exhibit the same (dramatic) separation of the red and colorless corpuscles:

> But the eye of the observer hardly has time to catch all the details of the picture before it is fettered by a very unexpected occurrence. Usually it is a vein with the typical peripheral arrangement of the white corpuscles, but sometimes a capillary, first displays the phenomenon. A pointed projection is seen on the external contour of the vessel wall; it pushes itself further outwards, increases in thickness, and the pointed projection is transformed into a colourless rounded hump; this grows longer and thicker, throws out fresh points, and gradually withdraws itself from the vessel wall, with which at last it is connected only by a long thin pedicle. Finally this also detaches itself, and now there lies outside the vessel a colourless, faintly glittering, contractile corpuscle with a few short processes and one long one, of the size of a white blood-cell, and having one or more nuclei, in a word, a *colourless blood-corpuscle.* (56, p. 250, 1889)

This diapedic event takes place simultaneously in different portions of the veins and capillaries. A large number of the colorless corpuscles emigrate to the exterior of the vessels and their place in the peripheral layer of the vessels is immediately occupied by others. This phenomenon may develop (after the vessel is exposed to air) with different velocities.

At one time the earliest *emigration* very quickly succeeds the pavementing; at another an hour or more may pass without anything happening to draw attention to the contour of a single vein or capillary. In any case the final result, after six or eight or more hours have elapsed, will be the enclosure of all the veins, small and large, of mesentery or wound of the tongue with several layers of colourless blood-corpuscles. These fence in the veins, in the interior of which the previously described conditions continue, namely, the peripheral arrangement of the colourless cells and the central unbroken flow of red blood-corpuscles. (56, pp. 250–251, 1889)

Arteries exhibit no such analogous phenomenon, whereas capillaries, which have both red and white corpuscles in contact with the vessel wall allow both cell types to emigrate. Thus, whether white or red corpuscles pass out of the vessel lumen "depends solely on the numerical relations of the cells accumulated in its [blood vessel] interior" (56, p. 251, 1889).

Keeping pace with this *exodus, emigration,* or, as it is also called, *extravasation* of corpuscular elements there occurs an increased transudation of fluid, in consequence of which the meshes of mesentery, or the tissue of the tongue, are infiltrated and swell. But this is not all. The extravasated colourless corpuscles distribute themselves, in proportion as their numbers increase, over a larger area, forsaking the neighbourhood of the vessels from which they were derived. The tissues become more and more densely packed with them, while the red cells, which have not the power of independent locomotion, remain seated in the vicinity of their capillaries, yet these also may be carried off by the stream of transudation. Soon a moment must arrive when the products of exudation and transudation can no longer be accomulated in the tissue. They now gain the free surface of the mesentery, and should the transuded fluid coagulate, as is the rule here, the final result of the processes just described will *be the deposition on the mesentery,* as well as on the intestine, *of a fibrinous pseudomembrane, densely packed with colourless blood-corpuscles, and interspersed with isolated red cells.* (56, p. 251, 1889)

The same appearances were observed after painting the smooth surface of the frog's tongue with croton oil (56, pp. 251–253, 1889).

We will discuss later how Cohnheim's views in regard to the possible interpretation of the leukocytes' mobility as spontaneous changed between 1867 and 1877. However, it is already obvious that this description of diapedesis in no way claims to define the essence of inflammation. Cohnheim organized the whole exposition of his observations in such a way that the reader's attention is drawn not to the possible spontaneity of leukocyte mobility, but to hypothetical "molecular" vessel changes in the vessel walls. Apparently, he did not want the idea of leukocyte spontaneity to shadow the idea of the molecular vessel changes that determined, from his point of view, the essence of inflammation. Starting with speculations about the gradual transition from life to death, Cohnheim inferred that there must be such stages of transition that are not observable optically and that could be detected only through secondary effects. Thus, his observations of diapedesis are embedded in the semantic context determined by this speculatively born question:

If such alterations [the molecular alterations in the vessel walls] occur we are justified in asking—*what effect have they upon the circulation?* (56, p. 247, 1889)

It seems that in this particular case, Cohnheim exposed his hand. Noting that the tissues surrounding the vessels became increasingly packed with the colorless corpuscles, he observed:

The red cells, which have not *the power of independent locomotion* [emphasis added] (*waehrend die rothen, denen die Faehigkeit der selbststaendigen Locomotion fehlt* [56, p. 199, 1877]), remain seated in the vicinity of their capillaries, yet these also may be carried off by the stream of transudation. (56, p. 251, 1889)

We will see further that Cohnheim explicitly denied the idea of leukocyte spontaneous mobility. However, he does not propose here any explanation for the expression, "the power of independent locomotion." Did he truly intend to assign the white cell a power the red cell did not possess? Or perhaps he simply meant that the white cells are more easily carried (i.e., passively) by the transudation stream than the red cells and that "the power of independent locomotion" then refers to nothing more than absence of resistance. In this case, power is nothing but a metaphor for the hypothetical assumption that the white cells are passively carried, and Cohnheim's observations appear to favor that assumption. As we noted, he placed special emphasis on the correspondence between cell adherence to the vessel wall and subsequent emigration, concluding that diapedesis was not a function of a spontaneous mobility of white corpuscles, but resulted from plasma transudation owing to some molecular alteration in the vessel wall.

Serious studies of the microvascular features associated with the inflammatory process date from the end of the eighteenth century. Rather states:

[already] by 1832 C. F. Koch could write an extensive review of the findings harvested by these microscopists, all of whom worked with the living blood-vessels of frogs, salamanders, fish, rabbits and other small animals. In Koch's review almost every finding—with one exception—now regarded as part of the inflammatory vascular reaction is described, in spite of the fact that most of the work antedated the introduction of corrected lenses. This one exception was the passage, during the course of the inflammatory process, of white blood corpuscles through the intact walls of small vessels into the extravascular tissues. (23, pp. 6–7)

We will postpone discussion of this last issue and note here that in 1877 there was no difficulty for Cohnheim to identify the vascular changes as corresponding to the phenomenon of inflammation, providing that the term designated the famous complex of symptoms, *rubor, tumor, dolor, calor:*

The sum total of these events, together with their consequences, have been for ages comprised under the notion and name of *inflammation.*

On calling to mind the signs which make their appearance in a part of the body, in which the circulation and transudation has undergone the disturbances so often described, we find they are as follows. Such a part will be (1) *reddened,* owing to the overloading of all its vessels; this condition being complicated in severe forms with small, but numerous, haemorrhages. It will be (2) *swollen,* because of the increased vascular fullness, but especially because of the great increase of transudation. (3) It will be *painful,* owing to the pressure on, and dragging of, the nerves of sensation by the overfilled vessels and abundant transudation. (4) It will, if situated superficially, be *warmer* to the touch, because a more than normal amount of heat is supplied to it from within by the increased supply of blood. Lastly, (5) its function will be *deranged,* both by reason of the pressure to which the terminations of the motor and secretory nerves are subject from the transudation, and the so essentially altered blood-circulation, in particular the retardation of the capillary stream. Now these five symptoms are nothing more or less than *the cardinal symptoms of acute inflammation,* of which the first four—the fifth, the *functio laesa,* is in reality less symptom than a resulting condition—had been already established by Celsus: and, despite the advance made in our knowledge of the processes, still serve best to characterize the condition of an inflamed part. (56, pp. 261–262, 1889)

What does this microvascular picture of inflammation add to the understanding of inflammation? Despite agreement as to which phenomenon was designated as inflammation (namely, what was described for centuries as the complex—*rubor, tumor, dolor, calor*), there was still no generally accepted consensus concerning the nature of the phenomenon.

For Cohnheim, the explicatory basis of inflammation was the central issue of all medical systems:

> Indeed, one is perhaps justified in saying that it is the interpretation of inflammation which has formed the starting-point and goal of all the systems and schools of medicine that have, in the course of centuries, succeeded one another. (56, p. 281, 1889)

Only a few of these theories, as Cohnheim stated, "have been able to maintain a footing up to our time" (56, p. 281, 1889), of which he believed the most prominent was the so-called *neurohumoral* theory; the central thesis was that the circulatory disturbances lead to hyperemia and the retardation of the bloodstream. There were two forms of the neurohumoral theory, an *ischemic* and a *paralytic* version. According to the ischemic theory (here Cohnheim refers to the works of Gottfried Eisenmann, Joseph Heine, Ernst Bruecke), the excitation of sensory nerves reflexively calls forth the contraction of the afferent arteries, which leads to circulatory disturbance, in particular to the slowing of the capillary stream. According to the paralytic theory (here Cohnheim refers primarily to the works of Jacob Henle [57]), a reflex initiates relaxation and dilatation of the arteries with resultant inflammatory hyperemia. From Cohnheim's point of view, both versions of the neurohumoral theory were wrong. He objected on the basis that when an irritant was applied the arteries might undergo contraction, dilatation, or contraction followed by dilatation. But

> *with inflammation, however, these phenomena have nothing to do,* for it can be shown in the most positive manner that they may be present without subsequent inflammation, and—what is still more decisive—that inflammation very often sets in the absence of these antecedents. (56, p. 282, 1889)

Cohnheim presented Virchow's cellular theory of inflammation (58) as a popular alternative to the neurohumoral school:

> According to it, the events connected with the vessels are far from being the main element in inflammation. They occupy only a subordinate place, and are to be regarded as secondary; while the genuine central point of the entire process must be sought in the *tissue-cells* of the affected part. These are supposed to swell and enlarge on exposure to the inflammatory irritant, and then to give birth to new cells, the pus-corpuscles. The necessary material is of course abstracted from the increased stream of transudation, which itself is explained by a sort of *attractive influence,* supposed to be exerted by the tissue-cells on the vessels, or their contents. The cells which the irritant had caused to enlarge induce the neighboring vessels to dilate, and to allow an increased transudation. (56, pp. 285–286, 1889)

This "attractive influence" forms, from Cohnheim's point of view, the weak point of the theory.

> This theory . . . introduces into physiology a principle discovered *ad hoc,* and having
> no analogy elsewhere—that of *an attraction of the tissues or tissue-cells on the vessels
> and their contents.* (56, p. 286, 1889)

As we have already mentioned, presence of both white and red cells in the inflammatory site was for Cohnheim a result of the transudation stream that, in its turn,
he considered as resulting from the molecular change of the vessel wall. Ironically,
the molecular changes he proposed were purely hypothetical, but apparently fulfilled
his criteria for the scientific and mechanical requirements of a model. Hence, the
absence of a physical analogy placed Virchow's assumption in a compromised
position.

> An attractive influence of this kind could at most relate only to fluids, in the case of
> which we are acquainted with certain analogies in the phenomena of diffusion. But
> how the tissue-cells are set about enticing the colourless or red corpuscles out of the
> vessels, passes, as I told you, at least my comprehension. (56, p. 286, 1889)

This last argument not only carried a physical ornament, but is also essentially retrospective. Virchow's paper, "Cellular Pathology," in which his new doctrine was
stated for the first time, was published in 1855 (59), and the first edition of his book,
carrying a similar title, appeared in 1858 (60). His pupil, Cohnheim, published (in
Virchows Archives) his observations of diapedesis only in 1867; these were in apparent contradiction with Virchow's theory (61). Hence, at the time of its formulation,
Virchow's theory did not introduce the "attractive influence" (at least in relation
to the blood corpuscles) as an *ad hoc* proposition. The real defect of the theory was
not the emphasis on this hypothetical attractive activity of the inflammatory cells
(whose activity was alledgedly more speculative then Cohnheim's own assumption
of molecular changes), but the disparity between the theory's predictions and
Cohnheim's direct observations of diapedesis. From this point of view, Cohnheim's
accusation of Virchow's theory as an *ad hoc* assumption might be interpreted as
an attempt to protect himself from similar accusations—in fact, these would have
been justified!

In any case, Cohnheim stated, no one including Virchow could now argue the
cellular theory in its pure and unadulterated form and deny the independence of
intravascular events. On the other hand, no one should doubt that "the processes
connected with the vessels are sufficient to bring about the aggregate phenomena
characteristic of inflammation" (56, p. 287, 1889). Cohnheim concluded:

> This being the state of affairs, the only question that can be debated at present is
> whether, side by side with the circulatory disturbances, Virchow's so-called nutritive
> and formative changes of the tissue-cells at all occur in inflammation, and in partic-
> ular *whether by means of these changes exudation—or pus—corpuscles, arise.* (56,
> p. 287, 1889)

Of course, Cohnheim continued, as "living beings with a metabolism," the cells of
the inflammatory site cannot be but affected and altered by inflammation, for example, the disorganization and degeneration observed in an inflammatory locus. But
the question is whether or not those changes, which Virchow called progressive, and
which lead to formation of new cells (pus corpuscles), in fact do occur.

An assumption of this kind was not merely permissible, but even enjoined, at a time when the capacity of the pus-corpuscles for locomotion, and especially their emigration, was still unknown. Nothing then appeared more natural than that the pus-cells found anywhere should be the descendants of the tissue-cells of locality. Since an acquaintance with cell extravasation has become common property, this assumption is no longer necessary, for we now know that prodigious quantities of colourless cells can be furnished by the vessels of an inflamed area. Under these circumstances the question whether, in addition to these, a certain number of pus-corpuscles are produced by the tissue-cells, is as regards the inflammation itself, of really subordinate importance. (56, pp. 288–289, 1889)

Until the 1870s, Cohnheim continued, pus corpuscles, being seen among epithelial or other cells, were assumed to have arisen *endogenously* because of the division of the surrounding cells. Since then, improved histological methods permitted finer recognition of cells, and it was established that pus corpuscles could wander through tissues into every part of the organism. Thus Cohnheim could write:

We accept the *new formation* of a pus-corpuscle as demonstrated, only where we have seen it take place directly under our eyes, or where—and this appears the utmost concession we can make—strict proof can be offered that the pus-corpuscle in question cannot have traveled from some other place. *No one has so far succeeded in observing the formation of a pus-corpuscle. . . . Moreover the second mode of proof has not so far been attended with success* [emphasis added]. (56, pp. 289–290, 1889)

It is interesting to compare this opinion with Virchow's, as expressed in his *Cellular Pathology* of 1858 (60). Referring to William Addison and Gustav Zimmerman's equation of white blood cells and pus corpuscles, Virchow asserted that they had "imagined they had found colorless blood corpuscles when they were really looking upon pus" (60, p. 527, 1971). And he continued that to distinguish between a colorless blood corpuscle and a pus corpuscle "there is no other criterion than to determine whether the cell arose at a spot where a colorless blood corpuscle might be expected to arise, or at one where it ought not be produced" (60, p. 527, 1971). It might appear as if the difference between Virchow and Cohnheim's views simply corresponded to two successive stages in the directly observed data. Virchow's position seemingly compensates with forced (but cautious) speculations for lack of supportive data as well as reflecting on the restrictions imposed by insufficiently developed methodologies to address the question more directly. (Virchow must surmise whether or not a colorless blood corpuscle might be *expected* to arise at a given locus.) Meanwhile, Cohnheim's position—argued from accumulated data acquired through direct observations over the ensuing two decades—appeals first to the facts that *established* how the colorless blood corpuscles can wander into every part of the body and then to the fact that the new formation of pus corpuscle had not been observed. There can be no doubt that this disagreement, in an essential degree, was conditioned by objective scientific progress, but there were other implicit philosophical differences between Virchow and Cohnheim.

Metaphysical Considerations

Although there is no evidence that Metchnikoff was ever consciously interested in the metaphysical assumptions that had influenced the inflammation theories of his immediate predecessors, in order to appreciate the novelty of Metchnikoff's position in the field we must explore this area. Virchow's dependence on the traditional speculative tropes of *naturphilosophie* and romantic medicine has been admirably demonstrated by Walter Pagel (62). The so-called naturalistic school of medicine, which Virchow closely followed, was a late branch of Romantic medicine, which in its turn, was conceptually structured by *naturphilosophie*. In this school, disease or the pathological was determined by a specific interpretation of the organism concept and the relation between organisms and their environment. From the *naturphilosophie* point of view (i.e., Dieterich Georg Kieser, "Novalis" (Friedrich von Hardenburg), Lorenz Oken, Johann Reil, Johann Wilhelm Ritter, Friedrich Wilhelm Joseph Schelling, Ignaz Paul Vitalis Troxler), the nature of the relationship "organism/external world" is ambivalent. The organism in order to support its integrity must keep its independence and spontaneity, but being a finite entity, it cannot exist independently and must sustain certain relationships with the external world. The ambivalence was designated by the naturphilosophers as *polarity*. The striving to the first pole presents the "egoistic," or "positive," tendency of life, and the striving to the second pole determined the "cosmic," or "negative" tendency (63). The egoistic, which sustains self-equality of a given living form, leads to annihilation of the other forms relating to the organism. The cosmic tendency leads to participation in the life of the external world; the extreme of the tendency, death, is a transformation into other forms of existence. Life is this struggle between life and death: the final victory of the cosmic tendency is death. There must be an intermediate stage between life and death, which is fulfilled by disease.

Perhaps more than direct observations, this philosophical speculation structured Virchow's basic belief (64): pathological processes and physiological processes are identical in essence.

> However much I herein differ from many of my living contemporaries, however positively the peculiar (specific) nature of many pathological tissues has been insisted upon during the last few years, I will nevertheless endeavour in the course of these lectures to furnish you with proofs that every pathological structure has a physiological prototype, and that no form of morbid growth arises which cannot in its elements be traced back to some model which had previously maintained an independent existence in the economy. (60, pp. 88–89, 1971)

And further, when discussing diversity of neoplasms, Virchow directly pointed at *naturphilosophie* as the source of his belief in a physiological paradigm for every such pathological form:

> Many attempts had indeed been made even before this to refer the apparently so irregular forms of new formations to physiological paradigms, and herein essential service has been rendered by natural philosophers. (60, pp. 89–90, 1971)

Thus, disease is different from the healthy state not in essence, but only in respect to quantitative characteristics of certain phenomena as well as their location and time order. On the other hand, the essential equality of physiological and pathological processes is just another expression of the fact that the cosmic, or negative tendency, being considered in relation to organismic integrity, is nothing but deviation from the positive or egoistic pole—the deviations being always complementary to the positive (self-sustaining) tendency (i.e., the tendency that continuously restores the positive pole—organismic self-equality). That is why, in this perspective, any patholog-ical process is thought to be complementary through the efforts of the "healing power of Nature."

It is apparent that the idea of healing power is quite different from Metchnikoff's future idea of immunity. The former does not imply, as does the latter, that the heal-ing power is exercised by a special subsystem in order to restore integrity of the organ-ism. On the contrary, it implies that the integrity, as an essence underlying particular physiological processes, acts on behalf of the processes. After Metchnikoff, the immune idea argues for a special activity (a subsystem) of the whole that performs the functions of a personal physician in respect to the whole. The normal activity of this special part takes place when the normal (the integrity) is violated. Quite oppo-site to that, the healing power of Nature is nothing else but the expression of the whole on behalf of its parts (in order to prevent their extreme deviation under the influence of cosmic tendency). Using the same analogy, the whole is the physician of its own parts. It was also an expression of the teleomechanistic program with which Virchow found close affinity (65). This school, which included von Baer, Johannes Peter Mueller, Liebig, and Schwann, opposed the Romanticism of *naturphilosophie,* but structured its scientific approach under the same guiding principle of the domi-nance of the whole over the constituent parts. (Von Baer's *Bauplan,* the universal form, is one such manifestation of the teleomechanistic school.) In this respect the Romantic interpretation of the healing power is no different from that of Galen, for whom the restoring forces of organism and the forces supporting health are identical (66).

Pagel further illustrates how Virchow's localistic medicine is connected (through the philosophy and medicine of Ferdinand Jahn) with this understanding of the heal-ing power. It is from this philosophy that Jahn came to a conclusion that proved crucial for Virchow, namely, the assertion that the ability of the whole to sustain its wholeness is the ability to restore the parts (67). One possible conclusion is that the wholeness must be intact to have the capability of curing injuries in the parts. If the whole is damaged only partially, this seemingly means that not its wholeness has been damaged, but just a part; on the other hand, the damage of the wholeness means nothing else but that the organism has ceased as organism, that is, such damage means death.

> If disease is an expression of the struggle of the individual against annihilation, it cannot involve the whole body at once which would make such struggle impossible as it is incompatible with life. Hence disease must of necessity begin as a local affair. (62, p.14)

Another possible conclusion from this philosophy is the notion of the relative inde-pendence of each organ and even each "fibre." Every such unit is, in this perspective, a "relative totality." Disease, as local aggression, separates the totality of the organ-ism from the "relative totality," and thus "doubles life" in the body or "breaks life in itself." Pagel concluded:

> The two concepts of disease-location and the cellular theory of disease seem to emerge in Virchow's work as the product of *empirical* research. In reality they are part and parcel of a *philosophy.* (62, p. 17)

Pagel also demonstrated (67, pp. 17–25) that the fundamental direction of young Virchow's research was determined not by the concept of cellular physiology and pathology, but by the tendency to localize disease and by the opposition to the particular wholistic ideology of humoralism and constitutionalism. This tendency, Pagel continues, conditioned Virchow's belief that "it is the formation of a local blastema and not the emigration of cells through the vascular wall which accounts for cellular proliferation or pus" (62, p. 15). The very idea of cellular pathology was predetermined by the search for ultimate units as the centers of life's functions in health and disease (68).

Thus, there were certain philosophical positions that forced Virchow to view cells as relatively sovereign entities—the seats of the basic functions of life in health and disease. Does this then mean that Virchow shared Metchnikoff's concept of organism as a multiplicity of sovereign, interacting centers whose harmonious coordination was viewed not as something provided, but rather as one of several possible evolutionary and ontogenetic outcomes? Emphatically not. The idea of relatively independent units of organism was always in good agreement with the idea of preestablished harmony. In this respect, Virchow's ideas could be traced back at least to the philosophy of Gottfried Leibniz, who asserted that the sovereignty of the final units of reality (the monads) required a preestablished harmony. Virchow wrote:

> There is no reason to fear that our many vital units will let us lose the unity of the living organism. It is true that we are unable to demonstrate it in the sense of Neuro-Pathology. The Spiritus rector is missing, it is a free state of single beings equal in right, though not equal in endowment, a state which keeps together, because the individuals depend upon each other and there are certain centres of organization, the integrity of which ensures the necessary nutritive material reaching the individual parts. (59; Pagel's trans. [62], p. 20)

Romantic as well as the Naturalistic schools of medicine structured their nosological systems in accordance with the ancient idea of three levels of organization: the system of "vegetative life," the system of "animal life," and the system of "sensitive life." Virchow's adherence to the same tradition can be seen in his classification of the elementary pathological processes as "formative," "nutritive," and "functional" disorders. These disorders correspond to the three main aspects of cellular activity that, in their turn, are nothing else but the relics of the classification proposed by the Naturalist school: the vegetative life as devoted to plastic reproduction and secretory production, the animal life as devoted to the distribution of blood and "irritability," and sensitive life as presented by nervous activity (60). We saw that Metchnikoff also willingly used the opposition of the organs' system of the vegetative life versus the organs' system of the animal life. Again, it may appear as if there is an essential similarity between the philosophical ideas underlying Metchnikoff's biology and pathology with those of Virchow's and his Romantic predecessors. But although, for Metchnikoff, the very fact of coexistence of these systems creates organismic disharmony, it is obvious that for Virchow and his predecessors disharmony might arise in the relations of systems or in their respective functions, but coexistence of the systems as such express a coordinated unity rather than a given organismic disharmony (69). Thus, Virchow's idea of the sovereignty of cells in no way excluded the idea of the preestablished harmonized unity of the organism. On the other hand, Metchnikoff's use of the same notion, which pertains to the ancient traditional description of organismic integrity, does not mean that the approaches of Metchnikoff and his predecessors to the problem of integrity were essentially similar (70).

Roux Versus Metchnikoff

In 1881, Wilhelm Roux published *Der Kampf der Theile im Organismus* [*The Struggle of Parts in the Organism*] (71). The goal of the book, as Roux proclaimed, was to explain organismic expediency *(die Zweckmaessigkeit)* not as something "deliberate but as becoming, as arising not teleologically but in a natural-historical, mechanical way" (71, p. 2). Roux saw the theoretical basis of his undertaking in Darwinism.

> As it is known, Ch[arles] Darwin and A[lfred] Wallace discovered not just the new principle of the struggle as the cause for the mechanical becoming of expediency, but they demonstrated also that this kind of struggle must take place as a result of organism's multiplication in geometrical progression, and that further, as a result of the continuous variations of the organism in all its parts, there are possibilities of changes for the better. (71, p. 3)

Roux explicitly acknowledges that it is Virchow's idea that permits him to apply Darwinism to the problem of individual development. The theme of the second chapter, which has the same title as the entire book, *Der Kampf der Theile im Organismus,* is posed by the words, "It is almost thirty years since Virchow has pointed to the sovereignty of cells (71, p. 65). It is interesting that in 1892 Metchnikoff published (in Russian) an essay under almost an identical title—"The Struggle for the Existence of Parts of the Animal Organism" (72)—in which he expounds his favorite topic, the inherited disharmonies of organisms. Despite not having found in any of Metchnikoff's writings a direct reference to Roux's book, it is likely that Metchnikoff knew of it. Roux's work was well known, and its topic—individual development in perspective of the selection theory—was (in the 1870s and the early 1880s) Metchnikoff's principal theoretical concern. Because Roux was among the most prominent students of Haeckel (with whom Metchnikoff was in bitter debate since the mid 1870s), it is likely that Metchnikoff was aware of Roux's views. Finally, the similarity of the titles is an unlikely accident. But the shared titles hardly reflect an essential agreement of opinions on the problem of organismic integrity. Metchnikoff's view of disharmonies and Roux's teaching concerning the struggle between parts of the organism had a different philosophical relationship to Virchow's theory. Metchnikoff's originality is well illustrated by these differences.

We argued in the preceding chapter concerning Metchnikoff's evolutionary opinions that, as in the case of many morphologists of his time (who in their discussion of evolutionary issues were interested not in adaptive variations of given structures, but rather in evolutionary realization of the processes that led to formation of the structure), Metchnikoff's vision of variability was much more saltative than Darwin's vision of the phenomenon (73, pp. 137–142, 1950). Contrary to Darwin, he believed that crossbreeding would not allow for preservation of small variations (73, pp. 139, 191, 1950). He supported Fleeming Jenkin (73, p. 182, 1950) and asserted:

In order to be able to start to act, it is not sufficient for natural selection to have merely individual deviations; it is necessary to have a certain sum of individuals who have changed in advance in a similar way. (73, p. 183, 1950)

Correspondingly, Metchnikoff believed that the most important and bitter forms of struggle occurred between species or between a species and its abiotic environment (73, p. 146, 1950). There is nothing original in this position, which is quite similar to that held by Koelliker, Naegeli, Askenasy, Mivart (all of whom are analyzed at length in the "Essay on the Question Concerning the Origin of Species" [73]). The source of Metchnikoff's originality (as we have striven to demonstrate) is his reinterpretation of the recapitulation idea. From his point of view, recapitulations do not provide a clear-cut parallel between ontogeny and phylogeny, but rather to ontogenetic coexistence of different integrities pertaining to different stages of phylogeny. This coexistence creates the basic disharmony of individual development, and this disharmonic relationship Metchnikoff designated as the struggle between the organism's components. No semblance of this concept is encountered in Roux. The central thought of *Der Kampf* is orthodox Darwinism: struggle originates in individual variations. Darwin was seemingly indebted, when he referred to the work as "the most important book on development that has appeared for some time" (74). However, the metaphysical basis of Roux's book is formed by the trivial assumption that there are no two entities that would be equal in every respect. The basis of the struggle between the organism's parts is the principal inequality of those constituents (the molecules, the cells, the organs) (71, p. 69). The relationships between unequal components then turns into struggle when the inequality pertains to vital aspects of an organism's life (71, p. 67). Roux was apparently comfortable that having intended to explain what is vital to the organism in terms of struggle, he then offered an explanation of struggle in defining vitality. It is not surprising because, as Wilhelm Roux frequently cites in *Der Kampf,* he followed Heraclitus in interpreting the concept of struggle ("The struggle is the father of everything"), and he believed that Darwin and Wallace simply continued in the same metaphysical tradition (71, p. 65). Thus, in spite of the "new mechanical, nature-historical" approach proclaimed by Roux, he professed an ancient metaphysical vision of the organism's integrity. However original was Heraclitus semimythological exposition of the concept of "struggle", it was, after all, quite typical of the classical understanding of disharmonies (or tensions between oppositions [75]): the very fact of disharmonies manifested the underlying cosmic unity. In this context, it is important that Metchnikoff frequently stressed the radical difference between his own understanding of organismic integrity and that of the ancient Greeks (76, pp. 1–16, 166–199).

We will show that to some extent, Metchnikoff's theory of inflammation may be considered as having adopted certain features of both Virchow and Cohnheim's respective theories, but here two points must be stressed. First, both Metchnikoff's metaphysical and scientific vision of organismic integrity, which constituted the background of his theory of inflammation, was radically different not only from Virchow's original theory, but even from the later Darwinian reinterpretations. Second, in order to understand Cohnheim's hidden polemic with Virchow, we have to keep in mind that the conflicting ideas reflected not just results of pure empirical observations, but they had been structured by a strongly emergent reductionist orientation embedded (this may appear paradoxical) in the old holistic idea of organism. In this case, consciously or not, Cohnheim's opposition to Virchow's ideas carried a certain metaphysical potential. Where then does Metchnikoff fit in the confusing currents of biological theory to which Virchow and Cohnheim represent opposite poles?

Metchnikoff's Conceptual Novelty

There is no doubt that Cohnheim's work had a strong experimental orientation, but the difference between his theory of inflammation and that of Virchow cannot be reduced to an empirical versus a speculative approach, respectively. As Russell C. Maulitz argues:

> It is not sufficient, however, to "explain" Cohnheim's arrival at his new notion of inflammation solely in terms of the techniques, experimental apparatus, and tissue preparations available to him. These technical features, after all, had been available by and large to von Recklinghausen as well. The idea stated by most historians of pathology, that Cohnheim was the most experimentally oriented pathologist among Virchow's immediate successors, is of some help [77, p. 51]. But even this is not quite the missing link in the explanation, since others indulged in experiment with less innovative theoretical results. (78, p. 178)

It is true that Virchow's assistant, Friedrich von Recklinghausen (whose vacated position in Virchow's Berlin Pathological Institute was filled by Cohnheim), had already approximated Cohnheim's future conclusions in 1863. As Rather noted (23, p. 156), von Recklinghausen's predecessors (Wharton Jones, Casimir-Joseph Davaine, George Buck, T. H. Huxley, Johann Lieberkuehn) described the movements of the colorless corpuscles in blood as contractile rather than locomotive. In 1863, von Recklinghausen described (33) locomotive movements of pus corpuscles and certain cells of connective tissue. These movements allowed these corpuscles and cells to travel relatively large distances. Working from 1858 to 1864 as Virchow's assistant, von Recklinghausen could not have been unaware that this result somewhat contradicted Virchow's theory, which demanded that only local cells at the inflammatory site gave rise to pus. But von Recklinghausen did not present an alternative (i.e., nonlocal) origin for pus cells and avoided research in this area. Rather writes:

> The reader may perhaps wonder why von Recklinghausen, after having shown that colourless lymph corpuscles tagged with vermilion dye migrated into bits of corneal tissue suspended in the lymph sacs of frogs, after having identified lymph, pus and white blood corpuscles on grounds of both appearance and behaviour, and after having expressed doubts as to the origin of pus corpuscles at inflammatory sites, did not take the obvious next step, namely, to tag the amoeboid cells of blood and lymph and then induce corneal inflammation in the same animal. If the tagged cells then made their way to the inflamed corneal tissue, the obvious inference could have been drawn. (23, p. 159)

Why von Recklinghausen was unwilling to proceed in this direction is unclear:

> Perhaps the step was not as obvious as it appears in retrospect. Or von Recklinghausen may have felt that he had already come close to treading on the toes of his master. In any case his interest lay not in the subject of inflammation but in the existence of the tissues and fluids of animal bodies, up and down the scale of life, of a widely distributed group of cells sharing the common property of mobility, the "wandering" cells, as they came to be called. (23, p. 159)

Rather believes that von Recklingausen's failure was due to psychological factors, that is, the next step could have been taken without essential reconstruction of the basic intellectual framework, but was prevented by an unwillingness to precipitate a personal disagreement with the master as well as by a reluctance to proceed with a topic—inflammation—that was not one of his own primary interests. Maulitz reconstructs the case and indicates that the failure was due primarily to von Recklinghausen's positive adherence to Virchow's localist tradition and, consequently, that he viewed the conceptual apparatus of Virchow's theory as essentially restrictive of progress in this area, "He was too consummate a histologist in the localist morphological tradition, and too loyal a follower of Virchow, to superimpose on his experiments an outlandish holistic approach." (78, p. 175).

In any case even if von Recklinghausen had anticipated the experiment performed four years later by Cohnheim and had surmounted these psychological obstacles, he would have required, as the next step, to explicitly surmount the restrictions of Virchow's localist theory. Therefore, in Cohnheim's case, we would expect some special circumstances that allowed him to adopt a holistic perspective. Maulitz argues that Cohnheim's switch from the morphologist–localist position to the physiologist–holist position was influenced by the physiological chemists with whom he collaborated in Virchow's institute. The most notable was Willy Kuehne, an *assistant* in chemistry from 1861 to 1868, who was to become Cohnheim's principal biographer (78). If so, then Cohnheim's thought, which appears as strictly positivistic and motivated by concrete experiments and sober observations, achieves an additional intellectual dimension. In 1867, Cohnheim believed that the active amoeboid movement of the colorless blood corpuscles accounted for their passage through the intact vascular wall (61). But later (79), he accepted Simon Samuel's opinion that passage of the cells through the vessel walls was conditioned not by their active movement, but by hypothetical changes in the walls and by an increase in lateral pressure within the vessels (80). In his *Lectures,* Cohnheim even expresses a bewilderment at those who supported that "obsolete belief" in active movement of white cells, "The exit of the colourless cells does not depend on spontaneous movement, as I myself formerly supposed, and as is, oddly enough, still maintained by [Karl] Binz and other writers" (56, p. 293). This shift in Cohnheim's opinion could be understood as a manifestation of the ascendent reductionist influence of the period, but another possible explanation—that in no way excludes the first, but rather points to another dimension of the same intellectual process—is the notion that spontaneous cell movement might have appeared to Cohnheim as too closely associated with Virchow's idea of cellular sovereignty. Depriving cells of spontaneity, Cohnheim reestablished the holistic sovereignty of the organism. In this case, a mechanistic perspective was closer to the holistic-physiological approach than to Virchow's localistic-morphological concept.

We have noted how important, from Cohnheim's point of view, the concept of inflammation was in various medical theories throughout history. As Rather explained:

> The concept of inflammation was, from the first, not merely a complex of signs and symptoms—the redness, heat, swelling and pain of Celsus in the first century A.D., so familiar to the readers of today's textbooks of pathology—but rather a theory of

the way the body and its component parts "worked" during a particular set of circumstances. Consequently the concept had to change whenever ideas of the structure and function of the body underwent change. (23, p. 2).

The opposition of structure and function as a basic construct reflected the nineteenth-century's opposition of morphology and physiology. The term *structure* pretends to replace *form,* or *morphe,* of earlier periods. In its turn, *morphe,* which expressed in the Aristotelian tradition, organismic identity and integrity, carried a meaning inseparable from both structural and functional aspects of the organism. Thus Rather's observation of how concepts of inflammation changed reflects the effects of evolving concepts of organismic integrity: interpretation of inflammation thus changed whenever the fundamental idea of organism was altered. In this respect, Metchnikoff could hardly find novelty in Cohnheim's treatise. Even if he was conscious of metaphysical integrity, it was the old idea of an underlying unity. As we believe, Metchnikoff's own theory of inflammation was connected with the problem of *evolving integrity,* an issue totally absent from Cohnheim's concern.

The same issues are raised with Ernst Ziegler's work (81). Here, as with Cohnheim's text, Metchnikoff could find rich material pertaining to the activity of the wandering cells, detailed descriptions of Cohnheim's results, and the same criticism of the neurohumoral and cellular theories of inflammation. The general conceptual framework of Ziegler's exposition bears the traces of Virchow's philosophy, reduced by the 1880s to a set of introductory ritualistic sentences:

> *Life* is known to us only in the concrete. It is indissolubly bound to a material substance. This substance, the basis of all the vital processes, is fashioned out of cells and their derivatives. . . .
>
> The vital activity of the cell is of a threefold kind. It is directed in part toward its self-preservation, in part toward its propagation, and in part toward the ordering of its outward relations. Virchow distinguishes these severally as the nutritive, formative, and functional activities. (81, p. 1, 1883)

Ziegler attempts caution and avoids any clearly defined "nature" of inflammation, rather referring to "a complex of many elements":

> *Inflammation* is a term implying a whole series of processes partly vascular and partly textural: and these processes admit of a great variety of combinations. Inflammation being thus a complex of many elements, we are unable to give a definition of it that shall be brief and at the same time exact. We might say, indeed, that one or other element (such as that relating to vessels) is characteristic of inflammation; but the whole content of the term cannot be fully indicated without describing the process to which the term is applied. (81, p. 137, 1883)

And then Ziegler satisfies himself with the classical symptomatic definition of inflammation:

> From the time of Celsus, *i.e.,* from the first century A.D., four cardinal symptoms of inflammation have been recognized: namely *rubor, tumor, dolor, calor*—or redness, swelling, pain, and heat. To these we may generally add a fifth, the *functio laesa, i.e.,* impairment or arrest of the function of the inflamed part. (81, p. 137, 1883)

And of course, the mechanism of inflammation is associated for Ziegler first of all with injury to the vessels:

> The causes of the alteration in the vessels are thus the causes of the inflammation. In other words, the alteration in the vessels is the direct or indirect consequence of the injury which excited the inflammation. Or still more accurately—any injurious agency which is capable of altering the blood-vessels, in a particular way is capable of producing inflammation. It is clear then that the number of agencies capable of exciting inflammation is indefinitely great; they are beyond enumeration or separate discussion. All we can say is that mechanical, thermal, and chemical agencies (and especially the latter) may act so as to alter the vessels and produce inflammation. (81, p. 143, 1883)

It may appear as if Metchnikoff occupied a compromised position between Virchow and Cohnheim: like Virchow, he recognized a certain degree of cellular sovereignty; like Cohnheim, he held a physiological-holistic approach rather than Virchow's morphological-localistic orientation. Cohnheim died before Metchnikoff published the phagocytosis hypothesis, but Virchow recognized an affinity between his own position and that of Metchnikoff. In 1885, Virchow published "The Struggle Between Cells and Bacteria" (82). In this paper, he predicted Metchnikoff's auspicious undertaking. Why was he so attracted by a theory that was apparently so far from his own? It is obvious that Virchow found in Metchnikoff (quite correctly from our point of view) a cellularist, who opposed Cohnheim's views on inflammation, which by the mid-1880s, in turn, had pushed aside Virchow's own version. From Virchow's vantage, Metchnikoff's interpretation of inflammation was connected primarily to the concept of a particular group of cells possessing a special activity, and the inflammatory reaction could not be simply reduced to the damage produced by harmful factors. "The poor little cells!" Virchow exclaims, "In fact, they fell for a time into oblivion" (82).

Ultimately, however, Metchnikoff's theory expressed a radical novelty that cannot be reduced to the combined views of his eminent predecessors. From Virchow's point of view, inflammation is a local disturbance of the *nutritive* relation between blood and tissues. The disturbance might be caused by internal or external injuries; Virchow called such a disturbance irritation *(der Reiz)*, a passive event, which, in its turn, provoked a reactive disturbance in the local cells to induce basic cellular processes (e.g., nutrition, reproduction). Any salutariness of the inflammatory processes is, for Virchow, highly doubtful. Virchow's understanding of cellular activity as a reactive intensification of certain basic functions has nothing in common with Metchnikoff's vision of mesodermal cellular activity as representing a basic form of activity of an ancestoral organism. It is true that Metchnikoff's theory was "more physiological" than Virchow's and that in this respect Metchnikoff was more closely related to Cohnheim. But we must remember that diapedesis does not have any protective function in Cohnheim's theory. More than that, the biological meaning of diapedesis was never posed by the theory: Cohnheim concentrated his attention on the vessels and the hypothetical damage to their walls; thus no inflammation without vessels (61). In explicit opposition to this position, Metchnikoff coined his own motto: "There is no inflammation without phagocytes" (83).

In a certain sense, the phagocytosis theory may be considered as a novel synthesis of these previous theories, but there is no possible combination of Virchow and Cohnheim's ideas that would result in Metchnikoff's hypothesis. These theories had been utilized by Metchnikoff in a dimension that neither predecessor would have suspected. The same can be said concerning the defensive activity of the colorless blood corpuscles. Rather writes:

> A protective, policing role had been attributed to cells even before the rise of the germ theory of disease in its modern form. The belief that pus contained a "concocted" *materia peccans,* i.e., digested and rendered ready for discharge from the body, rests on a Hippocratic basis. With the discovery that pus contained "corpuscles" together with the partial identification of free cells in multicellular organisms and free-living unicellular organisms it might easily have occured to someone that the pus corpuscles themselves were engaged in the disposal of the *materia peccans.* And in fact we find Virchow in 1847 rejecting as anachronistic precisely this view. "We no longer," he wrote, "regard the pus corpuscles as gendarmes ordered by the police-state to escort over the border some foreigner or other who is not provided with a passport." (84)

If we are inclined to reduce the real content of Metchnikoff's theory to only asserting the protective or salutary properties of the phagocyte, then there is no *principal* difference between this theory and those of his predecessors. But we argued that beyond the apparent similarity between Metchnikoff's idea and those who previously suggested protective properties of the colorless blood cells a radical difference lay in both the respective metaphysical and general experimental positions. For Metchnikoff's predecessors, in full agreement with the Hippocratic tradition, in the protective properties was the particular (in this sense, metaphorical) expression of the general healing power of organism. Thus, the real nature of the phenomenon was always viewed parenthetically and remained (as the wholeness of the organism) beyond this particular phenomenon. The idea of protective activity was thus destined by its very essence to remain as another metaphorical expression of self-sustained *physis.* On the other hand, Metchnikoff saw in the phagocytosis process, not a manifestation of an underlying wholeness, but recapitulation of a basic function of an ancient organism. This very fact introduced the theme of the mesodermal cells' protective activity as immediately embedded in two possible research programs: (a) comparative evolutionary studies of this activity and (b) the role of phagocytic activity in individual development. None of Metchnikoff's predecessors possessed anything similar to this general biological vision; his idea of a protective activity was thus thoroughly novel.

Of course, there always is a temptation to interpret Metchnikoff's theory without this metaphysical exposition. Is it not sufficient to note that Metchnikoff was only more consistent than others in combining an old idea of a putative protective function with: (a) the newly established bacteriological etiology of disease and (b) the Darwinian struggle between different species (in this case, between the host organism and the parasitic bacteria). Recall from chapter 4, the attempt to identify the host–parasite relationship, taken in terms of the interspecies struggle, as the paradigm for the idea of protective phagocytosis (85). We argued there that from Metchnikoff's point of view (between the late 1870s and the early 1880s), selection, being understood as the result of the interspecies struggle, could not account for the processes of individual development and that correspondingly such a concept of selection could not serve as the basis for discrimination between progressive and regressive evolution. The search for a criterion for this discrimination reflected Metchnikoff's concern with the problem of organismic integrity in his morphological studies. Metchnikoff's studies of parasitism may only be properly understood within this context.

The Problem of Parasitism

Metchnikoff's interest in the phenomenon of parasitism may be traced to his first studies as a morphologist (e.g., to Leuckart's laboratory in the 1860s [see chap. 2]). In 1874, Metchnikoff's "General Essay on Parasitic Life" was published (86), wherein he presented parasitism from the morphologist's perspective: parasites are interesting as the main representatives of regressive evolution. Here he also asserts that natural selection favors a decrease in organization rather than an increase. Metchnikoff asserts that lower organisms have more opportunities for victory in their struggle for existence than those that are comparatively more highly organized. In contrast, Metchnikoff's idea of immunity hinges on the organism's ability to mobilize its forces in order to protect its integrity against the intruders that have obviously lower organization. In the 1870s and the early 1880s, Metchnikoff saw in the phenomenon of parasitism further proof of his pessimistic belief that inasmuch as the struggle for existence is responsible for a given relationship, the lower forms were more likely to triumph over the more complex (87). This pessimistic orientation animated his efforts against the beet weevils *(Anisoplia austriaca)* of southern Russia. Metchnikoff wrote in "Illnesses of the Larvae of the Beet Weevil":

> The entire sum of scientifically acquired facts leads to the conclusion that lower parasitic organisms are actually the most powerful enemies of animals and therefore can be used to relieve man of harmful insects. (88, p. 340; Todes's trans. 85, p. 92)

But in what way can this practical idea be considered as paradigmatic in regard to the phagocytosis hypothesis? Metchnikoff does not refer to internal protective forces of the cultured plants that are attacked by these beetles. He does not consider special protective mechanisms that could possibly defend the beetles against the fungi. He saw in the situation what he usually saw in the relationship between hosts and parasites: the lower organisms were favored in their struggle against higher organisms. The situation reflected his general pessimism, but in this particular case, the situation may be turned to man's benefit. Neither in this essay nor in the series of essays written on the same topic in 1880 (89) can be found the idea of active host defense. We do not discern any hint of a special system in the host that could play a role in active defense. Thus we question Todes's conclusion:

> For Metchnikov this interpretation [the phagocytosis hypothesis as the interpretation of the facts pertaining to the functions of the amoeboid mesodermic cells] followed logically from an understanding of parasitism, evolutionary theory, and the struggle for existence. (85, p. 95)

What followed logically from Metchnikoff's understanding of parasitism, evolutionary theory, and the struggle for existence was the belief that the host organism might win its struggle with a pathogen only by chance, not because it was able to protect itself, but because the parasite failed to succeed on other terms (90). The only general idea Metchnikoff expresses in these works on parasitism, and that pertains to the interspecies struggle, is that lower forms are the usual victors in the struggle with more complex species. Thus, a host's protective mechanism appears in no guise and is not suggested by Metchnikoff's understanding of parasitism as interspecies struggle. Disagreeing with Todes, we do not imply that Metchnikoff's studies of parasitism did not influence his future formulation of the phagacytosis hypothesis, but we believe that (1) the host–parasite relationship did not play a *paradigmatic role* in Metchnikoff's formulation of the hypothesis and that (2) the primary theoretical focus of Metchnikoff's studies in parasitism was not to analyze the phenomenon as a demonstrative example of interspecies struggle. The main point was to study the phenomenon that demonstrated clearly (as Metchnikoff believed) that radical morphological transformations (in this case, regressive ones) that determine the systematic positions of organisms *could not be caused in any manner by the struggle for existence.* As we have argued, the general theoretical goal in relation to Metchnikoff's interest in parasites revolved about the typology of organizational levels. The facts supporting the rejection of unilinear evolution, for Metchnikoff, correlated with the failure to establish a single scale of such a typology. (Were such a scale available, it would be possible to construct the "main" direction of evolution and to interpret all others as deviations from the only "correct" one.) This search for an organizational typology fully correlated with Metchnikoff's search for principles according to which it would be possible to determine integrity of a given organic form.

As we have already discussed, the primary problem which Metchnikoff sought to solve was the identification of developmental structures in his comparative-embryological studies. The logic of the task guided him in his search for organismic integrity. In this context, to admit failure in establishing a general criterion of biological progress only reflected the absence of a general objective scale of progress. It was equivalent to conceding that individual development could not be universally interpreted as revealing a provided unity. Correspondingly, it may be possible that an organism in the course of its ontogeny surmounts its own initial state of disharmony and establishes its own integrity. Evolution might preserve success, but there is no guarantee that evolution would provide such an integrity or preserve it once achieved. The supposed regressive evolution of parasites was viewed as the best proof of the lack of concern that evolution demonstrates in such a relationship. Traditionally, morphology saw in individual development a *revelation* of integrity. From Metchnikoff's point of view, it was possible (but only in some cases in which development does not have a regressive nature) to consider developmental processes as *establishing* integrity. But then it becomes possible to consider processes that restore or defend integrity. Parasites (especially in cases where the larvae form have a higher level of organization than the adult form) demonstrate a counterexample: their development may illustrate the realization of a provided unity that degrades and thus loses its initial integrity. The idea of development as establishing integrity (by surmounting an initial lack of integrity, i.e., disharmony) creates a metaphysical space for the idea of a special system that is charged with protecting integrity. The idea of parasitic regressive development creates the metaphysical antiworld, the horizon of the nascent phagocytosis theory. Only in this intellectual configuration do we see the true significance of Metchnikoff's studies in parasitism for his future formulation of the phagocytosis hypothesis.

It is a widespread opinion (in part owing to his own retrospective rationalization) that Metchnikoff's great virtue was a "consistent" application of Darwinian (original or revised) ideas to the problems of inflammation and immunity. For example, Rather valued Metchnikoff's *Lectures on the Comparative Pathology of Inflammation* as "one of the great medical and biological classics of modern times":

> And this is not because, as is sometimes said, Metchnikoff introduced the comparative biological method into medicine. Anyone familiar with the nineteenth-century medical literature, with the work of Johannes Mueller and Koelliker in Germany, for example, or of [William] Carpenter and [George] Gulliver in England can hardly accept that claim without qualification. What Metchnikoff did do was to apply the comparative method, in the light of evolution and natural selection, to the study of a particular set of pathophysiological events traditionally grouped under the heading of inflammation and by this means define the essence of the process. No one before him had so thoroughly shown the connection between extracellular and intracellular digestion and the relation between digestive, protective and immune processes. (84)

What Rather ignores here is the fact that Metchnikoff reconciled himself with natural selection as the basic evolutionary principle only *after* his formulation of the phagocytosis theory. And it was only then that he performed the revision of his theoretical beliefs on the basis of the new theory. Metchnikoff's originality lay not in his ability to see the phenomenon of inflammation in the light of evolution and natural selection, but rather in his ability to see evolution from his specific mesodermal perspective. If insensitive to Metchnikoff's complex perspective, it is but natural to conclude that he differed from the others only in that respect to which he succeeded more thoroughly to demonstrate the relationship of digestive, protective, and immune processes. This qualification is not necessarily unfair. But this kind of quantitative characterization (e.g., scientist *A* demonstrated something more/less thoroughly than other scientists) does not adequately reveal what was truly accomplished. Rather asserts that others, prior to Metchnikoff, considered inflammation as possibly protective and that some even attempted to apply the selection theory to the problem, but none were as consistent or successful in this undertaking as Metchnikoff. But, in fact, the issue of protection did not constitute the core of Metchnikoff's theory! The protective effect of phagocyte activity was a secondary phenomenon. *Ironically, Metchnikoff arrived at his theory of inflammation and immunity because he was not concerned with the issue of protection.* As we argued, protection was connected with the idea of activity of the whole that patronized its parts; Metchnikoff's theory of inflammation arose from the idea of a subsystem taking responsibility for organismic integration. The theory is rooted not in the idea of protection (self-protection) of an underlying unity, but in the idea of *establishing* that unity. Thus, the primary biological meaning of phagocyte activity is not protection, because there is no entity to protect antecedent to the activity: phagocytosis establishes the self or in its less radical formulation at least shares responsibility with other possible processes for establishing integrity that, as soon as it has been established, may become the object of protection. If, in discussing the origin of "immunity" as an idea, we emphasize the concept of "protection," then, quite fairly, we can assert that all elements of Metchnikoff's theory had been more or less anticipated in the preceding history of pathology and that Metchnikoff differed from his predecessors only by the scope of his undertaking. But Metchnikoff, in fact, established a new science, immunology, which characterized a special subsystem, whose function defines the manner in which the organism deals with the problem of integrity and identity, that is, selfhood. So, in characterizing the novelty of Metchnikoff's theory, we cannot be satisifed by simply asserting that none of his predecessors so thoroughly connected protective, digestive, and immune processes. The cardinal point is simply that none could perform such a connection, for none dealt with *this* idea of immunity, self-definition.

The enchantment with the protection idea misleads us in our attempts to appreciate the evolutionary dimension of Metchnikoff's inflammation theory. Todes, for example, writes of Metchnikoff's *Lectures on the Comparative Pathology of Inflammation:*

> Originating as a series of addresses at the Pasteur Institute in 1891, Mechnikov's *Lectures* reflected his conclusion that resistance of his theory was rooted in medical theorist's lack of a broad evolutionary perspective. To remedy this he proposed a new field, comparative pathology, which was a branch of zoology charged with examining the relations between infectious agents and their hosts. In *Lectures* Mechnikov traced such interspecific conflicts through progressively more complex forms, beginning with the struggle of unicellular organisms against invading bacilli and continuing through simple multicellular forms, metazoans, coelenterates and echinoderms, orthropods and mollusks, and finally amphioxus. (85, p. 99)

From Metchnikoff's previous research, only one step was required to arrive at his idea of immunity: to recognize that the only adequate formulation of the problem of organismic integrity resides with the organism itself. In this perspective, Metchnikoff's comparative approach to pathology reflects the deepest intellectual sources of his theory and in no way may be considered as a tactical ploy. But taking Metchnikoff's theory of inflammation as primarily a theory of protection, Todes is forced to see in Metchnikoff's idea of comparative pathology nothing more than an attempt to support the phagocytosis theory by the idea of the interspecies struggle. As we have demonstrated, this retrospective rationalization does not reflect the true chronology of the history, nor its intellectual development.

In 1891, comparative pathology was not a new field for Metchnikoff. In 1883, Metchnikoff published "Studies Concerning the Mesodermal Phagocytes of Some Vertebrates" (91). He presented his observations of some Mediterranean invertebrates and of tadpoles and tritons obtained in a southern Russian village, Popovka. But he used the same materials in his Russian publication (in *Reports of the Society of Odessa Physicians,* vol. 5, 1883–1884) under the remarkable title "Materials for a Comparative Pathology of Inflammation" (92). This is not only a trivial issue of an altered title, for it sufficiently rids us of the syllogism that prejudices (in most cases subconsciously) our reading of Metchnikoff: his theory of inflammation essentially coincides with the theory of immunity; any theory of immunity is a theory of organismic protection, hence the essence of Metchnikoff's theory is the interpretation of inflammation as a set of processes that protects the organism against harmful agents and external pathogens. This syllogism does not allow us to see that *inflammation, from Metchnikoff's point of view, is primarily a normal physiological phenomenon* and not a protective reaction against pathological factors. The syllogism impairs the recognition that pathological inflammation, as a protective reaction against harmful factors, is in Metchnikoff's theory only a particular case of those physiological processes that play a constitutive role in normal individual development. In "Studies Concerning the Mesodermal Phagocytes of Some Vertebrates," Metchnikoff reports his observations on inflammation in different stages of amphibian metamorphosis: he noticed that the concentration of mesodermal cells at inflammatory sites in triton larvae was accompanied by an insignificant emigration of leukocytes from the vessels (a not so subtle attack on Cohnheim's inevitable connection of inflammation as a consequence of a damaged vessel wall) and a more marked diapedesis in tadpole metamorphosis. He then generalized by noting that he never observed an exudation at the site of inflammation (reiterating his anti-Cohnheim position). On the basis of these ontogenetic and phylogenetic observations (i.e., the comparative approach), Metchnikoff concluded, "So-called serous inflammation presents a relatively later phenomenon, but the concentration of the phagocytes corresponds to the earlier primary period of inflammatory reaction" (91). Several years later in his *Lectures* (Number 7), he returned to this topic with a more detailed discussion in light of more extensive comparative data. The role played by wandering cells in *the active atrophy* of muscles and nerves remained a prominent interest for another decade, publishing with J. Soudakewitch, in 1892, "Muscular Phagocytosis" (93).

It is of particular note how Metchnikoff introduced the theme of protective phagocytosis in his famous paper of 1884 "Concerning the Pathological Meaning of Intracellular Digestion" (94). He began by describing mesodermic cellular activity (as responsible for intracellular digestion) in coelenterates, and he then discusses the role of these cells in the metamorphosis of echinoderms and amphibians and points to the striking analogy between these processes and the atrophy of muscles and nerves. (This latter topic will preoccupy his later musings on senility as the disharmonious— and in this sense, pathological—final stage of the *normal* order of individual development.) And only after these observations does he present his true theme of the pathological, "Every time a certain tissue has been affected by a traumatic or any other disturbance, it is eliminated, devoured by the mesodermic cells" (94). And finally, Metchnikoff turns to the theme of protection against intrusive foreign invaders, "External bodies, in their turn, share the same destiny: regardless of the way they have penetrated into the mesoderm, they become in any case its prey [i.e., of the mesoderm] (94).

Summary

Metchnikoff undoubtedly was more energetic and consistent than others in promoting how amoeboid mesodermic cells served as defensive agents, but this does not explain what he really did and why he was successful. We have argued that assigning a protective function to phagocytes was not the issue of his concern. He saw in the activity of amoeboid mesodermal cells the recapitulation of the basic activity of an ancient organism; this then generated the question of how this primeval activity might be integrated within the functions of later evolutionary origins. In its turn, the question naturally developed into a dual ontogenetic-phylogenetic research program. Thus the evolutionary dimension of Metchnikoff's theory of inflammation is not a later device adopted to provide an external theoretical support, but rather one that served as a foundation of the theory. On the other hand, no less essential for understanding Metchnikoff's position is to recognize the ontogenetic basis of the program. The fact that the theory arose from the problem of organismic integrity is reflected first of all in Metchnikoff's preoccupation with the phenomenon of inflammation as the basic factor of individual development—as demonstrated by metamorphosis, active atrophy, and senility. Inflammation then became a specific expression of harmony/disharmony. As a modeling factor of ontogeny (i.e., as a harmonizing factor), it became a normal physiological process. But disharmonies are also biologically normal; in some cases (e.g., senility), the normal process might be disadvantageous for the organism. The normal is not always opposite to the pathological. In this case, pathological inflammation, as a phagocytic reaction against external harmful factors, is only a particular case of *physiological inflammation.* Finally, immunity was considered as a particular case of inflammation—a kind of nonlocalized inflammatory reaction. In his first publications, dealing with the phagocyte response in models of infectious disease (starting with "Ueber eine Sprosspilzkrankheit der Daphnien" [95]), it is plainly evident how the modern concept of immunological research was based on this *biological* understanding of inflammation and the comparative approach to the problem.

Starting with the belief that the general immune response is "a diffuse inflammation," Metchnikoff began his studies of the phenomenon with *Daphnia* and then in the next work continued in succession with experimental models in frogs, lizards, turtles, guinea pigs, and rabbits (see chap. 6). We saw that the problem of the digestive activity of amoeboid cell recapitulation on different "levels" of evolution coincided for Metchnikoff with his primary problem—identification of the second embryonic layer as the mesoderm. Metchnikoff believed that there were enough facts in general pathology and in pathological histology to accept the new phagocytosis theory. On the other hand, those observations from vertebrates offered a complex array of mixed functions of various structures, and the data did not easily reflect the most basic processes constituting the phenomenon of inflammation. But in his preparations of *Bippinaria* larvae and other invertebrates, Metchnikoff was able to demonstrate to Virchow (already at Messina in 1883) that he "had set up the phenomena of inflammation without the assistance of nervous or vascular systems" (22, p. 519). Metchnikoff appreciated the significance of his simple model and extrapolated it to the complexity of the inflammatory reaction in higher animals. "It occurred to me," he wrote in *Immunity* "that a comparative study of inflammation in lower animals of simple organization would certainly throw light on the very complex pathological phenomenon in the Vertebrata, even in the frog which had served as the starting point for Cohnheim's remarkable experiments" (22, p. 578). Metchnikoff correctly understood his success as a result of choosing the right model, although he never used the word *model,* at least in its modern epistemological meaning. What was so natural for Metchnikoff was not at all natural for pathologists. For instance, that very Ziegler, from whose book Metchnikoff had acquired his extensive knowledge of the pathology literature on the role played by leukocytes in resorption (22, p. 513), vigorously opposed the phagocytosis theory. Unfortunately, the application of a model always presents an implicit difficulty—interpretations of results are dependent on the reasons for which the model has been chosen. Beyond Metchnikoff's choice of the "simple" model there was his understanding of the problem of the relationship between phylogeny and ontogeny. His *Comparative Pathology of Inflammation* was both a comprehensive substantiation of the choice and an elaboration of a succession of such models as an approximation of the pathology of inflammation of vertebrates. The stage was thus set for a tumultuous debate.

CHAPTER 6

The Phagocytosis Theory and Its Reception

The Setting

Metchnikoff's theory of active defense by phagocytes was novel not only in assigning a new function to these cells but also in offering a revolutionary concept of immunity. Competing theories were all passive as labeled by Ernst Sauerbeck in a 1909 summary, *The Crisis in Immunity Research* (1), in which various other hypotheses of the period were also considered. Pasteur's depletion theory (2), the retention theories of M. von Nencki (3) and M. A. Chauveau (4)—and their physicochemical variants—as well as lingering forms of mithridatic theory each viewed the pathogen as acting autonomously in the process of immunization. This in contrast to Metchnikoff's "active" theory of a responive host accounting for the immune state. The theory proposed by Pasteur in 1880 pertaining to the exhausted crucial nutrient state of the host was based on an extrapolation from the in vitro studies of bacterial growth in which specific nutritional requirements were an important focus of microbiology. Pasteur proposed that recurrent infection (at the time he was studying fowl cholera [2]) would not occur if a nutrient was exhaused in the first infectious episode. Earlier depletion theories were based on observations that blood possessed some power to inhibit putrefaction. Timothy R. Lewis and David D. Cunningham in 1872 (5) and Moritz Traube and Richard Gscheidlen in 1874 (6) showed that blood drawn under sterile conditions would not become putrid even if bacteria had been injected into the animal twenty-four to forty-eight hours prior to phlebotomy. The original thesis was that the antiseptic qualities were correlated with the state of erythrocyte oxygenation (an orientation shared by W. Grohmann [7]), thus anticipating Pasteur's general depletion notion; in the case of the observations cited in 1872 (5) and 1874 (6), an exhausted inhibitory factor, not an active defensive reaction of the host, accounted for sterility. At the same time, von Nencki proposed the converse hypothesis, namely, that deleterious substances known to accumulate with bacterial growth in culture (e.g., phenols, phenylacetate) might accrue in vivo and inhibit pathogen growth in the host. In this case, specificity was due to the peculiar substances produced by each organism. Chauveau extended the theory to juvenile sheep, who sup-

135

posedly acquired anthrax immunity from their mothers by placental transfer of these noxious substances.

Before von Behring made his antitoxin discovery, he proposed a theory analogous to these retention hypotheses. Drawing a parallel between blood pH and its ability to sustain growth, he suggested that the alkalinity resulting from bacterial growth would impede further multiplication in the host (8). His own antitoxin experiments refuted this position. It is interesting that in his second antitoxin paper (9), von Behring considered it important to discount mithridatic adaptation as an explanation, noting that the immune mice received protection by passive means and had no opportunity to encouter (adapt) diptheria toxin prior to the experiment.

Baumgarten continued with the physicochemical approach, arguing that by altering the osmotic environment, the bacteria, in fact, induce an inhospitable milieu for their continued viability and would suffer osmotic lysis (10). He incorporated the antibody data only to the extent that these humoral factors made the microorganism more susceptible to osmotic destruction, a position he held at the same time Metchnikoff published *Immunity,* obviously never converted to the cellular theory. An extrapolation from in vitro bacterial-growth experiments was effectively discarded when Daniel E. Salmon and Theobald Smith demonstrated immunization with dead microorganisms (11)—and even more forcefully with the discovery of toxic humoral factors.

In this intellectual setting, we can understand both the hostility and resistance evoked when Metchnikoff first proposed his phagocytosis theory, which was immediately attacked by German pathologists and microbiologists. Led by Baumgarten and Ziegler, criticism was levied against the hypothesis in three general respects: (a) Can an analogy truly be established between leukocyte phagocytosis and the feeding of monocellular organisms? (b) What is compelling about the phagocytic process as a universal defensive activity? (c) General philosophical objections, centered on the accusation of a teleological formulation. Underlying the argument was the rejection that the response of phagocytic leukocytes was truly causal in the successful response to infection. The humoral school of immunity was not established until the years 1888 to 1890, and the early debate between Metchnikoff and his detractors was not over an alternative theory of an active immune response—there was none. With the development of the humoralist position, in direct response to Metchnikoff's formulation, a true dialogue about immunity in the modern context of active host response was initiated. The debate at this point changed to issues of mechanism (cellular vs. humoral effectors), and the relative importance of defining innate versus acquired immune processes.

The humoralist's position can be traced to Joseph Fodor, a Hungarian investigator, who in 1886 while studying the bactericidal power of blood came to the conclusion that the organism was "protected against the spread of bacteria by an unknown vital power of blood" (12). He formulated the conclusion as an argument against Metchnikoff's hypothesis. When Wyssokowitsch considered the disappearance of bacteria from blood as only reflecting movement to parenchymal organs (13), Fodor countered with an in vitro experiment in which he mixed anthrax bacilli with whole blood and showed bacterial diminution on culturing (14). The criticism that the microorganisms were entrapped in the clotted specimen was answered promptly by George

Nuttall (1888), who repeated the basic study with defibrinated blood and further showed that the bactericidal capacity of the blood was destroyed by heating to fifty-two degrees centigrade for ten to thirty minutes (15). Not only was this the basic discovery of complement, but Nuttall acknowledged phagocytic function in addition to humoral bactericidal factors, a duality Metchnikoff rejected. Buechner's studies of the same time, confirmed the bactericidal capacity of blood and showed this activity in cell-free serum (16). Emil von Behring's classic studies—those with F. Nissan (17) showed that only immunized guinea pigs would kill *Vibrio metchnikovi* (!) (named by Metchnikoff's friend Nikolai Gamaleia); those with Kitasato (18) showed that organisms immunized with tetanus (and Behring on his own simultaneously published parallel work on diptheria [9]) generated a humoral factor to neutralize exotoxin; and those with E. Wernicke (19) showed that protection was afforded by passive transfer of immune serum—firmly established the humoralists position by 1890 (20, 21). Hans Buechner had coined the term *alexine* (I defend) for this humoral factor(s) (22) (later renamed *complement* by Ehrlich), thus authoring the first of the various humoral theories that claimed to account for host defense. The vociferous debate with the cellularists was chronologically and conceptually a response to Metchnikoff. Those critiques offered *before* the humoralist position was firmly presented in 1890—seven years following Metchnikoff's crucial discovery and theoretical formulation—accentuate the novelty of the phagocytosis theory. First we will examine criticism by Baumgarten and related critiques, independent of the humoralists counterarguments. We will then consider in chapter 7 the debate with the humoralists, where the rigid, and essentially weak position Metchnikoff assumed unnecessarily polarized the discipline and limited his participation in directing the course of immunology, on the one hand, and reflected a more subtle rejection of his conceptual understanding of organism and its definition in evolutionary principles, on the other hand.

Metchnikoff's First Immunological Studies

The wandering mesodermic cells refer not only to blood leukocytes but also to the amoeboid cells of the connective tissue. Metchnikoff was struck by the similarity between the reaction of invertebrate mesodermic cells against foreign bodies and the complex processes of inflammation in vertebrates, thus formally initiating his comparative pathological approach to inflammation. In his first presentation of the phagocytosis hypothesis, given in an address ("The Curative Forces of the Organism") before the Congress of Naturalists and Physicians in Odessa (and later published), he set forth his theory concerning intracellular digestion as the basis of the healing process. He hypothesized, based on phagocyte distribution that the spleen was the most important organ for healing, followed by the lympahtic glands, bone marrow, liver, and the kidneys. As Metchnikoff wrote much later, these publications did not attract the attention of the medical public, "These investigations had a character that was too zoological to be noticed by pathologists" (23, p. 521). But his subsequent publications, in which he reported observations of phagocytosis in experimental models of infectious diseases and wherein he argued that the phagocyte functioned as a defensive agent, immediately aroused severe criticism. Note that Metchnikoff, from the beginning had prominent early supporters: Virchow and Carl Claus each published Metchnikoff's initial studies, the latter providing the Greek equivalent to *fresszellen* (devouring cells), *phagocyte* (*phagein* [to eat] and *kytos* [cell]).

In 1883, Metchnikoff published his work "Research on the Intracellular Digestion of Invertebrates" (24). First, reviewing research of invertebrate intracellular digestion, he focused his main concern on digestion of food by the mesodermic wandering cells. He stressed the general physiological role of these cells—the absorption of microbes was merely part of their multiple activities:

> It has also been shown that one function of amoeboid mesoderm cells is to eat up those parts of the organism which have become useless, and also any foreign bodies which may have pierced through the ectoderm; or, if it be not possible to eat up such bodies, to surround and isolate them. (24, English trans. p. 102)

Metchnikoff compared his findings with R. Koch's observations of tubercle bacteria in giant cells and anthrax bacilli in leukocytes; in a cautious and hypothetical fashion, Metchnikoff presented the idea of phagocytosis:

> So that throughout the whole animal kingdom the wandering cells of the mesoderm make use of their ingestive power for the destruction of bacteria and similar organisms, which need for their development a suitable (necrotic) nidus. (24, English trans. p. 107)

Metchnikoff's research of infected *Daphnia* followed upon Koch's classic study of 1876, which described the natural history of the anthrax bacillus in several species, including the frog (25); Koch carefully described the presence of bacteria within granulated leukocytes:

> This appeared to be the first clear demonstration of ingestion of schizophytes by ameboid white blood cells. It had been believed previously that these cells ingested micrococci, but it had been difficult to differentiate between the micrococci and the cytoplasmic granules. (25, English trans. p. 77)

One must wonder if Koch's later resistance to Metchnikoff's conclusions was not, in part, based on a sense of frustration that the same observation yielded the modern theory of immunity, whereas Koch's own observation was satisfied with establishing the anthrax developmental cycle and etiology of the disease. Koch recognized the unanswered issue, leaving the problem of host resistance to others:

> Factors concerned with hindering or preventing penetration of the bacilli and spores into the blood and lymph vessels should also be investigated. (25, English trans. p. 77)

Metchnikoff explicitly, in the *Daphnia* paper, published seven years later, drew direct parallels between Koch's studies and his own, concluding that the earlier experiments suffered from in vitro artefacts (bacteria-laden leukocytes burst, freeing anthrax) that were inoperative in the in vivo examination of *Daphnia,* and thus the true function of the phagocyte was overlooked (26). It should be noted, however, that Metchnikoff, at this juncture, was not dogmatic, "I believe that the bacilli are destroyed by the phagocytes, although the influence of other factors that may hinder their development is not eliminated" (26, 1884, p. 191). This caution was swept aside in the ensuing debate with the humoralists and by 1901, a defiant Metchnikoff proclaimed, "There is only one constant element in immunity, whether innate or acquired, and that is phagocytosis. The extension and importance of this factor can no longer be denied" (23, p. 543). How he arrived at this extreme position may be traced in the difficult polemic in which he was engaged. The early stages of the criticism did not appeal to any humoralist immunologic alternatives (27); those facts, which Metchnikoff's opponents erected in this early stage of the debate, were organized into a theoretical alternative only several years later.

Metchnikoff dealt with the defensive behavior of phagocytic cells in three papers published in 1884. In the first, a description of fungal infection in *Daphnia* (26), Metchnikoff reported his results of continuous microscopic observation of the water flea (a comparatively small and transparant animal) infected by a fungus that he first employed and named *Monospora bicuspidata*. Metchnikoff observed that in the *Daphnia* gut, the asci fungal spores penetrated, by their ponted ends, the intestinal wall (partially or entirely), entering the coelomic cavity. At that time, the amoeboid white blood corpuscles attempted to capture the intruders and Metchnikoff thought, destroy them. There were three subsequent possibilities:

(a) The leukocytes would succeed in devouring all invading spores, leaving neither spores nor candida, and the *Daphnia* would remain healthy and free of infection.

(b) If the fungus was not contained, for example, an overwhelming number of microorganisms would invade and the uncaptured spores would proliferate candida and spread through the blood system. Although the candida might also be seized by blood and connective tissue phagocytes, the struggle would fail. Some overloaded cells would burst, others (apparently by a chemical effect produced by the fungus) would be destroyed. Under these conditions the disease would flourish. (Metchnikoff viewed the process as a struggle between competing organisms, an affair that had an unpredictable outcome.)

(c) In this instance, Metchnikoff noted the presence of spores surrounded by phagocytes in the body cavity without any sign of disease, signifying a stable parasitism. Thus Metchnikoff differentiated between disease and infection (apparently it was the first such distinction). Further, Metchnikoff saw a correlation with Koch's observations of anthrax bacilli within giant cells, thus interpreting Koch's results in accordance with the phagocytic hypothesis.

In the second paper, "Concerning the Relationships Between Phagocytes and Anthrax Bacilli" (28), Metchnikoff began his studies of vertebrate immunity, working with frogs, lizards, turtles, guinea pigs, and rabbits. A solution of anthrax bacilli was introduced under the dorsal skin of frogs known to be immune. The first group was kept at room temperature and Metchnikoff observed that the bacilli were engulfed in large number by leukocytes. After several days, the engulfed bacilli were destroyed; some were contained within vacuoles resembling the digestive vacuoles of Infusoria and Rhizopoda, which he noted normally appeared during intracellular digestion. The injected anthrax lost their infective properties when injected into non-immune animals, a fact Metchnikoff interpreted as proof of the hypothesis that the organism mounted an active host response against foreign intruders. Although animals of this first group did not demonstrate any signs of anthrax disease, a different picture was observed with the infected group of animals who were warmed to thirty-seven to thirty-eight degrees centigrade. All of these frogs became sick with anthrax disease. In these animals only a small number of bacilli were found within leukocytes, the majority remaining free in blood and tissues. Similar observations were obtained with lizards and turtles, but these animals were also resistant to anthrax at the higher temperatures. In his experiments with guinea pigs and rabbits (two groups of animals that are susceptible to anthrax), Metchnikoff saw only a few blood and tissue phagocytes carrying the bacilli, with most microorganisms remaining external to the cells. When rabbits and guinea pigs were inoculated with attenuated bacilli, leukocytes that gathered at the site of inoculation contained numerous engulfed anthrax bacilli, demonstrating the same process of destruction observed earlier in the frog. When these warm-blooded animals were inoculated with virulent anthrax bacilli, again Metchnikoff observed the bacilli within leukocytes gathered at the site of injection, albeit fewer than in the case of attenuated bacilli. Finally, Metchnikoff attempted to investigate the leukocyte reaction of those animals that had been previously vaccinated by Pasteur's protective inoculation. The immunization was successful only with one rabbit. In this case, the samples taken two hours after injection demonstrated complete lack of free bacilli and an increase of bacilli-containing leukocytes. Unfortunately, the animal died as a result of an injury three days after the vaccination, but an autopsy revealed absence of free bacilli in blood and tissues (29). In cases where artificial immunization had failed, there were fewer leukocytes engulfing bacilli and a correlative increase in the number of free microorganisms was observed.

Metchnikoff considered these results as supporting his phagocytosis hypothesis of active defense. In order to explain the observed difference in phagocyte activity, he assumed that the anthrax bacilli secreted varying amounts of inhibitory poisons at different temperatures. Either increasing or lowering the temperature below normal homeostatic levels reduced resistance. The unexamined assumption served to explain the resistance of cold-blooded animals to anthrax under normal conditions and a weakening of that resistance at a higher temperature. The effect of preventive vaccination, Metchnikoff explained by the assumption that the phagocytes of warm-blooded animals gradually became accustomed to the secreted poison and, as a result, developed the capacity to digest even virulent anthrax bacilli in large amounts. (This position was markedly altered in the mature summary of his theory written in 1901 [23].) But the entire argument was obviously an *ad hoc* proposition with no scientific evidence, a recurrent construction that even his most ardent admirers today must view with chagrin. He never could admit to unsolved paradoxes or inconsistencies, as we will further have occasion to note. When he dealt with the problem of acquired immunity, at this point in his development, Metchnikoff simply attempted to incorporate the same construct that he formulated for innate immune mechanisms, not recognizing that the immune reaction might differ according to presensitization.

The similarity of the results, which he observed in his experiments with *Daphnia* and the vertebrates, Metchnikoff extrapolated to the data presented in the concurrent literature. He analyzed Koch's research in tuberculosis and Neisser's research in leprosy and concluded that their results were in harmony with his own and therefore might be interpreted in accordance with the phagocytosis hypothesis. He criticized some data (contradicting his opinions) of Victor Cornil concerning *Staphylococcus* infection. Metchnikoff asserted that because phagocytosis is a result of evolution, there are different forms and stages of adaptation both on the side of the phagocytes and the invading bacteria. He even admitted, "that some of the captured organisms were able to resist digestive activity and finally, instead of becoming food, became a parasite of the digestive organ or a symbiot" (28). As we will discuss, this position was vigorously attacked (the critics would not allow for phagocyte failure), and Metchnikoff was forced into a dogmatic posture, wherein the natural struggle of competition was subordinated, during his fiery defense.

In the third paper "Concerning the Pathological Meaning of Intracellular Digestion" (30), Metchnikoff gives a short review of his general biological opinion concerning the genealogy of the mesodermal phagocytes, their general physiological and pathological roles:

> It is possible to state as a general principle that the mesodermic phagocytes, which originally (as in sponges of our days) acted as digestive cells, retained their role to absorb the dead or weakened parts of the organism as much as different foreign intruders. (30, p. 563)

Metchnikoff continued, for higher animals, the differentiation of these functions from digestive activity has been realized in forming a specialized phagocytic system, including such structures as the lymph glands and the spleen. This phagocytic reaction constitutes the basic process of inflammatory phenomena. Although in sponges there is no significant difference between their inflammatory reaction and normal digestive process, other lower invertebrates differentiate the normal capture of food by endodermal phagocytes, but irritative invaders are seized by mesodermal phagocytes. Higher invertebrates substitute (completely or partially) intracellular digestion of food with extracellular enzymatic digestion, whereas mesodermal phagocytes practice their original activity in inflammatory processes and in normal and pathological atrophy of tissues. If the reaction of connective-tissue phagocytes is not sufficient, vertebrates invoke recruited blood leukocytes. This process is possible because of an intimate relationship between the connective-tissue phagocytes and the endothelium.

With these three papers, Metchnikoff quickly established the cardinal pillars of his phagocytosis theory:

(a) Mesodermal amoeboid cells had a diverse, but functionally aligned, purpose analogous to their original intracellular digestive function, namely, to engulf and devour atrophied or unnecessary host tissue or invading microorganisms.

(b) Tissue and blood leukocytes were functionally equivalent.

(c) Host defense was based on the successful containment of pathogen by phagocytes.

(d) The inflammatory reaction revolved about this phagocyte–pathogen struggle.

His leads were quickly followed by other investigators (31), but the theory was soon attacked.

Paul Baumgarten

In order to understand Metchnikoff's early detractors, and consequently, to approach the intellectual atmosphere in which the birth of the theory took place, we will carefully consider at first the earliest criticism by Paul Baumgarten (1848–1928, a leading microbiologist and professor of pathology at Koenigsberg, later Tuebingen) and his students, who were the most serious and severe critics of the phagocytosis theory in this early stage of the polemic against Metchnikoff. In 1884, Paul Baumgarten published (27) a critical review of Metchnikoff's first publications (26, 28, 30) on the phagocytosis theory of immunity. What Baumgarten characterized as a "strictly objective" critique, Metchnikoff ironically accepted as more "strict than objective" (29). Perhaps Metchnikoff's caustic comments were fair in a deeper sense than he could recognize at the time. Baumgarten's disagreement was directed not so much against the objective data provided by Metchnikoff's observations and not even against the hypothetical nature of Metchnikoff's interpretations, but rather against the intellectual basis implicitly underlying Metchnikoff's hypothesis. Baumgaretn did not argue from a standpoint of an alternative theory of an active immune response. There was none. The first alternative theory—formulated by von Behring and other humoralists—was only presented several years later. Of course, Baumgarten recognized the phenomenon of acquired immunity, but if we understand immunity and natural resistance of organisms to infection as the *active* measures that the host organism takes in its defense, then we could say that Baumgarten argued against a theory of immunity as we understand the concept.

Metchnikoff and Baumgarten considered the same data. But the first was inspired by the hope that he had found an active source of self-healing. The second believed that the attempt to combine Metchnikoff's idea of self-healing with the pattern of reasoning accepted by contemporaneous pathological research was fundamentally flawed. The early argument between them (1884–1888) can help us appreciate the radical difference in their respective general intellectual assumptions, and the principal novelty of Metchnikoff's hypothesis. But at the same time, their debate was not purely philosophical. The argument stimulated Metchnikoff in respect to extending his experimental research and in articulating the general principles of the immunological theory.

Baumgarten's arguments against Metchnikoff's theory may be divided into five groups:

(a) It is not self-evident that foreign bodies captured by leukocytes, undergo the process of intracellular digestion, in the sense observed with feeding amoebae.

(b) If leukocytes are destined to protect the host organism, why then are they inactive in certain instances of greatest danger?

(c) Why should we accept the hypothesis of active capturing and destruction of microorganisms if it is just as likely that we are observing the natural death of virulent bacteria owing to the limits of their host environment?

(d) Active phagocytosis is not a universal response and may not be extended to a broad generalization of host defense.

(e) Objections of a general philosophical nature.

Of Baumgarten's first objections, the issue of a parallelism between feeding amoebae and phagocytosing leukocytes, he wrote:

> The author [Metchnikoff] indeed demonstrated doubtlessly, that *Sprosspilzes* spores causing *Daphnia's* disease had been directly destroyed by the effect of the engulfing amoeboid cells, and if it is possible to argue against something it is whether this process of destruction (which really had taken place) can be equated with true intracellular digestion. (27)

Why does Baumgarten doubt that this is an example of intracellular digestion? He offers no concrete argument. But a possible indication is contained within his quite amorphous explanation of how he understood the phenomenon of intracellular digestion:

> We understand under digestion an assimilation of substances which were taken in, a utilization of the substances in favor of someone's interest, a process similar to that we observe in the intracellular digestion of true amoebae. (27)

And Baumgarten concludes without any explanation, "It is impossible to speak about this kind of circumstances in the case of *Daphnia's* blood corpuscles, which contain the spores of the *Monospora bicuspidata*" (27). Baumgarten does not argue why "it is impossible," but he appears to connect the concept of "digestion" with a vague idea of acting "in favor of someone's interest." Thus, if intracellular digestion by leukocytes is observed, it follows that these cells (as part of the whole organism) must act in their own interest to protect the host and assume the responsibility for an organism's integrity. But Baumgarten associates this responsibility only with the idea of the organism (unicellular or multicellular) acting as a whole, and in no way could he allow such a function for any constituent. Thus, Baumgarten's first criticism rested on an intuitive orientation that reflected not so much his special interest in pathology, but patterns of reasoning in general biology of the time, that is, a newly emergent mechanoreductive model of scientific reasoning.

Baumgarten continues:

> It is very questionable that the amoeboid cells of the higher animals really have [owing to atavistic heredity] this high degree of independence inside of the whole organism. [It is just as questionable that the leukocytes] could satisfy their nourishment impulse spontaneously or by the instincts of a true unicellular organism. In any case, the assumption [Annahme] cannot be proven by remote outer resemblance, which compares, on the one hand, the process of taking up foreign corpuscular elements by wandering cells and, on the other, true intracellular digestion. (27)

Baumgarten is intuitively correct in noting that there is something novel in the presuppositions of Metchnikoff's theory, but he does not discern its intellectual roots. It appears to Baumgarten as if Metchnikoff made an *ad hoc* assumption (about the leukocyte's capacity to digest) in order to strengthen the explanatory power of his hypothesis concerning the defensive role of white blood cells. Although the assumption does support the phagocytosis theory, Metchnikoff arrived at his conclusion by an opposite route: digestion led to defensive phagocytosis, not vice versa.

As we have detailed earlier, Metchnikoff had an extensive research program to establish genealogical relationships between metazoans. He examined the intracellular digestion of multicellular organisms from the vantage of comparative embryology to define the evolutionary destiny of the primary embryonic layers and, more specifically, the comparative study of the functions that amoeboid mesodermal cells perform in ontogenetic development. He began with studies of ontogenetic formation of the mesoderm of lower animals, from which he believed the endoderm had been formed as a specialized organ of digestion. He then proceeded to study the modification of that function in the ontogeny of higher animals. In the publication by which we date the beginning of his immunological theory, "Research on the Intracellular Digestion of Invertebrates" (1883), Metchnikoff stresses the general physiological function of mesodermal cells and their role in ontogenetic development, describing their protective role only as one of many modifications of their general physiological function. "They engulf both excessive parts of the animal's body itself and the particles which penetrate from outside, or at least if it is impossible, to surround to keep them" (24). Metchnikoff's immediate post-1883 studies were to examine in parallel both the resorptive properties of leukocytes and their defensive role against invading pathogens. Baumgarten views the subject as a pathologist. He did not recognize the general biological dimensions of the problem. Without Metchnikoff's perspective, Baumgarten poses a formal and, in some sense, restrictive question: How can we verify that the process in question is true intracellular digestion?

> His [Metchnikoff's] method (to comprehend a complicated pathological phenomenon in its own essence, which he traces through the whole realm of animals down to the simplest organized creatures) should be recognized as a witty and, in principle, legitimate view to which the author has arrived. . . . [but it] cannot be conceded, in the reviewer's opinion, as more than having value as a witty hypothesis. (27)

Metchnikoff's theory was born in his understanding of the developmental history of leukocyte function. He arrived at his hypothesis in the context of his embryological methods and that methodology was an experimental realization of the development of a broad theoretical construct that Baumgarten did not appreciate. Where Baumgarten saw only a metaphor of leukocyte protective behavior, Metchnikoff recognized a long history of a research problem devoted to the development of an understanding of the ontogenetic and phylogenetic role of amoeboid mesodermic cells.

The inability to recognize Metchnikoff's theoretical issues led Baumgarten to certain unfair objections. The most interesting question from Metchnikoff's point of view was the differentiation of mesodermal cells and how they assumed new functions in evolution. Baumgarten totally ignored that issue and therefore failed to discern differences in the general properties of phagocytes from the specific phagocytic activity of freely mobile white cells. Metchnikoff wrote:

> When Baumgarten, criticizing my views, speaks only about the white blood cells, he obviously does not want to take in consideration that I never identified [all] phagocytes with leukocytes, the point of view which is often and completely unfairly attributed to me. In all my works, I speak of different phagocytes (by the way, those also of non-mesodermal origin [i.e., ectodermal phagocytes]) of which the white blood corpuscles and cells of mesodermal tissue are predominant. (29, p. 236)

Arguing against Metchnikoff's theory, Baumgarten appeals to the example of recurrent typhus:

It is not known whether the recurrent spirilla were ever captured by the white corpuscles. On the contrary, one sees the former always lying free or moving in the blood, yet recurrent typhus ends with recovery in most cases. It follows from this that the living organism can manage with the energetically growing parasites without any help from the phagocytes. (27)

Metchnikoff sees in the argument the example of the same mistake of equating all types of phagocytes with mobile white blood corpuscles. He believed that if blood leukocytes did not phagocytose spirilla, then tissue-based phagocytes would be responsible for containing the infection. As recurrent typhus mainly strikes parenchymal organs, and spirilla disappear from blood shortly before crisis, Metchnikoff first hypothesized that they might gather in the spleen where the bacteria would be captured by the numerous tissue phagocytes found there (29, pp. 234–236). And in the next paper (32), he reported that in monkeys, in fact, the absence of spirilla in blood was associated with their concomitant phagocytosis in the spleen. Of course, this preliminary research could not satisfy Baumgarten's original objection: How do we know that engulfing leukocytes are digesting microorganisms? Indeed, how do we know that the splenic phagocytes "act on their own behalf"? Metchnikoff's reply does not directly answer him because intracellular digestion for the two opponents had different meanings. But Metchnikoff's early results obviously demonstrated the predictive power of his general theory.

The second group of Baumgarten's arguments may be defined by the following:

If the amoeboid cells were really destined [*bestimmt*] to protect the living bodies of animals against infective organisms, it would be possible to expect that they develop their work most actively in those cases when the former are seriously threatened by the latter. Something exactly opposite takes place! (27)

If we suppose that an activity, or phenomenon *A*, is responsible for the appearance of phenomenon *B*, and that at the same time, in some cases, the presence of *A* is not followed by the appearance of *B*, we can choose one of two conclusions: either our supposition is wrong and there is no such activity of *A*, which generates *B*, or in this particular case, *A* did not perform this kind of activity. Speaking formally, there is no advantage in either conclusion. The argument between Metchnikoff and Baumgarten may be reduced to this schema, for where Baumgarten sees evidence against the phagocytosis theory, Metchnikoff invokes that evidence to confirm his hypothesis. Baumgarten wrote:

In the case of leprosy [cited by Metchnikoff as a proof for his opinion], and moreover in the case of the bacilli-septicemia of mice, the parasites lie mainly inside of cells, despite the fact that leprosy and mouse septicimia are absolutely incurable diseases. (27)

Naturally, from Metchnikoff's point of view, this argument could have no power:

After all, the most essential thing is weakening and killing of parasites and connected with it, suspension of their damaging activity in the host. If [the parasites] are only engulfed by the leukocytes but not digested [destroyed], it cannot be the cause of healing. Baumgarten's case of mouse septicemia corresponds completely to my own data about candida of yeast fungi—the disease of *Daphnia,* whose data speak in favor, not against, the phagocytosis theory. (29, p. 237)

The main ideological objection that inspires Baumgarten's critique is allegedly the teleological nature of Metchnikoff's theory. And he builds his argument in correspondence with this assumption: "If the amoeboid cells were really destined to protect the living bodies of animals against infective organisms, it would be possible to expect . . . ," and so on. Metchnikoff objects that the argument is valid only in relation to Baumgarten's own teleological formulation of the question, but does not have any validity in relation to the phagocytosis theory. He argued:

At this point the whole formulation of [Baumgarten's] question is indeed teleological, but it does not have anything in common with the principles of the phagocytosis theory. In accordance with the latter, the amoeboid cells by no means are *destined* for healing activity, but the latter is a *result* of their capacity to engulf and digest different foreign bodies. The activity, which has a long history, is based upon the digestive function of sponges and other animals possessing intracellular digestion. From this point of view, the danger to an animal does not seem to be predestined in advance, but appears as a result of the phagocytes' inactivity, conditioned by one or another cause. (29 pp. 237–238)

It is interesting that both Baumgarten and Metchnikoff agree that a lack of perfection is an argument against the teleological nature of a function. This very implication pushes Metchnikoff to object to any attempt to approach his theory from a teleological position. But, in fact, Baumgarten argues not against teleology, but against the very possibility of accepting any idea of an active protective response on behalf of the host. Here we see the profound novelty of Metchnikoff's theory, for it represented the first formulation of active host defense.

We now turn to the third group of Baumgarten's arguments: Why should we accept the hypothesis of an active protective phagocytic response instead of proposing that virulent bacteria might be killed by some accidental or external effects? Indeed, what would change in Baumgarten's argument if he read Metchnikoff's thought in a slightly different manner? For instance, instead of reading the idea in terms of teleology: "amoeboid cells are destined to protect the animal," he would read the issue (as Metchnikoff himself prefered) in cause–effect terms, "a protective effect is a result of active phagocytosis." The formulation would not change anything in the logic of Baumgarten's argument; in this case, he would repeat the same syllogism: Why should we accept the hypothesis of phagocytosis as a cause of healing if there is evidence that some incurable diseases are associated with active phagocytosis? It is clear that we could draw out of the syllogism a much more general conclusion: How would it be possible to suppose any protective mechanism if there are incurable infective diseases? Metchnikoff quite clearly recognized this weak point of Baumgarten's argument. He wrote, "Apparently, it is easier for my critic to suppose that pathological microorganisms perish 'by themselves' " (29, p. 236).

And it is true that Baumgarten again and again returns to the same thought—the virulent bacilli could not be killed by protective forces of the host organism. Thus, speaking about the changes of the anthrax bacilli that Metchnikoff observed in the leukocytes of vaccinated guinea pigs and rabbits, Baumgarten noted:

There is no proof that the same changes do not have place for that weakened bacilli which could also be found outside the cells. Because of it we may put the question: is it really impossible that the bacilli had been changed in their form (as we see the change inside of the leukocytes) before they were captured by the cells? . . . The same can be said about the bacilli inside of the frog's leukocytes. . . . It remains unclear whether the loss of the infective power is conditioned by the capturing in the cells or also (or only) by other causes. (27)

In order to appreciate the value of Metchnikoff's theory as the first modern theory of immunity, we have to recognize that by opposing Metchnikoff, Baumgarten did not defend at this stage of the polemic (i.e., several years before the formulation of the humoralist position) the possibility of an alternative mechanism of protection against infection, but only asserted that there could be different reasons why parasites were unable to survive in the host organism. In fact (as we have previously noted), he argued against the phagocytosis theory not because this model of defense seemed too teleological, but because the very idea of defense appeared teleological.

The fourth group of Baumgarten's arguments disputes Metchnikoff's right to generalize certain observed phenomena because they were not found in all cases. It is clear that this group of arguments is closely connected with the above-mentioned second group: If the leukocytes are destined to protect the host organism, why do they not perform adequately in all instances? But accusations of this fourth category forced Metchnikoff not to a philosophical defense against accusations of teleology, but rather forced him to perform specific experiments of each disputed case in order to justify his right to generalize. In certain instances, he directly answered the opposition (e.g., in the research in recurrent typhus), which was, in part, influenced by Baumgarten's arguments that there was no evidence of active phagocytosis during this disease. Another example, Baumgarten's assertion that he could not observe any degenerative changes of ingested tubercle bacilli in the phagocytes of rabbits was answered by asserting that rabbits were very sensitive to the infection and, correspondingly,

> from the point of view of the phagocytosis theory, it is not just that the victory of the phagocytes or the death of the bacteria is expected for this kind of animal, but something opposed should be presupposed. If [Baumgarten] took less sensitive or immune animals (for instance, dogs, rats, frogs) to study the fate of the tubercle bacilli in the organism, he would perhaps, come to completely different results, which I hope to expound in my work on the phagoctye activity in tuberculosis. (29, p. 239)

That work was published in 1888 (33), establishing that giant cells of resistant tubercular animals were capable of engulfing bacilli, which then underwent degeneration. But we must note, there were instances where Metchnikoff's rebuttal rested on *ad hoc* assumptions.

The fifth group of Baumgarten's arguments—shared by Metchnikoff's other early critics—explicitly shows that the rebuttal was inspired not by an alterative program in host-defense research, but rather by what the critics viewed as an idiosyncratic hypothesis. Baumgarten wrote:

> We have to emphasize that an inquiry in natural sciences [*Naturforschung*] should presuppose as the ultimate goal to reduce [*zueruckfuehren*] phenomena of life to mechanical and chemical laws and so far it can not be taken as progress when Metchnikoff endeavors to put his openly teleologically breathing conception in place of physio-chemical attempts to explanations which Cohnheim endeavored to propose for the gathering of inflammatory cells, and especially for the penetration of the colorless blood corpuscles in inflammation. (27)

There is nothing strange in this positivistic-scientific declaration, being a reflection of the prevalent Zeitgeist. But if we remember that the same Zeitgeist inspired Metchnikoff himself, who from his school years and until his death professed the German mechanistic-positivistic phylosophy (34), his answer is somewhat unexpected:

> I cannot share Baumgarten's opinion in accordance to which any physico-chemical explanation has to be of a greater significance than a biological one. If the possibility to reduce all phenomena of life to mechanical and chemical laws was the final goal of studies of nature, it would not yet follow from this that a preliminary physico-chemical formulation of a question has to signify a success in solution of the given question. (29, p. 238)

But the way in which we formulate our questions is the most intrinsic characteristic of the structure of our thinking. This answer to Baumgarten defines the course of development through which Metchnikoff passed in his biological studies prior to the phagocytosis theory. That development, without which it would have been impossible to overcome the metaphysical horizon that delimited Baumgarten and, conversely, that allowed Metchnikoff to reformulate the metaphor of protective forces into a theoretically articulated experimental research program was characterized by a broad perspective on biological processes and the power of synthesizing divergent phenomena into a unified theory. Further, seemingly inconsistent data were effectively incorporated into his construct. For instance, what he saw as exceptional or anomalous to the basic principles (i.e., that twenty percent of *Daphne* could not resist infection or that anthrax spores were resistant at the same time the bacilli were sensitive to phagocyte killing) were incorporated into the broadest understanding of the theory. He further understood that the conditions of study were obviously critical in Koch's observations of isolated granulocytes as well as in the choice of which frog species was innoculated (i.e., at room temperature, frog resistance to anthrax was uniform, whereas at thirty-five degrees centigrade, only certain species were resistant). Later, Metchnikoff appreciated that the choice of bacterial strain was also crucial (i.e., when others showed that variant bacteria that grew well at low temperatures overwhelmed leukocyte defense, thus demonstrating phagocyte function was dependent on exogenous factors [e.g., temperature]). Further, Metchnikoff recognized from the frog model that resistance to cholera vibrio was not sufficient for defense because the elaboration of the toxin would result in fatality if prompt destruction did not ensue. Thus Metchnikoff understood the complexity of the phagocytic struggle, where variation of microorgansms, host, and pathophysiology of disease each contributed to the outcome of infection. With all these provisos, he adamantly insisted on the primacy of the phagocyte in host defense, staunchly defending the core concept against the vagaries of experimental design and what he understood as anamolous exceptions. He would not allow the growing reductionism in biology deviate his organismal orientation, where his theory, a dynamic and vibrant understanding of evolutionary biology, constructed the data comprehensively and creatively into a new theory of immunity. If there was a central defect in Metchnikoff's defense, it was the exclusiveness of his point of view. But we have to recognize that his single-mindedness cannot be explained as a peculiar personality feature or, at least, it was not the only basis of his polarized position. For many years, Metchnikoff's posturing in the debate was stimulated by objective issues of the scientific arguments.

Other Early Critics

Perhaps the first experimental work aimed against Metchnikoff's hypothesis was published in 1887 by John Carl Christmas-Dirckinck-Holmfeld (35), who reexamined Metchnikoff's studies concerning the fate of anthrax in warm-blooded animals. He found many dead and weakened bacilli outside the leukocytes. He concluded that the effect "should be ascribed rather to chemical-biological relations than to the ability of the cells to capture corpuscular elements." But how did Christmas-Dirckinck-Holmfeld understand these possible chemical-biological relations, which he believed played a more important role in the destruction of the bacilli than phagocytosis (if the latter plays any role at all)? He supposed that the cells accumulating in the locus of inflammation limited the supply of oxygen and this depletion process was the real cause of bacterial destruction. That inflammation might have curative (albeit secondary) effects had been previously expressed (e.g., by Ziegler whose treatise Metchnikoff cited as the immediate source of his knowledge concerning the pathology of inflammation) prior to 1883. How little Ziegler's notions had in common with the idea of active host defense is seen in the German's vigorous opposition to Metchnikoff's theory (discussed later).

A similar posture was assumed by Rudolf Emmerich (36), who injected anthrax bacilli, together with *Staphylococcus,* into rabbits (intravenously and intradermally). In many cases, he observed recovery as well as a certain degree of immunity against a second anthrax infection. Observing degeneration of bacilli exterior to the cells, he thought the effect could be explained by assuming that the host's cells had been irritated by the injection and, as a result, engaged in a higher activity of food consumption. In a nonspecified fashion, Emmerich proposed that the invading bacilli could then be used as a food source. He also considered that the host's cells, being in a more active state, might release a product that would directly damage the bacilli; but Emmerich did not ascribe to the phagocytes any role in the annihilation of the bacilli. In another publication (together with Eugeneo di Mattei) (37), Emmerich stated that contrary to Christmas-Dirckinck-Holmfeld's assertion, he never observed in staphimmunized animals any pus formation at the site of anthrax injections. Nevertheless, the bacilli died in a short time, and the authors concluded that bacterial killing was independent of inflammatory cells. In this discussion, we are searching for a trace of an alternative immunological idea to that of Metchnikoff's active host-defense theory. Therefore, we are not considering Metchnikoff's theoretical and experimental objections that he promptly published in reply to almost every publication aimed against his hypothesis. (Extensively reviewed in *Immunity* [23].) For the same reason, we have not considered his supporters. For instance, Alexsandr Dmitrievich Pawlowsky (38) performed experiments similar to that of Emmerich and came to different results: investigating bodies of the animals after three days, he observed many anthrax bacilli inside the cells, especially in the macrophages of the spleen, where most of the bacilli demonstrated the signs of degeneration quite clearly. Again, there is no notion of a reactive response on the part of the host. The recurrent debate with the prehumoralists was hampered by the absence of a shared theoretical construct; these critics simply could not confront Metchnikoff on his own turf.

The crucial immunological debate truly began with George Nuttral (a young

American working in Earl Fluegge's laboratory), who in 1888, confirmed Metchnikoff's key finding in the anthrax-infected frog model, namely, that phagocytized bacilli were destroyed.

> However, from then on my findings essentially deviate from those of Metchnikoff in respect that I observed as many, if not more, bacilli that had undergone complete degeneration outside of the leukocytes, as with captured ones. . . . The fact that under the frog skin, anthrax bacilli were destroyed outside phagoctyes also in great number is the most important evidence for a judgment about the activity of phagocytes as a protective equipment of the organism. (15, p. 366)

Employing microscopic examination of blood from several species and various bacteria, Nuttall observed both phagocytosis and confirmed Fodor's (12) report of blood's bactericidal capacity, and for the first time demonstrated the serum factor's heat lability. Variation of conditions, time course, tissue fluids, and species contributed to diverse observations, but Nuttall made the first observation that led others to show that opsonins participated in the complex killing process.

> Indeed, we have been led by all these observations, to the conjecture that all these [bacteria] captured by leukocytes were not completely normal and some real factor, hostile to bacteria, should be sought in the liquid surrounding the cells. (15, p. 383)

Karl Fluegge, relying on the results of his assistants (Gennadii Smirnow, Vasilii Nikolaevich Sirotinin, Heinrich Bitter, George Nuttall) had come to the conclusion that phagocytosis occurred only after the bacteria were fatally wounded, that is, a post facto scavenger process. (39, 40)

Now, one hundred years later, the idea of immunological self-defense is so obvious for us that it distorts our perspective on this early debate. From our vantage, in the reexamination of the initial history, we are inclined to accept every new experimental result (or hypothetical assumption) confirming the phenomenon of the bactericidal capacity of blood as another argument in favor of an alternative humoralist theory of host defense. But that was not the issue for Metchnikoff's early opponents. In 1889, when there was already a significant corpus of results supporting the future humoralist alternative, Baumgarten wrote an extensive critique (41). Regarding Metchnikoff's notion of leukocyte behavior on behalf of the host, Baumgarten denied the impression that "the cells' power is the healing power," offering instead that "nature puts death upon life as an unsolvable bond, death, but not killing." Thus, in Baumgarten's view, the microbicidal process is innate to the bacteria, not a causal result of active host defense. This obscure poetico-metaphysical statement is the only "theoretical" argument that Baumgarten uses against Metchnikoff. The specific attack centered on Metchnikoff's experiment with the spirilla, where Baumgarten asserts that splenic phagocytes were able to engulf the bacteria only when the latter had been already killed or weakened:

> But if the spirilla really were actively moving in blood until the last moment and they must be alive, from where can Metchnikoff find a refutation of the opposite opinion that they died *by themselves (von selbst)* [emphasis added]? (41, p. 36)

In the next sentence, Baumgarten directly characterizes the spirilla's fate as "the independent dying" *(das selbstandige Absterben).* Not only Baumgarten launches this logic against Metchnikoff, but exactly the same argument is found in Carl Weigert's objections:

> Why the phagocytes [of the spleen] engulfed the spirilla only then when the latter had multiplied numerously and had already been presented in an enormous number? If they have the capacity to destroy this large mass of spirilla and prevent their further propagation, why then can they not do the same with less number [of the spirilla] presented before it? (42, p. 734)

Weigert concludes that it is not clear from the presented observation how the splenic leukocytes serve as the crematorium of spirilla weakened or killed by unknown factors. Does this reference to unknown factors mean that Weigert assumed an alternative (nonphagocytic) mechanism of possible host self-defense? Or maybe he is referring to some secondary effects, which might result in self-poisoning of the microorganism or its failure to find in the host a favorable environment? In another paper (1888) on the same subject (43), discussing Metchnikoff's theory of giant cells, Weigert writes that there is no doubt that active tubercle bacilli have been taken up by the cells and were involved in a "struggle for existence" with the host.

> The only question is in what way the struggle takes place, whether the mysterious force of phagocytosis is at the disposal of the human and animal's organisms . . . or another [force] independent from it, no less mysterious one can be supposed. (43, pp. 809–810)

Of course the struggle for existence does not necessarily mean that in order to protect itself, an organism takes some measures of active self-defense in reaction to a particular encounter with a competitive organism. Thus, Weigert's references to a mysterious force of the host, which might be responsible for the microbicidal process, in no way can be considered as an assumption of an alternative mechanism to that proposed by Metchnikoff.

In 1889 Ernst Ziegler published an essay under the very promising title, "About the Cause and Essence of Immunity of Human Organism Against Infective Diseases" (44). Note that Fodor published his first results in 1886, Nuttall, Fluegge, and Bitter in 1888. (In the modern historical retrospective these publications are usually viewed as the initiation of the humoralist alternative.) In his essay, Ziegler refers to each of these publications as well as to those supporting Metchnikoff. It would be natural to expect that having this background, Ziegler would attempt to formulate a substantive statement concerning the cause and the essence of immunity. We might expect that being an irreconcilable adversary of the phagocytosis hypothesis, he would offer a counterhypothesis of the mechanism of self-protection. But nothing in this regard is found in his essay. Ziegler rejects Pasteur's depletion theory of immunity (2) because of the well-established fact that a sterile supernatant from culture growth of diphtheria or tetanus was immunogenic (11). More seriously, he then considers the self-poisoning theory: bacteria produce substances in the host organism that could be damaging to the microorganism itself. (Notice that both hypotheses offer explanations for the phenomenon of immunological specificity without any assumption of an ability to recognize and differentiate self from other, the ability that mediates the host response. Both hypotheses are formulated in terms of an immediate response or an immediate effect of a bacterial activity.) But Ziegler does not accept the poison theory either. It does not seem to him likely that a poison could be preserved in a host organism as long as some forms of acquired immunity last. He writes:

> I have to agree with Emmerich, Mattei and Fluegge when they assume that [immune] protection is provided, not through the poison itself, which is produced by the bacteria, but through their [bacterial] presence, entailing reactive processes in the tissues, which concluding from the observations of Emmerich and Mattei, possibly release chemical poisoning substances. (44, p. 431)

Thus we can see that the entire hypothetical explanation of acquired immunity is reduced to the idea that immunity is a result of an unspecified interaction between invading microorganisms and the host. Ziegler's scientific approach demands comprehension in chemical terms; *chemical* is the key word of the essay, but the theoretical construct is vacuous. The phenomenon of acquired immunity and immunological specificity receive a tautological explanation. Acquired immunity lasts because the interaction that generates the phenomenon has a lasting effect. Immunological specificity is explained by assuming that the interaction produces a specific effect, and so on. It is not surprising that Ziegler himself was not satisfied with this explanation. He (correctly) concluded that the variety and diversity of the bacteria–macroorganism interaction precluded any phenomenon as the only basis of immunity, and he would await further data, finishing the essay with:

> The time to set up a general and effective theory of the cause of immunity has not yet come. We are at the stage of just beginning particular investigations in order to undertake attempts to clarify particular cases. To gather new material for this is a rewarding task of the future. (44, p. 434)

In his caution, he had failed to grasp the cogent hypothesis offered by Metchnikoff. Moreover, neither Zeigler nor any of the early (or we might now refer to them as nonimmunological) critics offered an alternative immunological theory, nor did they wish to deal with one!

Summary

We can see that neither Ziegler (1889) nor Baumgarten's (1884) critiques were based on a specific immunological alternative to Metchnikoff's active mechanism of host defense. Although between 1884 and 1889 fundamental discoveries had been made that provided the experimental basis for the humoral mechanism of immunity, these observations did not alter the logic of Metchnikoff's critics in these early years of the polemic. The striking feature of the debate is not the inability of Metchnikoff's opponents to formulate an alternative hypothesis of an organism's self-defense, but their persistent unwillingness to accept the very possibility of interpreting the phenomenon of immunity in terms of a special protective mechanism. They firmly rejected a specific host response, seeing at best an undefined immediate reaction of the organism as a whole, or even less so, seeing only a failed environment for bacterial growth, a passive response to infection.

Metchnikoff himself, many years later, saw the issue correctly:

The pathologists who were adversaries of the phagocytic theory combined their efforts to demolish it, without troubling themselves to replace it by any other theory of defense on the part of the body which might more easily be made to accord with their principles and their statements. (23, p. 524)

We insist that the early critics of Metchnikoff's hypothesis were not inspired by any idea of immunity as self-defense. This is not to say that the humoralist experiments did not have an important impact on the development of the phagocytosis theory. Metchnikoff himself saw a radical difference between the critique of the pathologists (Baumgarten, Ziegler) and the criticism orginating from the bacteriologists (Fodor, Nuttall, Fluegge, Bitter). He wrote, "I must here confess at the outset that these attacks [of the bacteriologists] have been much more important . . . and have led to discoveries of the greatest value" (23, p. 525). In 1890, Behring and Kitasato (9, 18) clearly demonstrated that immunity to diphtheria and tetanus was mediated by a circulating humoral factor. The discovery came as the most serious challenge to the phagocytosis hypothesis. But the same discovery also proved a powerful challenge to the original opponents of the phagocytosis hypothesis. We must remember the historical context of the humoral studies and the true polemical issue between Metchnikoff's supporters and early opponents. From this point of view, Behring and Kitasato's publication appears as the tombstone of Metchnikoff's opponents. Although rivaling Metchnikoff's hypothesis, the humoralists obtained their own theoretical status only by adapting the most crucial metaphysical assumption of their opponent—immunity results from an active host-defensive mechanism. That position was not lightly won, but once obtained, the dialogue between cellularist and humoralist brought the debate concerning immunity to a new stage in the 1890s.

CHAPTER 7

The Phagocyte Eclipsed

The emergence of the humoralist position has been extensively discussed (outlined in the previous chapter and see, e.g., notes 1 and 2). For our purposes, it suffices to describe the principal studies that formed the challenge to Metchnikoff's cellular position in order to define the underlying logical basis of the controversy and to place it in contrast to the early debate. We endeavor to place the general development of the humoral position in the context of the phagocytosis theory by focusing on the studies of George Nuttall, Ernst Behring, Richard Pfeiffer, Jules Bordet, and Paul Ehrlich; at each turn we examine Metchnikoff's response.

Nuttal and Behring

George Nuttall, an American, went to Goettingen in 1886 to write a doctoral dissertation in the nascent discipline of microbiology under Carl Fluegge, whose laboratory had recently argued that bacteria were effectively dealt with by excretion in urine or bile; Nuttall however was intrigued by Fodor's report (3) that blood had a bactericidal capacity. The American's seminal paper, paid due homage to Metchnikoff, but it was highly critical:

> That phagocytic activity is the most important protective measure [that] must be weighed against the fact that anthrax bacilli under the skin of frogs are destroyed in large amounts outside phagocytes as well. It is clear that Metchnikoff's experiments suffer considerably by this finding. (14, Bibel, p. 163)

Nuttall initiated his studies, at Fluegge's request, to refute the signal role of the phagocyte, and he used the strategy that the leukocyte was a scavenger of already-damaged bacteria. Nuttall noted in the frog model that as many bacilli degenerated outside leukocytes as within, and he further complained of the inefficient phagocytic destructive process. In vitro, by observing anthrax in a thermostated microscope cabinet, Nuttall saw that the bacteria degenerated in serum alone, although he confirmed that killing was most efficient in whole blood that contained leukocytes. But he concluded, having examined several species, body fluids, and conditions that humoral factors played the crucial immunological role:

154

Without attempting to explain the antibacterial attributes of animal fluids, we can conclude with certainty that the destruction of the bacilli is not caused by the activity of the leukocytes. . . . It seems that the bacilli absorbed by leukocytes are not in their normal condition, and that the antibacterial agency is found in the surrounding liquid. The parallelisms, which in most of the experiments consist of the rapidity of the degeneration and the ingestion by leucocytes, support my assumption. The faster the degeneration appears, the faster the bacilli are taken up by leucocytes. If the degeneration is slow, the life energy of the leukocytes becomes lame and fades, and engulfment is only possibly in very small amounts. (4, Bibel, p. 165)

Metchnikoff noted that Nuttall's results and his own (5) were fundamentally opposed concering the ability of defibrinated blood to kill anthrax. In *Immunity in Infective Diseases* (6, pp. 150–152), Metchnikoff summarized supporting studies of his own position and in 1901 published a final rebuttal that again denied the bactericidal capacity of serum to kill anthrax, but he affirmed that a macerated preparation of microphages (neutrophils), but not macrophages, were efficiently bactericidal. Metchnikoff explained the effectiveness of serum as due to escaped leukocyte "ferments," a claim he reiterates in several contexts of his rebuttal:

The bactericidal substance, then, is essentially some substance which remains inside the uninjured phagocytes in the living animal but which escapes from these cells when they are injured, either in the body of the animal or outside in the blood withdrawn from the organism. (6, p. 193)

The first studies of leukocyte killing in the presence of specific antiserum were performed by Joseph Denys and J. Leclef, followed by Leon Marchand and Mennes between 1895 and 1898 (7–9). Almoth E. Wright was the first to quantify this phenomenon and strongly advocated its potential therapeutic importance (10). The so-called resolution of the humoralist and cellularist positions by showing their respective roles in the setting of enhanced killing in the presence of opsonins was popularized by Wright after 1903, although Metchnikoff acknowledged the stimulatory capacity of sensitized serum on phagocytic function in the case of acquired immunity.

We are thus compelled to accept the theory of an influence of protective serums not only on the micro-organisms but also on the organism of the animal into which they are introduced. As this influence manifests itself in the form of a strong phagocytosis, it is only natural that we should attribute it to the existence of a stimulating action of the serums of vaccinated animals on the phagocytes of the normal animals. The detailed analysis of the mechanism of the immunity acquired as the result of the injection of these serums, as we shall attempt to prove . . ., in many cases confirms this view. (6, p. 271)

In the case of natural (e.g., presensitized) immunity, he attributed no influence to humoral factors:

The phagocytes enter into a struggle against the micro-organisms and rid the animal organism of them without requiring any previous help on the part of the body fluids. Phagocytosis, exercised against living and virulent micro-organisms, is sufficient to ensure natural immunity. The bactericidal power of the serum, which for a long time served as the basis for a humoral theory of immunity, represents merely an artificial property, developed in consequence of the setting free of the microcytase of the leucocytes that have become disintegrated after the blood has been drawn. The agglutinative power of the normal fluids of the body plays no important part in the natural immunity. (6, p. 206)

Metchnikoff's hypothetical position that escaped ferments accounted for humoral immune factors and therefore of only secondary interest was in response to the 1890 studies of Behring and Kitasato, who demonstrated that serum factor(s) neutralized the toxins of tetanus and diptheria (11, 12). Although Pasteur had successfully vaccinated animals with attenuated bacteria (13), and Henry Sewall had achieved immunity to snake venom by gradual increase in dosage (14), the studies of Behring and Kitasato were unique in demonstrating (a) the protective capacity of immune serum in vivo and (b) the transference of that protection to another. The tetanus study (11), parallel to the one published by Behring alone on diptheria antitoxin (12), showed that cell-free serum conferred protection when it was either injected into a susceptible animal or the toxin was pretreated with the serum vaccine. The antitoxin was demonstrated to be stable and could be harvested only from immune animals. The experimental design employed an immunized rabbit, who was exposed to increasing doses of bacterial culture and was able to tolerate either tetanus bacilli or toxin injections at a dose twenty times that which would kill an unimmunized animal. Carotid blood of the immunized animal was injected intraperitoneally into mice, who twenty-four hours later were inoculated with tetanus bacilli. Control animals died within thirty-six hours, whereas the passively immunized animals suffered no ill effects. They showed tolerance was rendered by the serum component, that it could be used therapeutically after infection, and that its protective activity was directed against the bacterial exotoxin. The excitement of the potential of serum therapy was vindicated by successful treatment of a child the next year.

Metchnikoff's first counterargument, a position he took at the International Congress of Hygiene in London in 1891, rested upon viewing Behring's findings: "already accepted by everyone [as] a special [rather] than as a general phenomenon" (15, p. 531). But the debate flared when Behring extrapolated his findings to all cases of acquired immunity, to which Metchnikoff countered by demonstrating the limits of the humoral hypothesis in showing that immunity of rabbits against hog cholera did not generate protective serum factors (16). This demonstration—at least to Metchnikoff's satisfaction—proved that the bactericidal process was not dependent on humors and led Metchnikoff to conclude that a nebulous anti-infective property arose from stimulation of the phagocyte. In this context, he chose to interpret Richard Pfeiffer's cholera immunization studies (17) (showing humoral anti-infective properties but lacking antitoxic properties) as vindication of the cellularist position, by again invoking a cellular origin for these protective factors; for instance, he immediately embraced Buechner's suggestion that the alexines (which Metchnikoff termed *macrocytase* and Ehrlich later termed *complement*) were leukocyte products, elaborated during their defensive action. The general notion that humoral factors were escaped (i.e., secondary to leukocyte damage) or secreted phagocyte products remained the primary cellularist position throughout the polemic. In his scheme, immune humoral factors (what were later understood as complement and antibody) were classified with leukocyte ferments, including clotting and anticoagulating factors, digestive enzymes (i.e., amylase), and oxidases (for summary, see pp. 95–105, n 6). As noted, Metchnikoff maintained that these various factors were either secreted during the phagolysis process or released as an artefact when blood coagulated and serum prepared. It is noteworthy that when Pfeiffer, in 1894, cited Metchnikoff's counterargument in his famous cholera peritonitis paper (18) (discussed later), he naturally focused on the argument of least legitimacy: when Metchnikoff proposed that immunizing serum served as a specific irritant on the leukocyte, which then again was the final mediator of the microbicidal process, the hypothesis rested on no direct experimental data. Of course, Metchnikoff was ultimately correct: certain serum factors are generated by immune cells, but the argument was inferential and no significant research program attempted to establish that position. It is probably the best example of *ad hoc* fortifications that eventually were overpowered by the scientific course immunology chose to pursue.

We should note that Metchnikoff was received with cheers at the 1891 congress and that he did not stand alone (19). The most deliberate opinions conjured that more than one mechanism of immunity might be operative and the phagocytosis theory was not rendered obsolete by Behring's results. Lister, in his report of the proceedings remarked:

> The theory of immunity propounded by Metchnikoff did not exclude the possibility of there being other means of protecting the organism, but it affirmed that phago-cytosis had a wider sphere of action and was more efficacious than any other. It seemed to explain all the facts, and was, moreover, eminently suggestive.... Far from being shaken by the theories which were opposed to it, this theory of Metch-nikoff had gained by the opposition with which it met, and that was a guarantee of its soundness. (19)

But Metchnikoff, as we noted, took a highly defensive position, and we must acknowledge that he made no substantive scientific contributions as he defended his theory for the next ten years. In fact, his creative contributions to the development of immunology essentially ceased by the mid-1880s.

We must now turn to the core issue separating Metchnikoff from his detractors. The crucial statement of the Behring–Kitasato paper made in reference to Metch-nikoff's studies, condemns him as a vitalist and implicitly suggests a chemicoreduc-tive approach quite distinct from the cellularist's.

> Aside from the studies on phagocytosis, which seek to explain immunity in terms of the *vital activities* [emphasis added] of the cells, others have considered the bacteri-cidal action of the blood and the adaptation of the animal body to the toxin. (11, Brock, p. 138)

In reconstructing the debate against Metchnikoff, we must recall that the basis of the humoralist attack did not concern issues of specificity that became the focus of serol-ogy of a later period. What is glaring as a missing element is how the humors iden-tified their targets for destruction. In fact, during the nascent scientific debate, this crucial question of recognition was not explicitly formulated neither by Metchnikoff nor by his critics. One might argue that there was an implicit understanding of spec-ificity in terms of acquired immunity attained either by natural infection or by the development of vaccines (i.e., by Pasteur and his coworkers against fowl cholera, anthrax, and rabies), but the formal scientific problem did not exist until the mid-

1890s. Self versus nonself forms the basic biological axis of homeostatic control with the environment, nutritive/digestive activities, and preservation of self-integrity against pathogen invasion. Eat or be eaten was extrapolated by Metchnikoff to the theory of immunity, but the formulation of the basis of recognition as a scientific problem awaited others. The main attack, initially made by the Baumgarten school, centered on accusations of teleology and vitalism. Metchnikoff denied both charges, vigorously. As we noted, Behring characterized the phagocytosis theory as invoking vital activities, and he must have understood an active response of leukocytes as somehow autonomous. (What accounted for the acquired immunity-mediated by his humoral factors is not asked.) In invoking a cellular response on behalf of the host, Metchnikoff risked such accusation within a teleological orientation that was being rejected by a new reductionism in biology. He was sensitive to such attacks.

Metchnikoff was prepared for this accusation that had been hurled at him since his first presentation of the phagocytosis theory. Thus in the spring of 1891, shortly after Behring's December 1890 paper, Metchnikoff prepared a series of lectures at the Pasteur Institute that formed the basis of his first comprehensive summary statement of the phagocytic theory, *Lectures on the Comparative Pathology of Inflammation* (20). In the final chapter of that work, he dealth with the twin accusations of teleology and vitalism. Carl Fraenkel argued that the phagocytosis theory presupposed psychical activity to the leukocyte. Metchnikoff instead of refuting the charge, embraced it! He placed the "sensibility of the phagocytes" as the primordial expression of "psychical activities of man," a view that allegedly followed from the evolutionary process, that is, one cannot "maintain that the psychical acts of the higher animal are fundamentally different in their nature from the more simple phenomena peculiar to the lower organisms" (20, p. 193). He then turned to the charge of invoking a teleological argument, by again citing the evolutionary doctrine of preserved characteristics reflecting successful survival function:

> In consequence of this natural selection the useful characteristics, including those required for inflammatory reaction, have been established and transmitted, and we need not invoke the assistance of a designed adaptation to a predestined end, as we should from the teleological point of view. (20, p. 193)

Host defense is but a by-product of the digestive process employed by unicellular organisms. The basic process of the amoeboid leukocyte is the same, but it now takes place in the milieu of a complex organism, not the suspension of the sea. For Metchnikoff, the comparative zoologist, the harmony of this vision sustained him through all the experimental anomalies or, as others viewed them, contradictions. Precisely in the failure of the phagocyte would Metchnikoff argue the incontestable evidence of this expression of evolution's process:

> But the curative force of nature, the most important element of which is the inflammatory reaction, is not yet perfectly adapted to its object. . . . The phagocytic mechanism has not yet reached its highest stage of development and is still undergoing improvement. (20, p. 194)

Later, in *Immunity* (1901), Metchnikoff did not alter his position, but attempted to subsume his vitalism into an innocuous aspect of leukocyte function:

The theory of phagocytosis seeks to establish the part played by these cells in the destruction of micro-organisms. It maintains that the vital manifestation of the phagocytes, irritability, mobility, and voracity, constitutes an essential factor in ridding the animal of micro-organisms. (6, p. 539)

What Metchnikoff called the "stimulant action on the part of the phagocytes" (6, p. 532) was but an inherited property of their intracellular digestive role in early phylogeny; thus, the old accusation of invoking a teleological function was by 1901 simply brushed aside again by Metchnikoff's old assertion that not he, but evolution, had imprinted its mark on persistent activity characterized by phagocyte feeding behavior and a new assumed role in host defense. The earlier polemic reflected his fresh ardor, and his earlier impassioned comments in *Lectures* (1891) were probably closer to his true sentiments. But by 1901, he must have wearied of the battle.

Pfeiffer and Bordet

The third major assault by the humoralists on the cellularist position was Pfeiffer's phenomenon described by Richard Pfeiffer in 1894, then scientific director of the Koch Institute in Berlin. The reaction was found in studies of experimental cholera peritonitis, where a loss of mobility, granular degeneration and subsequent dissolution of bacteria within minutes was observed following their injection into the peritoneal cavity of immunized animals (18). He claimed the reaction was independent of leukocytes:

Immediately after the injection, all the vibrios stopped moving. After 10 minutes, many granules and swollen vibrios but almost no leukocytes were seen. After 20 minutes of the infection, all the vibrios disappeared and many granules remained. Approximately 95% of the granules were extracellular and 5% were in the protoplasm of the leukocytes. Before my eyes, the cholera vibrios were lysed free of phagocytic influence. . . . I obtained the same results with a passively immunized guinea pig. (18, Bibel, p. 199)

Learning that the bactericidal event was best obtained in vivo, Pfeiffer concluded:

The animal body plays a major and active role. It *reacts to the stimulus* [emphasis added] of the vibrios under the influence of the immune substances in serum to produce the bactericidal activity (18, Bibel, p. 199)

A few decades prior to this argument, Virchow's position against humoralism actually represented a revolt of the localist vision of medical theory against the holist view. Metchnikoff's argument with the humoralists can be considered in certain respects as a sequel of that previous dialogue: Metchnikoff presented the cellularist localist position, arguing for a sovereign activity of a certain cellular group; his humoralist opponents presented a holist position, defending the sovereignty of the organism over its constitutents. We argued that beyond Metchnikoff's immunological ideas, there was a very special formulation of the problem of organismic integrity. But who truly appreciated this novelty of Metchnikoff's thesis? Considering the argument only upon the axis of localists versus holists, Metchnikoff's position might appear more teleological than the position of his opponents. After all, Metchnikoff attributed to a group of cells the protective function in regard to the whole (i.e., the responsibility for organismic integrity). This seemingly means that not the present state of interactions between the elements of the whole system determines the behavior of the protective cell but that the interactions are somehow ordained by the idea of the desirable whole, that is, they are determined by the idealized future self: in short, an ideal whole would determine the protective functions of the amoeboid mesodermic cells. Not surprisingly, accusations of a naive teleology ceaselessly plagued the phagocytosis theory, despite Metchnikoff's attempts to dissociate teleology from his fervent arguments with the chemomechanical assault. These attempts were considered as only self-justifying and but another manifestation of his theory's weakness.

On the other hand, the holists, to deprive any constituent of its sovereignty, were satisfied in considering the part as only a particular mechanism, that is, the embodiment of a particular organismic function. The ancient metaphysical question concerning the essence of the whole that used the parts as its tools was pushed aside, irrelevant to the scientific thinking of the time. Included was any account of the activity that used the structure in question as its tools. In full accordance with the *Zeitgeist,* this scientific consciousness concentrated on describing function in physical-chemical terms. Under these circumstances, any reference to immunity in terms of activity was inevitably considered as loaded with (at least) excessive terminology. After all, if we are interested in a mechanism of a function, what kind of additional meaning could be carried by the expression, "the active immune response," as compared to the other expression, "the immune response?" The word *active* signified in this context apparently nothing but a relic of an ancient metaphysical position.

It is not surprising that Metchnikoff's early critics (e.g., Baumgarten) rejected, as a rule, any reference to "activity" as well as to the very concept of a special protective function. In the rejected metaphysics, the concept of self-protection coincided with the concept of organismic "wholeness," the *physis.* Hence, there was no room for a subsystem that assumed responsibility for the whole. Now, when arguing with Metchnikoff about concrete physiological (or chemical) processes, his holist opponents recalled this old terminology concerning *activity* and *protection,* which implicates their tacit (often unconscious) agreement with Metchnikoff that immunity could be discussed in terms of a special protective subsystem or special subset of protective functions among the whole set of physiological functions. The old metaphysics, which allowed reference to a protective activity, equated that activity with the whole. It did not allow a special mechanism (a special subsystem) of protection, but proposed, actually, only two options: either to refer to a protecting activity, ignoring the mechanism, or to consider a mechanism that ignored any interpretation of its possible relation to active protection. Combining these two perspectives in the discussion of protective mechanisms meant to actually accept the radical metaphysical shift that, apparently, had not been recognized by the majority of dissenters. Pfeiffer's phrase, "reacts to the simulus," in connection with his remark on "an active role" of the animal body in the immune response may well signify the acceptance of Metchnikoff's construction. No longer is active host defense a foreign concept, for its basic intuitions in the discussion of special processes of active protection are now common vocabulary. If in Baumgarten's critique, we witnessed the rejection of

Metchnikoff's central thesis of an active protective mechanism, then Pfeiffer's lexicon betrays that the scientific validity of the topic had now been recognized as self-evident.

To what extent did Metchnikoff's critics consciously engage his principle hypothesis, that is, the issue of active host defense? We have discussed the prehumoral position of, for example, Baumgarten, Ziegler, Emmerich, Fluegge, and so on, none of whom either offered an alternative immunolgical theory or understood this basic concept that served as the foundation not only of Metchnikoff's theory but also as the very basis of the modern concept of immunity. In the establishment of the humoral position, we note that Nutall's initial study was formulated in an attempt to refute the phagocyte's role as key to host defense. The underlying theoretical construct of those experiments is obscure: on the one hand, Nuttall (under Fluegge's sponsorship) sought to experimentally discredit Metchnikoff, but once doubt was raised concerning the role of the phagocyte, the mechanism of defense was left uncharted. Prior to 1890, the fundamental basis of host defense was left as a passive phenomenon: factors found in serum were protective, their origin and mode of action were obviously left for future study. We might consider Behring's experiments the true beginning of the humoral immunological theory, for in its experimental design, the implicit process of *induced* immunity suggested an active response. It is noteworthy that no explicit mention is made of that issue; in fact Behring concluded his paper with an offhand (ironic?) quote from Goethe, "Blut ist ein ganz besonderer Saft" ["Blood is a very unusual fluid."] We might well sympathize with Metchnikoff as Behring scoffs at the vitalistic elements of the phagocyte theory. However, with Pfeiffer's report, we find an explicit reference to an *active reaction.* It is only on the scaffold of active host defense that the cellular versus humoral theories of immunity become cogent. Metchnikoff would no longer be arguing in a monologue, but a true controversy over protective *mechanism* became dominant. Thus the importance of Pfeiffer's explicit allusion to the reactive component of the immune response must be emphasized.

The repercussions of Pfeiffer's assault on the cellularists resulted in typical rebuttal: Metchnikoff gave no quarter. Again, as he responded to Behring, Metchnikoff asserted Pfeiffer's phenomenon was observed only when (a) phagocytes were damaged and conversely (b) in body cavities where phagocytes were absent, the reaction did not occur (21). Out of this controversy, a more fruitful solution was offered by Jules Bordet, who as a member of Metchnikoff's laboratory, attempted to mimic Pfeiffer's experiment in vitro; in the process, Bordet differentiated the effects of complement (Buckner's alexine) and immunoglobin (sensibilising substance) (22, 23). As noted by Bibel, there is a quintessential irony that the single most significant contribution to serology and humoral immunity of this period came from Metchnikoff's protégé working in his laboratory (24)! Bordet drew a parallel between Pfeiffer's phenomenon and Buechner's earlier observation of immune hemolysis (25). Buechner had as early as 1892 considered the hemolysin the same as the serum bactericidal substance, a factor he called alexine. (Ehrlich mistakenly believed a single serum might contain several alexines, or complements, confusing the immunological specificity of immunoglobulin with presumed selectivity of complement [26].) Bordet established the dual factors of humoral immunity (complement and a sensitizing factor), the nonspecificity of complement that acted only on a sensitized target, and the parallel nature of hemolysis and bacteriolysis.

This 1898 article (24) served as a sequel to that of 1895 (22) in which Bordet had shown that immune serum contained two factors responsible for bacterial killing. In this study, Bordet demonstrated that (a) serum from immunized animals mimicked Pfeiffer's phenomenon in vitro, that is, the serum, when added to a bacterial (cholera) suspension, was microbicidal; (b) serum heated to fifty-five degrees centrigrade lost its killing power, but agglutination was unaffected; (c) fresh serum from nonimmune animals restored killing to heated serum; (d) these two factors were only "slightly bactericidal" alone. He then understood Pfeiffer's phenomenon as sensitized serum (immunoglobulin) activating complement for the bactericidal event. He was struck by the parallelism with Buechner's hemolysin studies, wherein the same distinction between clumping (agglutination) and lysis of erythrocytes or bacteria were evident. Thus in 1898, Bordet endeavored to demonstrate the universality of Pfeiffer's phenomenon with the hemolyzed erythrocyte system by injecting rabbit erythrocytes and heated antisera into the peritoneal cavity of unsensitized guinea pigs (24); after sensitizing guinea pigs with defibrinated rabbit blood, the immune serum was observed to agglutinate and lyse rabbit erythrocytes, a property lost if the serum was heated to fifty-five degrees centrigrade and restored with fresh nonimmune guinea pig or autologous serum.

Begging the question of the source of these humoral factors, Bordet's study inexorably shifted the focus of immunology to serology. Although the two disciplines do not entirely overlap (27), the ease and sensitivity of erythrocyte agglutination and lysis offered a powerful tool to probe issues of specificity. In fact, the resolution of the respective humoralist and cellularist positions only was mediated, in part, by the description of Almoth Wright and Stewart Douglas that humoral opsonins enhanced phagocytosis; that finding was reproduced with difficulty and led to a relatively minor access to the mechanism of immune effector function. It was truly Bordet's early decipherment of the Pfeiffer phenomenon that directed immunology into the new area of recognition. But Bordet reapplied Metchnikoff's predominant lesson. In his concluding statement concerning the parallelism between hemolysis and defensive immunity, Bordet reiterated Metchnikoff's masterful insight:

> What can be concluded from the group of analogies? It may be concluded that the properties which anti-cholera serum possesses have not been created by the body for merely an anti-infectious purpose, if we may so express it, but are due simply to initiate against the vibrio some preexisting functions that may be applied, if circumstances lend themselves, to some by no means dangerous elements, such as red blood cells. We can, in fact, inject into animals not just vibrios but very different corpuscles, red blood cells, incapable of constituting a serious danger for the organism, to obtain a serum that affects these bodies exactly as the cholera serum acts on the vibrio. *These properties do not arise spontaneously to defend against microbes, any more than phagocytosis, the hub of immunity, does not owe its existence to the struggle against an infectious agent. One of the most significant conclusions that is derived from the work of Metchnikoff is that immunity is a special case of intracellular digestion* [emphasis added]. (24, Bibel, p. 204)

Bordet, in one gesture, thwarted the lingering accusations of teleology directed against Metchnikoff's theory and at the same time methodologically oriented modern immunology from a descriptive discipline to a quantitative science. His studies closely approximated Ehrlich's standardization of antitoxins (1897) and the side chain theory (1900), which together swung immunology to a new commitment, immunochemistry (28). Metchnikoff was left to apply his phagocytosis theory to different bacteriological issues (especially syphilis) and to problems of senility, a problem with which he became obsessed. His active scientific career ebbed and his celebrity status rose as he popularized his philosophy of orthobiosis (29). But by 1908, when he shared the Nobel Prize with Ehrlich, Metchnikoff's scientific achievements were well recognized: the phagocyte was generally accepted as an element in immune effector function. But Metchnikoff maintained a more radical position: the host, through the vehicle of the phagocyte, asserts its integrity and strives for (in his terms) internal harmony, by *active mechanisms,* of which, as Bordet so clearly recognized, the immunological reaction against a pathogen was but one incidental example. That Metchnikoff failed to direct the tide of immunological research for the next half-century is clearly documented, but from our vantage, we must inquire: Why?

Ehrlich

Although Bordet seems to have accepted the principal Metchnikovian lesson, the ascendent wave of immunochemistry largely bypassed further exploration of the basic conceptual notion of active host response as a *biological* phenomenon. It is difficult, if not unfair, to assign a particular investigator or set of experiments as the fulcrum by which the vector of investigation swayed from immunopathology to the biochemistry of immunity. The key figures of the period reflected the ambivalence of immunology's conceptual focus. Ehrlich, who had begun his immunology research in Koch's laboratory (1890) by studying the antibody response to the plant toxins abrin and ricin (30) established the first practical method for standardization of diptheria toxin and antitoxin (31). In that seminal paper of 1897, he also first proposed the side chain theory of antibody formation. Here then, in the very same manuscript were seminal contributions to quantitative immunochemistry and the biology of the immune response. The side chain theory was an elaboration of Ehrlich's central thesis that various affinities were exhibited by chemicals, nutrients, or in this case antitoxins for target biologicals, that is, cells in the case of histochemical staining, chemotherapy for infectious microorganisms, and in the case of immune reactions, specific receptors for toxins. It was, in a sense applied chemistry. The function of the organism as a whole was not at issue; a grand synthesis of homeostasis was not of concern; the nature of how immune substances were elaborated or their pathological consequences were not questions that Ehrlich considered primary. His chief purpose was to apply *chemical* principles to biological phenomena in order to provide the vexing solution of quantitating toxins and their respective antitoxins. In laborious research, Ehrlich established (within a one percent error!) that

A molecule of toxin combines with a definite and unalterable quantity of antibody.
 ... It must be assumed that this ability to combine with antitoxin is attributable to the presence in the toxin complex of a specific group of atoms with a maximum

specific affinity to another group of atoms in the antitoxin complex, the first fitting the second easily, as a key does a lock, to quote Emile Fisher's well-known simile.

The compelling need to assume the presence of such matching groups in the toxin and the antitoxin, might well provide a clue to the way in which one might most easily comprehend the mysterious process of the origin of the antitoxins.

Most investigators probably accept Behring's view that antibodies are products of the living organism, and not products derived from the transformation of the injected toxin. The explanation, however, of the nature of such a reaction presents serious difficulties. If a chemist were offered the task of finding a physiologically and chemically inert antidote to an alkaloid or some other poison, which antidote must neither destroy the poison nor precipitate it in an insoluble form, but must, nevertheless, render any given quantity of it harmless, he would certainly refuse the task as chimerical.

Nevertheless, the living organism can perform this task easily, often within the course of a few days, and with a multiplicity of toxins. To attribute what could be called inventive activity to the body or to its cells, enabling them to produce new groups of atoms as required, would involve a return to the concepts current in the days of [an obsolete] natural philosophy. Our knowledge of cell function and especially of synthetic processes would lead us rather to assume that in the formation of antibodies, we are dealing with the enhancement of a normal cell function, and not with the creation at need of new groups of atoms. Physiological analogues of the group of the specifically combining antibodies must exist beforehand in the organism or in its cells. (31, English trans. p. 114)

What was true for a toxin would hold in parallel for antibodies: toxins bind to cellular side chains (now called receptors) by chemical avidity and, in turn, bind to antibody side chains by the same general process.

The side chain theory held three tenents: (a) antibodies were normal cell receptors, ready, on a best-fit basis, to bind antigen; (b) antibody specificity resided in chemical complementarity; and (c) antigen–antibody binding was a chemical and irreversible process. Following binding, the hypothesis predicted that the toxin would be assimilated and the receptor then freed for renewed function or regenerated; with massive toxin insult, cells presumably overcompensated for loss of cell-bound receptors and produced excess quantities, which would be shed, thus accounting for humoral antibody. This theory was closely related to Carl Weigert's (Ehrlich's cousin) law of overcompensation, which, in turn, had been applied to various pathological phenomena (32). Ehrlich's formulation was presentient in many crucial respects to our current theory: (a) the concept of receptor has had enormous importance in all areas of communicative cell biology; (b) the antigenic selective aspect of the theory was successfully revived in a modern version during the 1950s, with the clonal selection theory expounded by Jerne, Burnet, Talmage, and Lederberg (33); and (c) immunological specificity, conferred by the unique three-dimentional structure of antibody, was later confirmed. Soon, discovery of a plethora of antigens seemed to demand various forms of an instructional theory for constituting appropriate antibody affinities (34); in 1905, Karl Landsteiner suggested that novel products must account for immune recognition (35). And on the other hand, the diverse manifestations of immune phenonena, for example, agglutination, the precipitation reaction, and immune hemolysis required Ehrlich to present complicating *ad hoc* hypotheses: a first-order receptor (haptine) possessing a binding site for toxic antigens; a second-order receptor having two binding sites—one for the antigen, another for agglutination and precipitation (the zymophore group); and a third-order receptor accounting for binding of complement (36).

Of the various problems associated with Ehrlich's seminal theory, the criticism of Bordet is most crucial. On one level, they differed on the nature of the antigen-antibody bond: Bordet argued for an adsorptive, as opposed to chemical, binding (37). He used the widely used concept of "colloidal" interactions, which he viewed as reversible and implicitly less restrictive. They also differed on the mechanism of complement fixation and immune hemolysis; Erhlich's theory (we now know argues incorrectly for multiple complements with differing specificities) was ultimately eclipsed by Bordet's championing a single complement activity (38). Irrespective of the relative values of their argument about immune specificity, it seems clear that for Bordet the overall issues concerned the secondary physiological consequences of the immune reaction, not the nature of the primary antigen–antigen bond. In the argument over the nature of complement, Bordet's studies led to a series of important pathologically oriented discoveries in tuberculosis and whooping cough (37). Bordet (and Genjou, his brother-in-law) proved the unitarian view of complement in 1901 by showing that in the consumption of complement for bacteriolysis, none was left for hemolysis (38). Demonstrating uniformity of complement for both processes was crucial for the development of serology and, thus, paradoxically helped establish immunochemistry on a firm methodological basis. But Bordet was clearly an heir to the Metchnikovian orientation toward explicating pathological processes; viewing the immune reaction as a particular case of those processes that establish organismic integrity, cause–effect relationships were to be elucidated in the province of the physiology and chemistry, but the context and *meaning* of the chemical reaction was paramount to the chemistry itself.

In Ludwig Fleck's analysis of the development of the first serologic test for syphilis, he traces those studies as a direct result of these complement experiments (39). The Wassermann test, published in 1906, was one of the significant clinical applications of the newly emergent concept of immunologically oriented disease testing, and the assignment of immune reactants to pathophysiological states. Of these, the description of anaphylaxis in 1902 (40), the Arthus reaction in 1903 (41), and serum sickness in 1906 (42) suggested abnormal immune regulation as the basis of their respective pathologies. These conditions were regarded as "allergy," or altered reactivity. For example, that autoantibodies (antibodies directed at autologous tissue) were not a laboratory artifact, was first shown in 1904 by Julius Donath and Landsteiner. They demonstrated that a rare hemolytic anemia, paroxysmal cold hemoglobinuria, was caused by an autoantibody that binds to the subject's erythrocytes at low body temperatures and initiates complement-mediated lysis on warming (43). Arthur Silverstein notes that these early successes of immunopathology were followed by what he calls the "Dark Ages of Autoimmunity," for following the first decade of the twentieth century, little progress was made (or attention paid) in this area of investigation for forty years. The pendulum swing from a biological to a chemical orientation was reversed in the 1960s when observations in the diverse areas of tissue transplantation, tolerance, immunodeficiency and immunopathology demanded a more biological orientation (44).

Again, Ehrlich is viewed as having pivotal influence. He expounded the concept of "horror autotoxicus" as dysteleological (45)—"It would be exceedingly dysteleologic, if in this situation self-poisons, autotoxins, were formed" (see 1, pp. 160ff)—which is perhaps the clearest contrast between Metchnikoff and the immunochemists of the next generation. At the same time, Metchnikoff published *Immunity*, Ehrlich viewed with alarm the prospect of the immune reaction acting "against the organism's own elements":

> The organism possesses certain contrivances by means of which the immunity reaction, so easily produced by all kinds of cells, is prevented from acting against the organism's own elements and so giving rise to autotoxins ... so that we might be justified in speaking of a "horror autotoxicus" of the organism. These contrivances are naturally of the highest importance for the individual. (46, p. 253)

Silverstein cites Dietlinde Goltz as noting that Ehrlich did not disallow the formation of autoantibodies, only that they were prevented from acting (47). The general community of immunologists misinterpreted horror autotoxicus as prohibiting autoantibodies, altogether (48); that observation in itself is most revealing.

Why was autoimmunity viewed as dysteleological? From Metchnikoff's point of view, the immune reaction was based on warring disharmonious centers: the immune response arose from the disharmonic state. For Metchnikoff, phagocyte surveillance of disease, damage, or developmental metamorphosis was integral to "physiological inflammation," and immune mediation was but a special case. If antibodies were, in fact, only facilitators of these processes, then such autoantibodies were expected. In fact, search for such factors in Metchnikoff's laboratory were of great interest.

The experimental background of this issue was based on the first demonstration of an anti-antibody, that is, an antibody generated against another antibody. Two reports in 1898 (49) of an antibody against a hemolytic toxin of eel serum suggested to both Bordet and Ehrlich (with Julius Morgenroth) that a similar neutralizing antibody might be generated against a hemotoxic antibody found in the immunized serum of animals sensitized with erythrocytes. Experimental proof was shown by both groups (36, 50) and the data used for their respective arguments concerning the nature of complement (discussed earlier, and essentially resolved by Bordet's 1901 experiments). Because the studies employed whole blood, sensitization was not restricted to a particular antibody of specified activity, and the heterogeneous results were difficult to interpret (51). But each group found blocking antibody that inhibited the hemolytic activity of the immunogen: Ehrlich interpreted the data as evidence for multiple amboceptors and multiple complements; Bordet argued for single-complement activity because his rabbit anti-guinea pig hemolytic serum neutralized complement activity of guinea pigs, but no other species. Alexander Besredka, Bordet's colleague at the Pasteur Institute and Metchnikoff's adoring protégé, pursued the issue. Based on the logical extension of Metchnikoff's theory, he viewed existence of autoantibodies as the norm. These self-destructive factors were then postulated as being held in check by an anti-antibody to minimize self-attack (52). It is interesting that in 1901, when this proposal was presented, there was as yet no direct evidence of physiological or pathological autoantibodies, but when the Donath–Landsteiner hemolytic antibody was described in 1904, this theory accounted for that disease by the absence of the regulating autoantibody (35, 53). The weak experimental basis for Besredka's hypothesis has been well summarized by Silverstein:

Besredka justified his thesis by citing a series of experiments on hemolytic antibodies formed in species A against the erythrocytes of species B, utilizing complement from any other species. He showed that A anti-B serum lyses the washed erythrocytes of B, but that the addition of normal B serum inhibits this hemolytic action. However, sera from other species (C,D, etc.) exhibit no similar inhibitor effect. Furthermore, B's serum will inhibit the hemolysis of an anti-B-erythrocyte serum formed in any other species as well. From these data, Besredka concluded (1) that all normal sera contain anti-antibodies that protect their own erythrocytes from immune hemolysis; (2) that he had demonstrated the specificity of these anti-antibodies; (3) that the anti-antibody is not an anti-complement; and (4) that Ehrlich was wrong about the multiplicity of amboceptors—all anti-B hemolysins are identical, since they are all inhibited by the anti-antibody normally present in every B serum. (51, p. 264)

The argument from our modern perspective seems highly speculative, but then Ehrlich arrived at a similar position from the side chain theory. Again quoting Silverstein:

In 1899, Morgenroth had shown that animals inoculated with the enzyme rennin would invariably produce anti-rennin antibodies. But rennin is presumably one of the normal constituents of the animal's digestive tract, so the formation of an "auto-antibody" against a self-constituent could conceivably compromise the well-being of the host. Erhlich and Morgenroth returned to this question the following year and proposed a thought-experiment to explain the apparent paradox. Here is the logical extension of the side-chain theory in its most elegant form.

Suppose that a hypothetical antigen α is injected into an animal, then two consequences are possible according to Erhlich and Morgenroth. If the animal lacks group α, then the specific site α on the injected antigen will seek out its corresponding receptor on the surface of the host's cells, react with the combining sites on these receptors, and thus stimulate the formation of anti-α antibodies. This is the usual course of the immune response. Suppose, however, that the immunized animal possesses antigenic group α within its body, as is the case with rennin. Anti-α antibodies will still be formed, but these will now appear as "autoantibodies". But these circulating antibodies with combining sites specific for antigenic group α will themselves find cells with α receptors on their surface (i.e., presumably those cells responsible for the original production of that antigen). Such cells will be stimulated to produce additional α molecules for release into the circulation. But not only is α the original antigen, it is also functionally the autoanti-antibody able to combine specifically with the anti-α combining site to prevent its toxic action. Thus, an interactive network is established involving antigen, specific antibody, anti-antibody (= antigen), and so forth, all of which presumably reach a steady-state, self-regulated equilibrium to suppress autoimmune disease. (51, p. 265)

Despite the common conclusion that anti-autoantibodies were normally formed, Ehrlich projected this finding primarily as the means of thwarting a dysteleological condition, whereas Besredka (in fact, Metchnikoff) viewed phagocyte (immune) attack as normal, consistently teleological in the broader context of their true evolutionary function. Autoantibody in this latter case served as an opposing (in this case, harmonizing) the natural phagocyte activity. Thus, although the lesson of immune reactivity to pathogens and foreign insult was generally accepted by the immunological community by 1900, the metaphysical infrastructure of that understanding was certainly diverse. Beyond the different scientific traditions of descriptive biology versus chemicoreductionism, there resided a different orientation toward the basic teleological vector of the organism. Here we see Ehrlich invoking biological purpose in its most arcane form: How (or why) should an organism self-destruct? Metchnikoff had turned the question on its head: How (or why) are the disharmonious centers constituting the organism harmonized?

Metchnikoff and Ehrlich shared the Nobel Prize in 1908 "in recognition for their work on immunity," but to regard their concepts as complementary (as traditionally viewed) is an oversimplification. Ehrlich, in the first Harben Lecture, delivered in 1907, explicitly acknowledged Metchnikoff's dynamic scenario but offered an important alternate hypothesis.

> In the protean forms of the phenomena of immunity, of course, the action of haptines by no means excludes phagocytosis; destruction of the bacteria outside the cells and their assimilation by the phagocytes are processes which may take place alongside each other, and, by their simultaneous action, increase the protective power. A special proof of the importance of the study of haptines appears to me to be the fact that—as the opsonin theory, which we owe to Sir Almroth Wright, has made more evident—specific haptine reactions form the basis also of phagocytosis, which Metchnikoff has studied in so masterly a manner. The opsonins and cytotropic substances render the bacteria liable to attack by the phagocytes, and here we have a field in which humoral and cellular processes meet. One cannot, however, say that the possible causes of immunity are confined to haptine action and phagocytosis. Perhaps the athreptic view, by which differences of degree in avidity on the one side or on the other are presumed, is correct in many cases in which others are at work. (54, p. 117)

The athreptic view was a model of *passive* immunity! Ehrlich revived Pasteur's depletion theory by substituting the microbiologist's missing crucial element for growth, with an analogous defect—incapability of absorbing the essential nutrient. In this guise, Ehrlich proposed the concept of athrepsia, which he developed from his observations of cobra venom hemolysis and immune trypanosomicidal mechanisms, wherein resistance to destruction in both cases was understood as altered (lowered) affinity of the target receptors for the effector agents. What Metchnikoff understood as natural immunity, Ehrlich argued was only a starved condition:

> Probably the majority of so-called nonpathogenic micro-organisms, if introduced into the body of an animal, perish by this mechanism. It is not necessary to assume the presence of special poisons in the body, it suffices to suppose that the bacteria in question do not find the necessary means of existence in the body and therefore cannot multiply. This being the case, they cannot for any length of time remain alive in the body, for then the latter's defensive forces, its phagocytes, come into action and destroy the invaders in a nonspecific manner. (55, p. 123)

When dealing with pathogens, it was

> safer not to attribute too great an importance to athrepsia. But it is evident that micro-organisms can only be pathogenic for a certain animal if they find in it possibilities of nutrition. Yet, to my mind, quite a number of infections are characterised by the fact that the micro-organism, with the exception of only a few survivors, becomes athreptic. (55, p. 123)

He applied this concept to syphilis (lesions were found in the skin but not blood because of the localization of the nutritive factors), the change of virulence observed on the transfer of pathogens (e.g., streptococcus, smallpox) from one species to another, and finally to tumors.

> To my mind, the explanation of this phenomenon is as follows: every proliferation depends in the first place on the avidity of the cells for the nutritive substances. Normally, there are certain well-defined laws of distribution, which guarantee the proper working of the organic functions. The avidity of the tumor cells is increased, as compared with that of the body cells. The more energetically a tumour proliferates, the more powerfully does it attract the nutrient substances from the blood. In the case of a rapidly growing tumour it may therefore very easily occur that for such cells as are under very unfavourable conditions of nutrition, e.g., cells inoculated or metastatically carried away, there is an insufficient supply of nutrient substances, and that they therefore either perish from athrepsia or at least are unfavourably influenced in their growth. From this point of view it is also quite evident that slowly growing tumours can attain far greater dimensions than rapidly growing ones, since in the former the rate of consumption of nutrient matter, in spite of their size, is less than in the latter, and thus the entire organism is injured to a lesser extent. (55, p. 125)

The rejection of a mouse tumor implanted into a rat was explained by athreptic immune concepts:

> A far simpler and more natural explanation of all these phenomena is afforded by my concept of athrepsia. According to this, the mouse-tumour cells require for their growth not only the ordinary nutritive substances which the rat can also supply to them in ample quantity, but, besides that, some well-defined substance which is present only in the mouse organism. (55, p. 126)

Thus Ehrlich thought that the inability of certain tumors to grow in some animals was due to analogous exhausted nutritional requirements first postulated by Pasteur for bacteria: Tumors either failed to grow or regressed once the factors were depleted. He extended the side chain theory to bacteria and tumor cells, proposing that each had chemoreceptors for these growth factors. He even criticized Pasteur's original formulation by stating that a threshold level was required, not total depletion; the alternative was that the receptors atrophied. Tumors grew because they were more competitive for nutrients.

> It follows that the increased avidity of the cells for the food substances is the most important characteristic of the tumour cells. But this increase does not suffice to explain all the phenomena observed. Albrecht already insisted that for malignant tumours one must admit not only an increase but an alteration in the assimilation in such manner that the "structure materials", taken up from the surrounding media, must in some way be bound or laid up "until they had reached an amount sufficient for the division of the cells." Besides this increased food-absorption, the result of action of the receptors, remote chemiotactic effects must, to my mind, play an important role. (55, p. 127)

This hypothesis is in dramatic opposition to Metchnikoff's own musings of the time, when he viewed active phagocyte responses to diseased or altered tissue as the primary mechanism of host integrity. Metchnikoff admitted he did not know the "real nature" of malignant tumors, but regarded it "probable that the malignant tumors will soon come to be ranged with infectious diseases due to invasions by specific microbes" (56, p. 214). As such, he viewed cancer as arising secondary to the toxic influence of microbial substances that poisoned the host. So-called putrefaction in the alimentary tract supposedly accounted for the high incidence of cancer there (57), and his efforts to alter the microbial flora of the large intestine by substituting lactobacillus had a dramatic impact on the growth of the yogurt industry in France (58). His central theseis was that in a dynamic struggle between phagocytes and the more "noble" cells, the senile process (those general degradative phenomena) was hastened by microbial poisoning (57, 58, 59). The striking difference between Ehrlich and Metchnikoff in this seemingly tangential issue of cancer growth boldly illustrates their respective points of view.

Ehrlich now broadened the discussion of the host–parasite struggle by suggesting that the pathogen (microorganism, tumor) must find its proper ecological niche (modern parlance) to thrive on its own terms as well as to deal with the active immune rejection expected by the host for self-preservation.

> Thus in all cases the struggle lies between the adaptability of the parasite and that of the host. The one whose adaptability is the highest will become the victor.
>
> Of course this struggle is to a great extent influenced by indirect actions, consisting in the secretion by each antagonist of dissolved substances hostile to the vitality and receptivity of the other organism. On the part of the bacteria, these substances are the toxins and the dissolved intracellular substances; on the part of the body, the anti-substances.
>
> A further role is played by actions of a protective and defensive nature. Thus we have shown that bacteria congregate in those parts where they find the most favourable conditions of nutrition, whilst the organism, both by its phagocytes and by means of encapsulation, endeavours to render the pathogenic germs harmless and to eliminate them. You see, therefore, that this is a war waged in different spheres, but in which to every action there is a corresponding reaction. Three-fold battle is joined—in the sphere of variation of avidity, of variation of poison, and of localisation. (55, p. 129)

This would appear to be an echo of Metchnikoff's active host-pathogen struggle, but Ehrlich has added an important caveat—the dynamic immune battle is supplemented by passive processes—and he takes aim at those who would exclude athreptic function:

> Hence, an immunity of this type is simply explained as being due to the great energy of the cells of the body, which are able to appropriate nutritious substances for themselves, and in so doing to deprive parasites of them. The opposite condition must be due to a certain disposing influence, and immunity of the parasites must be a condition of the cause of infectivity. The bacterial cells may in the same way be immune against heptine substances, and may withstand the action of the serum.
>
> Thus there exist unstable relations between immunity and infection, and between parasite and host, relations which may depend on the most varying influences, and which lead up to the phenomena of reversible action, which calls for further study.
>
> One cannot, therefore, go to work in a one-sided way when analysing and judging the various forms of phenomena, but must carefully consider together all factors in question. (54, p. 117)

Ehrlich's thesis, in this discussion, is interesting in two regards: (a) he has again applied a simple chemical notion of avidity to explain a highly complex biological phenomenon, and (b) he assigns to *passive* athreptic immunity a central role in host–pathogen relationships. We will not dwell on the first issue, but it is of note that Ehrlich well recognized the unity of his own thinking:

As you can see, I have dealt with a number of apparently very different aspects of biology and pathology, which are, however, united by a common bond. What is operating is, in fact, a competition of the different entities for the nutrient material. (55, p. 127)

As to the role of athrepsis as part of the immune pantheon, we are struck by Ehrlich's assignment of a nutritive state to immunology at all. *Athrepsis,* as a term, was new, coined by Joseph Marie Jules Parrot in 1874 to describe malnutrition, especially in infants (60). The rising awareness of nutrition in health and disease and the concern to discover missing dietary factors was certainly in ascendancy. More fundamentally, application of chemical principles to biological phenomena was becoming the dominant scientific ethos of biology. Whether Ehrlich's concept of athrepsis has validity as a biological concept appears moot in its most general stance, namely, that pathogens may coexist with the host in a variety of parasitic relationships, even within phagocytes! (61), as a result of both passive and active behaviors. Metchnikoff also recognized this neutral state in his first *Daphnia* studies. The particulars of Ehrlich's argument have not proven useful, but we are addressing the broader issue as to how to place athrepsis in the same category with humoral and cellular immune function. The issue is simply whether athrepsis is a form of immunity. The question is more than semantic.

For Ehrlich, athrepsis fell under the rubric of immunity because it was simply an extension of the host–pathogen relationship. It arose quite consistently from the same general notion of affinities that gave rise to the side chain theory. Trypanosomes resisted arsenicals if their chemoreceptors had poor avidity for the poison; bird-pox would thrive in fowls [chickens] but not in pigeons because of the "loss of certain receptors which are absolutely necessary for nutrition" (55); syphilitic spirochetes found their nutrients in certain tissues, but not others, and so on. The simplest definition was that athreptic immunity results "from certain substances not being at the disposal of the parasite" (55). This truly is a passive theory in Metchnikovian terms; it does not replace active host mechanisms, that is, phagocyte defense or augmented antibody responses, but Ehrlich has added a second dimension to the immune reaction: the microorganism, by changing the avidity for critical substances, alters its susceptibility. In summary, both Ehrlich and Metchnikoff (61) recognized the dynamic struggle between host and pathogen, but the former viewed the issue in passive terms, whereas the latter was ever conscious of an active response. But the most salient difference was Metchnikoff's seeming indifference to the primary recognition problem of immunity: How does the host recognize nonself? What is the means of identification? If we understand the issue of specificity not as the discrimination between the self and the nonself, but as specificity in reactions to different nonself substances, then it is possible to say that the entire issue of specificity of the immune response was never scientifically posed in Metchnikoff's writings. The failure then to formalize the question of immune specificity is the central lacuna of Metchnikoff's later defense of the phagocytosis theory. In a fundamental sense this is an ironic indictment considering the intellectual genesis of his research. We must turn to his more explicit philosophical musings of this period to most consistently trace the extension of this mature thinking (29, 59). The emotional-laden defense of the phagocytosis theory placed him in a constricted posture, where the full flower of his hypothesis was muted; in turn, his influence was thereby limited.

The Aftermath

With the discovery of an augmented antibody reaction, autoimmunity, and diverse immunopathology, one might well ponder why the biology of these problems was not more actively pursued after the first decade of the twentieth century. If the issue was solely recognizing Metchnikoff's cardinal observation that the host mounts an active response to pathogens, we would predict that the debate would have continued over that mechanism, the relative role of cellular and humoral components, and the basis of humoral elaboration from immunocytes. But by 1900, those issues were dormant and the question of specificity became paramount. Silverstein observes:

> During its first 30 years, immunology had primarily been the domain of biologically and medically oriented individuals who were interested in its implications for disease prevention and disease causation. With the exhaustion of the search for vaccines against the most important pathogens, and especially with the decline of the phagocytic theory of immunity at the hand of the more readily available and manipulable circulating antibody, biologists were replaced by chemists at the leading edge of immunological research. . . . These investigators focused their attention on the molecule rather than on the whole organism. They were more interested in the size, shape, and structure of the antibody than in its possible role in the pathogenesis of disease. Thus, the conceptual foundations of the new *Denkkollective* were markedly different from those of the old one, and the guidelines for research and for conceptual advance that accompanied this change were markedly different. This shift is well illustrated not only by the types of study deemed worthy of pursuit and worthy of publication in journals of immunology but also by how immunological phenomena were being interpreted. (62)

Metchnikoff's original contributions are sparse after the publication of *Immunity* in 1901. In all respects, he had fought vigorously and from our vantage, creatively. He was an acknowledged leader of the early development of immunology, but as the course of research reflected, the central questions he posed were not of prime interest to other investigators. We suspect his views were not fully comprehended or, if understood, were not considered salient to the pressing questions of the day. Metchnikoff chose not to pursue those issues, and, in fact, his scientific contributions to elucidating the function of antibody in retrospect appear conservative at best and even recalcitrant or reactionary. His defensive posture for the exclusivity of the phagocytosis theory as originally presented, essentially unmodified in basic structure throughout his career, reveals not only a singlular devotion to his point of view but a highly defensive posture. He must have sensed the movement away from his dynamic approach to biology, in which organismal integrity, the primacy of form, and the evolutionary perspective of his thinking could not incorporate the restricted chemical approaches to biological phenomena. When Lord Lister described Metchnikoff's scientific chronical as truly a "romantic chapter," his description was more apt than he might have realized in 1896 (63). For Metchnikoff (as many apostles of positivism and nihilism of that time) truly was a nineteenth-century Romantic philosopher whose last fifteen years were devoted primarily in searching for his elusive orthobiosis through self-healing processes. In contrast, Ehrlich soon turned to other applications of his general affinity theory that had proven so successful in his first research on histological staining and later the side chain theory. He applied these principles to chemotherapy and is credited as a founder of scientific pharmacology. Important discoveries in the therapy of trypanosomiasis and syphilis established his reputation in yet another scientific discipline. In contrast to orthobiosis, warfare against infectious diseases with "magic bullets" (Salvarsan) was evocatively, and successfully, employed.

Elucidating the biological role of the phagocyte meantime made slow progress, and not until the 1960s, in elegant studies by Geore B. Mackaness, was an experimental basis established for the macrophage's direct function in tumor destruction and microbicidal processes (64). The so-called activated state of the macrophage represents recognition and immunological priming events that are necessary for subsequent immunopathological destruction of targets. The concept of immunological priming for effector function is closely linked to macrophage antigen processing (established in the 1960s and early 1970s), which is crucial for normal lymphocyte responses (65). The macrophage, by playing a crucial role in antigen presentation and secretion of immune regulatory substances (66), is now viewed as central to the immune response, whether cellular (lymphocyte or phagocyte) or humoral. Its cousin, the microphage has been relegated to acute inflammation—the polymorphonuclear leukocyte (or neutrophil) is essentially directed to bactericidal activities and autoimmune diseases, whereas the eosinophil participates in allergic and microbicidal activities against helminths and protozoa (see app. B). Until the 1960s, the phagocyte fell under the province of immunopathology or inflammation—areas of experimental pathology that were only tangential to the main body of immunology. How the discipline developed in the twentieth century has recently become subject to historical analysis (33), but falls outside our purview. Suffice to note that Metchnikoff's original formulation of active host definition of selfhood was an implicit tenant of immunology, and the role of the phagocyte was not significantly improved on from his original description until Mackaness placed it in the midst of immune recognition and its diverse regulatory functions were discovered in the 1970s.

From our vantage, we now see the false separation of humoral and cellular immunity, artefacts of the ideological orientation of the respective groups, in which the chemists sought to quantitate and define specificity and the descriptive cellularists were engrossed in the pathology of immunity. The two schools have essentially merged in the past thirty years, obscuring what now appears as an arcane conflict. However, we believe that the metaphysical controversy underlying this historical dialogue has not been solved or exhausted by modern immunology. It is perhaps more appropriate to consider Ehrlich as a true heir of the holist-humoralist tradition than to assign Metchnikoff as the promotor of the localist opposition. Owing to Ehrlich's influence, modern immunology remains closely aligned to the holist position: assuming the whole as granted, the focus of the discipline has been on the particular mechanisms protecting that whole. With these assumptions, questions concerning self/nonself discrimination imply that the self is provided in advance, that is, the whole or organismic integrity is given. Correspondingly, immune processes are thought not as those which establish (i.e., ontologically define) integrity, but serve "merely" as the processes of protection or recognition of the self. The immune reaction does not establish what is the self, but at best, it discriminates between self and not self. The history of Metchnikoff's theory reminds us that the very idea of a protective mechanism, or protective subsystem, appeared as a result of another idea of integrity. Old holistic intuitions of integrity are still tangible in our modern understanding of the immune mechanisms as homeostatic in their nature, and by equating integrity with a homeostatic system. In this perspective, the self is the structure that is supported and protected by homeostasis. Metchnikoff did not formulate his approach to immunity in the terms of self/nonself discrimination. However, if we attempt to define retrospectively the best candidate for the title "self" in the Metchnikovian vision, we must perceive that the term could not be ascribed to a provided, or established, integrity. In Metchnikoff's view, immunological processes are, first and primary, those activities that establish (constitute) organismic integrity, and it is only because of secondary phenomena that integrity is protected. Similarly, these processes cannot be reduced to recognition and protection of the self, but rather self-integrity, the self, arises from the dynamics of these activities.

CHAPTER 8

Epilogue: From Metaphor to Theory

Metchnikoff's achievement may be viewed on many levels, but we have focused on what we perceive as the fundamental reorientation he accomplished in our concept of organismic integrity. Specifically, the issue centers on the intellectual horizon of self-protection. In this respect, we view Metchnikoff as the first who shifted the question of protective forces from a metaphysical formulation to a scientific program, based on a well-prepared theoretical foundation. This theory had a radically altered orientation in its metaphysical construction, for the Metchnikovian concept of organism was a totally new view of integrity. We must now schematically define this metaphysical novelty.

Metaphor

To consider organism in terms of opposition the system/its elements (or the whole/its parts), we may view the role of the "elements" from two perspectives. In the first, any element of a system mediates "the other" of the system, that is, any given element serves as a means by which the system deals (produces, destroys, reproduces, eliminates, consumes, assimilates, etc.) with "the other." Of course, some "elements" may be considered from this perspective not as terminal effectors, but as the mediators of other means in a successive or hierarchical order. What is important for this perspective is the vision in which actions of the system proceed toward "the other." Correspondingly, elements of the system are considered as designed and oriented in accordance with this vector, that is, there are structures whose functions are to process "the other." In the second perspective, elements of the system mediate the system itself (in the system's relation to "the other"). The role of the elements in the latter case may be understood only when assuming their responsibility for the system's integrity. It is clear that the real meaning of "responsibility" and our interpretation of the concept "integrity" are mutually interdependent. But whatever concrete interpertation, the issue of integrity appears thematically in each particular case when considering the system from this second perspective. In the first approach, we are concerned with the means by which the system deals with "the other," but not with itself, that is, not with the system as such. Similarly, the idea of integrity forms a boundary of the first perspective rather than its theme (functioning as an intuition as opposed to an explicitly formulated idea).

We can hardly doubt that the idea of an organism's self-protection pertains rather to the second perspective than the first vision of the metaphorical opposition, the system/its elements. Regarding the historical and intellectual background of the immunity idea, we can assert that the concept (to the extent that immunity can be equated with self-protection) could appear only in the context of a primary concern with the problem of organismic integrity. We argued that the problem (in its various guises) formed the thematic center of Metchnikoff's life. We demonstrated that his morphological studies were organized primarily around the problem of embryonic integrity. We demonstrated how his devotion to zoology extended beyond considering his science as his life's business; rather he committed his entire life to the business of science. His research concerns with the problem of disharmony (organismic disintegrity) resulted both in elaborating a pessimistic personal philosophy and the tragic existential posture that led him to suicide attempts. On the other hand, the hope (generated from both personal and scientific developments after 1883) that he might solve the problem of integrity changed not only the direction and the field of his scientific occupation but also his philosophical ideas and apparently deeply altered his very personality. In this respect, we can argue that the phagocytosis theory was born from an obsession with the idea of integrity.

We further attempted to demonstrate that the traditional idea of organismic integrity was based on a metaphysical construction that primarily had a metaphorical nature. Integrity presented in this way excluded a scientific approach to the problem. To examine any element of the organism in its defensive function, a reformulation of integrity is required to allow scientific study. Without such an orientation, the very idea of studying a mechanism as a function devoted to host defense could not occur. Protection of the organism is not a product of reductionist thinking, but is within the agenda that views the problem of integrity as its primary concern. We do not mean that a reductionist point of view and the holistic concern with integrity cannot coexist in the same scientific mind; there are many examples of their complementarity. What must be emphasized, however, is that the idea of studying the mechanisms of organismic protection did not originate from a purely reductionist (mechanistic) posture of thought, and given the history of the idea, it appears natural that the scientific approach to those studies was first formulated by a man obsessed with the problem of integrity.

The problem of an organism's integrity is a *necessary* condition for formulating the idea of protective forces, but does that question guarantee the *sufficient* metaphysical condition for developing the immunity idea? We argued that there is an essential difference in the metaphysical infrastructures supporting the ancient speculations on the topic of the protecting and healing forces, on the one hand, and the idea of immunity, as it has been developed by Metchnikovian immunology, on the other hand. Not a holistic vision of organismic integrity, but a very specific one, prepared the birth of active host defense, namely, immunity. What is crucial in this respect is not just an abstract antireductionist posture, but the particular way in which the question about organismic integrity was formulated. We argued that the traditional expression of this question could not provide the metaphysical space for the immunity concept.

The difference lay in Metchnikoff's reoriented concept of integrity. Prior to him, integrity was given. The very meaning of the word *integrity* is the organization and the form of the organism. Thus, it is impossible to ask how integrity arose or was formed. From this position, formation of integrity is not truly a construction, but rather an explication of a potential order. Thus development appears as a natural metaphor from this perspective; organism appears as a metaphor of its own nature *(physis)*. Integrity may then be viewed as an actor changing roles, the scenery, or even the very stage, but not the nature of his identity: he may be absorbed in different "others," but he can not lose the self-equality that he carried within himself since his first performance.

How is it possible (within the limits of this vision of integrity) to formulate the question about mechanisms that form, protect, or restore the organism? It is clear that under these assumptions, any such mechanism does not establish integrity as such, but only provides a realization of the potentially given integrity upon a new stage or new challenge. On the other hand, any other physiological function could, at the same time and in the same sense, be considered as protecting integrity. Thus there are no ways to formulate the idea of a special protective mechanism. Whenever we describe a particular mechanism in this context, we invoke a means by which organism processes the "other," but not a particular way for its self-mediation. We find here the basis of the reductionist position: the whole can be objectively described only as a sum of its parts or, speaking more precisely, as a sum of functions, every one of which is processing its own particular "other." On the other hand, the same perspective provides the traditional holistic approach: the very fact that "the other" is always an object of mastery by the organism's means, refers then to each particular function as performing on behalf of the organism, that is, establishing the organism's integrity. But this self-mediating aspect of a particular function never can be thought of in objective terms because by describing the function in such a way, we describe not the organism's self-mediation but a particular way in which the organism mediates a particular "other." Thus integrity can never be described in terms in which its parts can be described. We find here the source of the ancient philosophical belief of the whole as something more than merely a sum of its parts. Correspondingly, integrity is viewed as being expressed in every function of the organism, but as this *expression* it refers to something other than it is: it becomes the self-mediation (self-determination, self-formation, self-protection, self-restoration) of the organism, but it *is* also the mediation (the mastery) of "the other." In full accordance with the metaphorical nature of the traditional understanding of the organism's integrity, *all* of the organism's functions could equally lay claim to perform those roles that were to become the functions of the immunological system(s), but only metaphorically. Any developmental processes as well as any forms of excretion, consummation, regulation, or mobility could be announced as the manifestation of the Forming and Healing Power of Nature. But the Power (or the Nature), as taken beyond a particular manifestation (a particular function as processing a particular "other"), remained only a metaphor of the organism's integrity.

Theory

Precisely from this metaphorical juncture, we were interested in Metchnikoff's undertaking. Asserting him as the author of the immunity idea, we do not mean to claim that he was the first among those who speculated on the topic of the organism's protective forces or who was the first to apply these speculations in their medical practice. The claim would be meaningless because both the speculations and their application began with the dawn of Western medicine. We do not claim even that Metchnikoff was the champion among those who ascribed protective functions to the colorless blood corpuscles. We claim that he was the first who interpreted the cells' activity in regard to their responsibility for the organism's integrity and then moved to elaborate the question from metaphorical to a scientific theory.

We sought to trace how the self-obviousness of *integrity* disappeared in Metchnikoff's research in comparative morphology. As a morphologist, Metchnikoff simultaneously followed two collisionary paths: on the one hand, as a traditional descriptive morphologist, he strove to clarify a typology of invertebrate development, that is, to explicate the organisms' integrity as something provided by nature; on the other hand, he was forced to doubt that integrity was provided in all cases, and it was not clear to him which criteria provided the basis of assessing integrity. He saw the self-evident object and natural goal of comparative morphology as the explication of a natural typology. At the same time, he doubted that there were objective (i.e., natural) criteria for such a typology. As we argued, this paradoxical situation resulted from Metchnikoff's interpretation of recapitulation, which was not transformation of a "logical" genealogical succession into a pattern of individual development. He viewed recapitulation as reproduction of ancient structures or even entire ancestral organisms in the course of individual development. But this reproduction did not define a logic of individual development, but only repeated a corresponding logic of genealogical succession. On the contrary, such a reproduction meant that every ontogeny was a kind of rewritten phylogeny in a new version. The idea of recapitulation rather put the question (How could an organism succeed its own history?) than explain how the history provided a pattern for individual development.

We argued further that this interpretation of recapitulation was closely connected with Metchnikoff's vision of the complementarity of the genealogical and descriptive embryological approaches in his comparative embryological studies as well as with his general approach to the problem of evolution. In the late 1870s and the early 1880s, Metchnikoff's attitude toward the idea of natural selection was in certain respects very close to those morphologists who saw in the mechanism of selection rather a source of physiological adaptations (to variations in external environments) of given morphological structures than the force that formed structures in the course of evolution. On the other hand, Metchnikoff's interpretation of recapitulation implied that identification of a structure as a true recapitulation involves descriptions of the structure as still presenting (in this particular ontogeny) the *whole* of the ancestral organism. The structure could be considered as recapitulated only if we succeeded in demonstrating that its primary functions (performed in a given individual development) manifested the biological meaning of the structure in an ancestral organism. Thus, within individual development, the relation between the processes determining morphological transformations and the processes of physiological adaptations received a new meaning: transformations of physiological roles of a conservative morphological structure appeared as the main source of those processes that shape the patterns of individual development. The genealogical approach to comparative morphology became, for Metchnikoff, actually identical with the physiological problem. The notion of Cuvier and von Baer that morphological structures could be properly understood only from the perspective of their functions, now received in Metchnikoff's studies a very special form: the pattern of individual development (for Metchnikoff, a type of organismic integrity) could be properly understood only in the complementarity of the genealogical (physiological) and the descriptive (embryological) approaches. Individual development could not be understood as simply a short repetition of a genealogical succession, but at the same time development required reconstructed succession. The latter could not be merely understood as an analogy with a self-obvious type of individual development, but neither could it be understood independently from reconstruction of such a type. Thus, integrity as the object of comparative morphology could not be viewed as having been naturally provided in one of these two approaches. Integrity was no longer self-obvious. Now, the only way Metchnikoff could define integrity was in the reality (as the object of comparative morphological studies) that was provided by the very complementarity of the genealogical and the descriptive embryological programs.

We cannot say that Metchnikoff himself fully realized the metaphysical novelty of his theoretical posture. He clearly saw that integrity of organisms could not always be accepted as naturally provided. But this does not mean that he clearly saw that the very concept "integrity" was not something given. Because integrity had turned out to be such an elusive object that could not always be grasped at hand, he implemented a complementary approach. But we can not say that he clearly understood that this approach predetermined an essential metaphysical shift in the very concept "integrity." In many cases, he desperately struggled in attempting to express his radically new intellectual posture in terms of the old metaphysics and the descriptive science of morphology. Such was the case with his theory of *orthobiosis*—the perfect accomplishment of the human life cycle. On the one hand, he always emphasized his opposition to the ancient teaching about human development as a revelation of an inherited harmony: integrity is not something naturally provided, it is rather an ideal. On the other hand, his theory provided the scientific recommendation for such an achievement. From his point of view, the rationale could only mean an explication of a naturally provided potentiality of harmonious development. Then, either his theory of *orthobiosis* was based on a tautology (harmonious development, i.e. integrity, is the realization of the potentiality of the harmonious development) or there was no difference between his idea of harmony and that borrowed from ancient Greek culture. Then what was this strange theory for? Why was he so attached to it? We believe the message, which he attempted to convey in the phagocytosis theory, was that integrity (the harmony), as the particular object of scientific studies, could not be considered as something naturally provided, it could not be studied in the manner of traditional morphology and physiology; the very question about integrity could be formulated only as the question concerning the mutual relationship of genealogical and morphological approaches of development. On the other hand, he did not realize, apparently, that this very posture abolished the self-obviousness of the concept "integrity." It appeared as if it were self-obvious for him: integrity meant harmony. What else could it mean? The true content of his scientific and metaphysical position could not be placed within the old metaphysical conceptual framework. The old opposition "harmony/disharmony" was, obviously, not quite suitable to convey this new intellectual posture.

Certainly, in many respects, Metchnikoff was a classical descriptive morphologist, whose object of study was self-evident. It is ironic that the very year Metchnikoff embarked on a new direction of his personal research, 1883, embryology was also undergoing a transformation in its experimental orientation. Weismann formulated the germ-plasm theory, and Wilhelm Roux hypothesized unequal nuclear divisions and speculated that these might lead to essentially different distributions of hereditary determinants. These theories reoriented developmental biology and heralded the appearance of experimental embryology. When in 1888, Roux published his experimental results and thus started his program of developmental mechanics *(Entwicklungsmechanic)* (1), Metchnikoff was already committed to immunological studies. Despite the classical facade of his descriptive morphology, Metchnikoff dramatically changed the concept of integrity as the object of his science.

We may consider Metchnikoff's entire intellectual evolution as a single process oriented toward revelation of the real meaning of "What is integrity?" As soon as he had succeeded in proposing the question, it became synonymous with another problem (only seemingly different): What is the intersection (the mutual mediation) of the two histories (the phylogenetic and the ontogenetic)? Or (as we discussed before), How can an organism succeed its own history? Now integrity has lost its a priori nature and its self-obviousness. The question refers then, not to integrity of the organism, in general, but is concerned with the organism only in respect to how mutual mediation of certain genealogical and developmental processes have been formulated as a problem. We attempted to trace how in Metchnikoff's work the question was gradually shaped into a specific focus on the mesoderm, that is, how the question of integrity became a question concerning the mutual mediation of the genealogical fate and the ontogenetic destiny of the mesodermic amoeboid cells. We saw that in order to identify the second embryonic layer, Metchnikoff implemented the idea of recapitulation. The idea demanded consideration of the layer as the carrier of an ancient biological meaning, clearly distinct from the function of the structures derivative from that layer. Specifically, individual development (to the extent that it is considered as inscribing a recapitulated structure into a new ontogeny) is viewed here as transforming the physiological role of the structure in question. This posture demanded a genealogical reconstruction in order to establish the primary biological meaning of the structure. For Metchnikoff, this intellectual course resulted in a demand to create a model of a primary multicellular organism, as a transitive creature, whose structure in question performs a function supposedly inherited from its ancestral past. In Metchnikoff's *parenchymella (phagocytella)* hypothesis, the primary function was intracellular digestion. The model demanded, first, that one consider the entoderm not as the true secondary layer, but rather arising from secondary differentiation of the genealogically primary parenchymal mass into the mesoderm and the entoderm; and second that one consider intracellular digestion as the primary function of the mesoderm, which inherited the function from the original parenchyma. If, on the one hand, the model was demonstrative and convincing in its assertion that intracellular digestion was the primary function of the mesoderm gradually to be replaced by evolution to cavitary digestion (as the primary function of the entoderm), on the other hand, the model left unanswered another question: How was the role of mesodermic intracellular digestion changed in the course of this evolutionary process? At the same time, the model was created to identify a developmental structure in the context of an ontogenetic transformation of its functional role. Thus, the next natural question concerned the role of intracellular digestion in the course of the developmental transformation. This led to Metchnikoff's studies of what he called "physiological inflammation." The problem was formulated and partially answered by his research (started in 1883) on the role of mesodermic phagocytes in the metamorphosis of echinoderms and amphibians. (Another reflection of Metchnikoff's concern with the same question were his studies of active atrophy and senility.)

By the very logic of Metchnikoff's position, identification of *any* developmental stage presupposed a corresponding genealogical reconstruction that, in its turn, created the perspective determining the second fundamental topic of his studies—comparative pathology of inflammation. This new field was, in fact, nothing more than the continuation of his *parenchymella* musings, complemented by the idea of "physiological inflammation." In the intersection of these two research avenues, organismic integrity appeared not as a plan to be explicated in the course of a particular ontogeny, but rather presented a particular formulation of the question concerning the essence of integrity: in what way(s) does this particular ontogeny master its own phylogeny? Phylogeny is still working within ontogeny. The ancestral organism (the amoeboid cells feeding by intracellular digestion) persists in its remote descendant. This ancient activity is (by its very nature) an aggressive and destructive power. This power, in the evolutionary retrospective of comparative pathology of inflammation, must be viewed as undergoing successive adoptions within the developmental process, that is, as going through different evolutionary stages of integration into different patterns provided by evolution. In this sense, the phagocytic activity is an *object* of evolution, as the process that elaborates integrity. In contrast, from the *pro*spective of "physiological inflammation," it is not evolution (understood as phylogeny providing the schema of ontogeny), but the seemingly destructive power of the phagocyte that is responsible for integration. This power then appears as the subject of development and is the obverse of the case when seen from the *retro*spective case of comparative pathology of inflammation. By evolutionary retrospection, the phagocytic activity is the *object* of mastery that establishes organismic integrity: this activity represents the phylogenetic origin of the organism as "the other" of the organism. In this case, the organism itself is actually equated here with the pattern within which "the other" is to be mastered. In the ontogenetic prospective approach, the same phagocytic activity appears as the *subject* of integration, that is, it appears to be "the self" of the organism—and in respect to "the self" the organism appears as "the other." In short, integrity is not a given entity, but a dialectical process. The two poles of this relationship are represented by the phagocyte switching its role between being the subject or object of the developmental process.

Metchnikoff has radically changed the classical intuition of integrity. Referring to self-mediation of integrity, we do not mean such mastery of "the other" that is an actualization of a potentially provided integrity. Integrity now can not be equated unconditionally with "the self" as opposed to "the (unconditionally external) other." The first "other" that is expected to be mastered here, is "the self" (the phagocytic activity). The first "self" that is to be mediated (self-mediated), is (not a potentially provided design but) the organismic structures that are to be *eliminated* or *transformed* in the course of ontogenetic development, in other words, self-mediation of integrity appears here as treating the organism itself as its own "other." Thus, elimination of "the other" then appears as the process of establishing integrity, but not in the same sense in which (according to the old metaphysical assumptions) any function, processing "the other," mediates (by the very virture of the processing) integrity. Only those processes take part in establishing integrity by processing "the other," and thus, in effect, alienate the organism from itself, that is, in treating the organism as "the other." Thus, a metaphysical space was opened for study of those special activities responsible for organismic integrity, and (as a particular case of this responsibility) for protection of the organism. As we noted, Metchnikoff did not derive his formulation of the idea of immunity because of an allegedly consistent and energetic pursuit of the idea of protective forces. A preoccupation with that idea presupposes, as a self-obvious assumption, that there is such a reality as organismic integrity that is to be protected. Metchnikoff came to the idea of immunity precisely because he was concerned *not* with protective processes, but with the question about what constituted organismic integrity. This question led him to erect the scientific (as opposed to metaphorical) horizons of his future studies in immunology, that is, the program of comparative pathology of inflammation and the developmental roles of the phagocyte.

Morphologists versus Darwinians, the Modern Debate

The schism between morphologists and Darwinians has continued to modern times. First, we must note that within the population biologists' own camp, a modern rigorous assault has been made on the Darwinians: Motoo Kimura's neutral theory of evolution (summarized in *The Neutral Theory of Molecular Evolution.* New York: Cambridge University Press, 1983) argues that chance effects are more important than natural selection as an evolutionary mechanism, and that most mutations at the molecular level are neutral, thereby allowing a high degree of protein polymorphism to persist. The postsynthetic theory will undoubtedly incorporate certain elements of his theory in a broadened perspective, allowing for Kimura's mutation clock, more complex mechanisms to account for speciation, as well as the role of developmental and other constraints. In this sense, the morphologists have been vindicated in asserting that the Darwinian argument was too restrictive to account for its problems. Metchnikoff's ongoing dialogue with Darwinism was essentially as a morphologist, whose criticism focused on the restrictions of natural selection theory to developmental processes. Metchnikoff's scientific descendents might well refer back to his initial resistance as a forerunner of current debate. The morphologists have reasserted their position principally in the debate on abrupt or punctuated speciation, although as we note, it falls into every arena of evolution theory.

The early difficulty Darwin had with the discontinuous fossil record has persisted to plague the Synthetic Theory. Despite strong support from modern paleontologists, a rigorous assault has been mounted from various quarters, and there are several threads to trace. First, the morphological record must be addressed. For instance, at the centennial of the *Origin,* E. C. Olson still felt compelled to assert the crucial role of morphologists in evolutionary biology, a testament today, that seems obvious.

Many who are not satsifed with current theory, the "synthetic theory", or simply "selection theory", are to be found in the ranks of the paleontologists and morphologists. This is true in spite of the fact that the role of the structural areas of biology, anatomy, and morphology have figured prominently in the development of Darwinian evolution, ... but it is of some importance, perhaps to re-emphasize that morphological information has provided the greatest single source of data in the formulation and development of the theory of evolution and that even now, when the preponderance of work is experimental, the basis for interpretation in many areas of study remains the form and relationships of structures. (1, p. 523–524)

The hegemony claimed by the synthetic theorists, especially Ronald A. Fischer, who wished to reduce evolutionary theory exclusively to change in genetic properties or mathematical exposition sought to exclude the morphologists from evolutionary debate. A strong defensive posture was then assumed:

> [These] definitions express a basic concept of the "synthetic theory" of evolution and, by the use of the definite article, imply that this is the—presumably the only—theory of evolution. The fact is, of course, as any of these writers would, I am sure, acknowledge immediately, that there are other possible statements of the theory of evolution. . . . The statement is made, in effect, that those who do not agree with the synthetic theory do not understand evolution and are incapable of so doing, in most cases because they think typologically. (1, p. 526)

Olson then delivered the recurrent criticism:

> The main objection to selection theory is that it cannot be disproved. Morphologists and paleontologists feel this, perhaps, more strongly than many other students of biology, since they, in particular, are concerned with structure, or the static components of the organic world. The origins of these structures are often "explained" by abstract models that derive their principal data from "laws" of genetics, "laws" which may be under dispute by the geneticists themselves. (1, p. 526)

Olson's complaints and the credibility of the modern morphologist's resistance have rung true and there is growing evidence for the breakdown of the all-encompassing synthetic theory. The debate ranges from the glib, "I do not think that the attempt to explain morphological evolution by species selection can survive. . . . But there never was much sense in the idea anyway" (2) to rigorous argument, that revolves now on how to interpret the saltatory nature of the fossil record. Stephen J. Gould well summarizes the situation:

> The modern synthesis drew most of its direct conclusions from studies of local populations and their immediate adaptations. It then extrapolated the postulated mechanism of these adaptations—gradual, allelic substitution—to encompass all larger-scale events. The synthesis is now breaking down on both sides of this argument. Many evolutionists now doubt exclusive control by selection upon genetic change within local populations. Moreover, even if local populations alter as the synthesis maintains, we now doubt that the same style of change controls events at the two major higher levels: speciation and patterns of macroevolution. (3)

Richard Goldschmidt (arguing in *The Material Basis of Evolution*) seems to have been prophetical in recognizing

> that geographic variation is ubiquitous, adaptive, and essential for the persistence of established species. But it is simply not the stuff of speciation; it is a different process. Speciation, Goldschmidt argues, occurs at different rates and uses different kinds of genetic variation . . . his explicit antiextrapolationist statement is the epitome and foundation of emerging views on speciation. . . . There is a discontinuity in cause and explanation between adaptation in local populations and speciation; they represent two distinct, though interacting, levels of evolution. We might refer to this discontinuity as the Goldschmidt break. (3)

Gould argues, the issues revolve around a hierarchical appreciation of evolutionary mechanisms in which macroevolution is "decoupled" from microevolution and evolutionary trends "use" species as their raw material. The morphological record then reflects a higher level process than speciation, representing a sorting out of speciation events. The laws governing such behavior are not well formulated, but we perceive that the resurgence of holistic, epigenetical, and hierarchical thinking has put the organism back as a necessary, but as yet unplaced, entity in modern evolutionary theory.

Richard Lewontin and Richard Levins have led the arguments for a dialectical approach to evolutionary theory. Starting from new premises, they write:

> As a preliminary analysis, the separation of organism and environment or of physical and biological factors of the environment—of density-dependent or independent factors, of consumable or nonconsumable requirements—has proved useful. But it eventually becomes an obstacle to further understanding; the division of the world into mutually exclusive categories may be logically satisfying, but in scientific activity no nontrivial classifications seem to be really mutually exclusive. Eventually their interpenetration becomes a primary concern of further research. It is in this sense that dialectics rejects the doctrine of the excluded middle. Opposed to the model in which an organism is seen as inserted into an already given environment, we note several aspects of the organism-environment interpenetration. (4, p. 53)

In fact, these are two theories of evolution, microscopic and macroscopic:

> The two theories can never make effective contact until the concept of relative fitness of genotypes within a population is connected to the fitness of populations and species in ecological communities. But this connection cannot be made until the dichotomy of organism and environment is broken down. The divorce between the relative fitness of genotypes and the fitness of populations arises from the fiction that new varieties are selected in a fixed environment, so that the only issue is whether, given that environment, they will produce fewer or more offspring. But in reality, a new variety means a new environment, a new set of relations among organisms and with inorganic nature. On the other hand, each mutational change cannot result in a totally new relation between organism and environment, or else no cumulative evolutionary change could ever take place. (4, p. 63)

Or as Lewontin writes:

> The organism cannot be regarded as simply the passive object of autonomous internal and external forces; it is also the subject of its own evolution. (4, p. 89).

In this view, development becomes a highly dynamic, responsive phenomenon:

> The view of development that sees genes as determinative, or even a view that admits interaction between gene and environment as determining the organism, places the organism as the end point, the object, of forces. The arrows of causation point from gene and environment to organism. In fact, however, the organism participates in its own development because the outcome of each developmental step is a precondition of the next. But the organism also actively participates in its own development because, as we shall see, it is the determinant of its own milieu. (4, p. 96)

And the organism actively determines its environment and ultimately its evolutionary fate:

It is impossible to avoid the conclusion that organisms construct every aspect of their environment themselves. They are not the passive objects of external forces, but the creators and modulators of these forces. The metaphor of adaptation must therefore be replaced by one of construction, a metaphor that has implications for the form of evolutionary theory.

... The incorporation of the organism as an active subject in its own ontogeny and in the construction of its own environment leads to a complex dialectical relationship of the elements in the triad of gene, environment, and organism. We have seen that the organism enters directly and actively by being an influence on its own further ontogeny. It enters by a second indirect pathway through the environment in its own ontogeny. The organism is, in part, made by the interaction of the genes and the environment, but the organism makes its environment and so again participates in its own construction. Finally, the organism, as it develops, constructs an environment that is a condition of its survival and reproduction, setting the conditions of natural selection. So the organism influences its own evolution, by being both the object of natural selection and the creator of the conditions of that selection. (4, pp. 104–106)

The issue, as formulated, skips a century of scientific development, but it is of historical note how the morphological position has fared in the contemporary context and how Metchnikoff's orientation has been both legitimized and proven valuable in the development of evolutionary science. The argument, of which Olson is but representative, is based on the assumptions of the geneticists as problematic, the unknown factors of development and environment, that is, the epigenetic factors that render the relative importance of selection in question, and the impossibility of morphologists to experimentally address the issues because of the time factor.

This same reformulation in terms of hierarchial organization has been offered by Marjorie Grene, who claimed a protected perspective as "a kind of ethologist (or epistemologist) watching the conceptual behavior of the other animals" (5). In "Two Evolutionary Theories," Grene (6) traces the morphological versus the Darwinian debate by contrasting the respective theories of George Gaylord Simpson and Otto H. Schindewolf—the former stressing continuity and adaptive evolutionary change, the latter seeing discontinuity and nonadaptive character of major changes: morphology and neo-Darwinism are incompatible, not on the basis of different factual issues or premises, but because the material is viewed in a diametrically opposed fashion. The two look at different aspects of their common subject matter: what is central for one is peripheral to the other. Simpson deals not with individuals, who do not evolve, but with populations that do evolve; Schindewolf, in contrast, attempts to relate unique individuals phylogenetically. It is the problem of defining what happened in individual development that underlies the abstract statistical relationship that population geneticists construct. "It is this underlying *real* change that Schindewolf is trying to envisage" (6, 1974, p. 138). Their respective visual aids or places of attention differ, for they pose different questions. One must explain discontinuity (G. G. Simpson), the other continuity (Schindewolf), from the discreteness of different morphological types.

The fundamental problem of adaptation highlights the different perspectives. Although all Darwinians abjure teleology, most assert that "all significant changes in nature are adaptive," a premise that is meaningful as structure is "explained away."

It is the shifting organism/environment relation, not the form of the organism itself, that is the basic unit. Organisms, already dissolved, from the perspective of evolution, into gene complexes, are themselves constantly changing as an (equally changing) environment plays upon them. Thus what changes is itself a product of two variables: average gene frequency and environment. There are no constants which would have to be assessed as patterns or achievements in themselves, only what Simpson calls the "splendid opportunism" of life.

This is indeed a brilliant perpetuation of Darwin's vision, and its persuasive force is compelling. Schindewolf's principles are simpler. He sees typical shapes, and he sees again and again what appear to be new shapes. Therefore he assumes that living things are able to originate novel types. Mutation, he agrees, must have been the mechanism by which they originated; but the adaptive control of mutation occurs only within, not between types. The basic pattern is of change from type to type, and always, as we have seen, with the more general appearing before its specialised subdivisions. (6, 1974, p. 142)

G. G. Simpson and Schindewolf represent closed, interpretive systems, alternative frameworks for understanding the data, which within limited issues can assimilate a theorem from the other, without endangering its total structure.

It is really a matter of choice whether we say that the higher categories come before the lower, or conversely, the lower before the higher. In fact, each of our two scientists, in this connection, explicitly concedes the other's position, Simpson admits that Archaeopteryx was already a bird and Schindewolf admits that though Archaeopteryx was definitely a bird, if there had never been any more birds nobody would have known it. Thus, on this particular point, each system can comfortably assimilate a theorem from the other, without endangering its total structure. So far as this particular case goes, we really can look at the matter either way. (6, 1974, p. 143)

Yet Grene noted, and the tumult in evolutionary biology confirms, that an inclusive theory accommodating both points of view is required. Darwinism provides a mechanistic explanation where its reductionism offers convincing power. Schindewolf's view of sudden origin of basically new types or organization implies the recognition of novel order

is distinct from the statistical manipulation of the conditions producing order. This, however, is to introduce a duality of logical levels: continuous and small-scale conditions *versus* discrete and comprehensive pattern; and that means to destroy the *unitary* character of the explanation. Again, to admit orthogenesis, or spontaneous direction in evolution, would be to deny the constant covariance of gene pool and environment, and thus to suggest as a third factor an inner dynamic in organisms, as distinct both from the non-directive control of random variation and the external steering "mechanism" of natural selection. But such a suggestion would deviate from the belief in the *automatism* of evolution. And again, it is precisely the double automatism of gene fluctuation and natural selection that *makes* the neo-Darwinian explanation a scientific explanation in the mechanistic sense. To say, therefore, that the "facts" suggest spontaneity in the origin and development of organic pattern is, for convinced Darwinians, not to offer scientific evidence at all, but to step outside the bounds of science. From the Darwinian point of view such "objections", which can be formulated only in non-mechanistic language, lie for that very reason beyond the scope of science altogether, and cannot therefore be taken seriously as scientific objections. (6, 1974, p. 146)

But are the criteria of mechanism adequae? As cited earlier, hierarchical appreciation of evolutionary mechanisms is becoming self-apparent, or as Grene concludes:

Some concept of biological organization, which implies a non-unitary logic, is indispensable to biological theory. Where, therefore, it is ostensibly dispensed with, it nevertheless creeps in again, either in the unformulated presuppositions of the biologist, or in some ingeniously contrived disguise. This kind of procedure: the pretence of understanding a subject matter in terms of fewer and narrower concepts than are in fact indispensable to its understanding, [Michael] Polanyi has called the fallacy of *pseudo-substitution*. It can be found, I think, at a great many places in the neo-Darwinian literature. (6, 1974, p. 147–148)

Ernst Mayr has also thoughtfully written of this issue, but from the other position. He considered the conflict between paleontologists (or systematists) and geneticists to explain species evolution as also arising from fundamentally opposed vantages. The former, studying populations and the phenotype, argued ultimate causes backward from species diversity, whereas the latter, examining individuals and the gene, argued proximate causes forward (7).

What form post–neo-Darwinism will take is as yet unclear, but from the perspective of Metchnikoff's vision, the philosophical problem as structured therein closely resembles his early formulation. Clearly, Metchnikoff had little influence over the concrete scientific debate as developed in the post-Mendelian period, but it is of interest to our appreciation of his critical acumen that he so closely identified the fundamental problems of Darwinism even from its infancy and without the benefit of our "sophisticated" vantage.

Perhaps the clearest path to trace Metchnikoff's scientific legacy as an evolutionist resides in his early polemic with Haeckel. As we noted, Metchnikoff was successful in supplanting Haeckel's theory of ontogeny recapitulating phylogeny with a more complex appreciation of ontogenetic development, rejecting a single pattern of gastrulation extrapolated from vertebrates to primitive invertebrates. Whether gastrulation occurs by invagination or by unipolar or multipolar introgression, the result is the same: a single bilayered, ciliated embryo incapable of further development is transformed into a two-layered organism capable of further movement via the ciliated ectoderm and of further development by the unciliated endoderm. Explaining this embryological strategy is a central problem in modern evolutionary theories, in which the modern synthesis (evolution and genetics) has omitted ontogeny (the synthetic theory of evolution is a "theory of adults") (8). As Leo Buss further explains, a single-celled protist must simultaneously express specialized modes of locomotion, feeding, and behavior and yet retain the capacity for cell division. Metazoans have no such constraint and have taken the strategy of differentiation and segregation of germ cells. At issue is the simultaneous need for an organism to move through fluid with cilia or flagella and to divide using a mitotic spindle. Unless a cell possesses microtubule organizing centers capable of performing both tasks or possesses multiple microtubule organizing centers per cell, the cell's functional range will be constrained. In certain protist groups, cell division and locomotion can occur simultaneously; in others, they cannot. Although many protist taxa overcome the ciliation constraint, those protists that give rise to metazoans did not. Metazoans inherited the constraint that limits simultaneous mitosis and ciliation; the movement and subsequent proliferation of cells from the blastular surface into the center of the sphere is gastrulation, a metazoan solution to the requirement of simultaneous movement and development (8).

There is a familiar parallel to Metchnikoff's orientation in modern biology: metazoan ontogeny is a sequence of cell lineages progressively denying their own capacity to increase for the collective interest of the individual (see Buss); on a more basic level, the same process is postulated to have occurred within cells by symbiosis, as argued by, Margulis (9). These notions of coevolved microbial communities, in which the eukaryotic cell is composed of several genomes from different sources (heterogenomic development, Margulis) or the strategies in which the metazoan collective of parent and variant daughter cells imposes constraints on cell lineages for the collective interest of the individual (Buss) are each closely related to Metchnikoff's original constructions, which were based on the conflict between the potentially opposing processes of various somatic elements and organisimal integrity. The existence of harmonious function in favor of the individual (and total) organism in Metchnikoff's original terms is an active process. How have organisms evolved so that some cells have abandoned their own capacity to replicate? The strategies are complex, but generally, patterns in cleavage and regulation are adaptations that serve the function of imposing selection at the level of the cell lineage. What Metchnikoff recognized—albeit in a poor and, from our point of view, unsophisticated manner— was that evolution must be understood by selective processes that operate on the interactions of cell lineages. "Evolutionary pattern has arisen not by selection on individuals alone, but by the interactive effects of selection operating at differing levels of biological organization" (8, p. 68).

The extension of this concept in the modern context results in a formulation that generates a highly evocative model for examining the immune system (10). Normal development in ontogeny proceeds not with every detail of cell interaction programmed, but metazoan cells must interact as a consequence of traits developed in the ancestral past; the genome encodes the relative competitive relationship of developing cell lineages. An epigenetic landscape was proposed by C. H. Waddington as a topography of undulating peaks and valleys, in which a ball placed above the ridges may proceed down any one of several pathways (11). Each valley represents the origin of a variant cell lineage in the course of ontogeny that competes with existing cell lineages. A particular ontogenetic expression then is but one of several potential pathways whose potential (i.e., mechanism of interaction) is programmed but whose final declaration is determined by the result of competition of cell lineages.

In this view, explanation of epigenesis must equally share with genetics an understanding of development, for "genes specify local rules, not global pattern. Above all, developmental events intervene between genotypic and phenotypic space" (10, p. 53). This alludes to hypothetical transformation rules developed by Lewontin (12). Selection acts on the phenotype, that is on forms that increase fitness, and the species evolves by changes in gene frequency in the population. To relate advantageous alteration in genotypic spaces as distinct from phenotypic space, four transformation rules have been assigned (a) to connect embryonic development to the mature animal that confers advantage, (b) ecological interactions in inter- and intraspecies competition, (c) gamete formation that enhances proliferation, (d) zygote formation and gene assortment. Recent study of cell surface proteins that confer recognition characteristics has been utilized for a new theory of epigenetic development, Edelman's morphoregulatory hypothesis. The basic formulation is that recognition proteins on cells and the extracellular domain allow cells to be addressed in time and space sequence for either division, movement, or death. The epigenetic component comes from the topobiological response to these molecules. Differentiation is, in contrast, controlled by historegulatory genes, another level of control. The link between the epigenetic and genetic components is tentatively proposed through inductive signals. The model is speculative in many respects, but highly evocative, and it represents a new molecular biological approach to the study of morphogenesis (13).

Current Views of Phagocyte Function

Phagocyte Metabolism

Metchnikoff's understanding of phagocytic function was essentially correct in regards to the basic concepts of immune effector function. He recognized the features of the phagocyte response in terms we still employ today; in many respects, he anticipated the main currents of modern investigation. As currently understood, there are two pathways by which the phagocyte interacts with the microbe: (a) relatively nonspecific mechanisms and (b) acquired or immune responses that involve complement or antibody. Metchnikoff implicitly recognized the distinction. In the first mechanism, phagocyte-pathogen binding is mediated by a carbohydrate moiety on the surface of the cell or the microorganism. The protein that binds the carbohydrate is a lectin, and the process is called lectinophagocytosis. This represents the first and probably most primitive modality of recognition; surprisingly, it is the least well-studied (and understood) mechanism of host–pathogen interactions. Clearly, it represents the first encounter and relies on a relatively crude or nonspecific interaction (1). In the second case, antibody (immunoglobuin) is generated to a specific antigenic structure and a target-missile analogy is erected. In either case, the microbe attaches to the phagocyte exterior membrane either through the "nonspecific" receptors or the specific receptors for immunoglobulin and complement. In the lectin case, the endogenous structures of the microbe serve as the vehicles of attachment; in the immune setting, the specified antibody recognizes the antigenic structure, attaches to that component on the surface of the microbe, and then the other end of the immunoglobulin projects outward to engage its phagocyte receptor. This so-called opsonization is what Almoth Wright recognized as the facilitative role of sensitized serum to the bactericidal process. The activation of complement is, in fact, the more primitive opsonin; certain carbohydrate structures on the surface of bacteria or fungi activate a cascade of linked proteins that results in the generation of a complement opsonin that acts much like immunoglobulin in that one end of the molecule is attached to the microbe, and its free end is now available to attach to the phagocyte. It is of great interest that complement has other roles in inflammation: one component is a chemoattractant for phagocytic cells recruited to inflammatory loci, another serves as a vasodilator and augments the tissue response to injury.

Once the microbe is attached to the phagocyte surface, it is engulfed and contained within a membrane-enclosed vacuole (2). This so-called phagocytic vacuole then serves as a directed site for the cell to discharge its granule contents of degradative enzymes to kill and digest the encapsulated pathogen. With the fall in pH and the elaboration of toxic oxygen-derived reactants, three modes of degradation serve as the killing mechanisms. Metchnikoff recognized the first two modalities; it was only in the 1960s that the third mechanism, oxidative destruction, was described. The so-called ferments have been identified as a complex array of lysosomal enzymes that have varied specificities for their degradative targets. Metchnikoff recognized the various phases of the inflammatory reaction as sequential processes: migration of phagocytes from the blood or congregation from tissue sources, phagocytosis of the microorganism and then its destruction by "ferments" or acidification. In many respects our current views of phagocytic function are but detailed commentaries on his construction.

Following adherence to the vascular wall, the directed migration of the granulocyte along a concentration gradient of a chemoattractant is the initial phase of extravascular cellular recruitment to an inflammatory site. The generation of diverse chemotactic factors (lipids, proteins, small peptides) by both immunological and nonimmunological pathways has been demonstrated. In fluid-phase systems, the activation of the classic and alternate complement pathways as well as the Hageman factor is complemented by the generation of chemotactic factors of defined cellular populations—recognized as a critical amplification pathway in the initial and subsequent mobilization of phagocytes. Activation of mast cells, lymphocytes, and neutrophils themselves has been shown to release chemotactic factors by both immunological and nonimmunological mechanisms. These factors from cellular and fluid-phase systems are structurally diverse and may interact with the neutrophil through unique receptors, or possibly with a single receptor, through different chemical mechanisms (e.g., net negative charge, hydrophobic domains).

Elucidation of cell activation has recently been advanced by appreciating that the neutrophil, like other secretory cells, shares a common signal transduction mechanism for translating receptor-ligand-coupled reactions on the plasma membrane to enzymatic effector function. Once the receptor is activated, a variety of membrane perturbatory events have been reported; the most important in the phagocyte is the guanine nucleotide-modulated protein system that is coupled to receptors of diverse structure and function but that share a common role of coupling receptor-ligand binding on cell membrane surfaces to intracellular enzymes that generate second messengers (e.g., inositol trisphosphate, or cyclic adenosine monophosphate [AMP]). These messengers, in turn, function to trigger metabolic events (e.g., increase in cytosolic calcium) that control the metabolic activities (e.g., phosphorylation) responsible for effector function. In the case of the neutrophil, an activation cascade leading from receptor binding of a chemotactic substance elaborated from gram-negative bacteria to activation of the enzyme complex responsible for production of toxic oxidative species has been charted.

The uptake of particulate material in a plasma membrane-derived vacuole is a complex process that may be divided for convenience into recognition and pseudopod assembly stages. As noted, nonspecific carbohydrate interaction in the so-called lectino phagocytosis interaction is distinct from the specific recognition mechanism employing humoral factors. Immunoglobulin G (IgG)—through its (Fc) receptor and C3b as well as other fragments of the third component of complement—mediate the binding of the opsonized particles by means of distinct receptors. Although IgG is most effective in stimulating particle uptake, a marked synergy exists between C3 and IgG that induces phagocytosis. Bordet's seminal discovery differentiating complement and antibody function has been confirmed by modern findings (3). Humoral defects associated with abnormal phagocytosis in many instances overlap with chemotactic abnormalities. Recent interest in this area is heightened by the observation that chemotactic factors enhance the expression of C3b and IgG Fc receptors on neutrophils.

Phagocytosis requires active cellular metabolism, again linked to receptor-coupled signals (4); actin, the major protein of the contractile skeleton of the granulocyte, forms a meshwork that is contracted by myosin, an ATP-dependent process. Other than to note that this meshwork is transformed from gel to sol forms, the actual process of vacuole formation in physicochemical terms is not well understood. The stimulation of the neutrophil results in movement of the various granules to the plasma membrane and discharge of enzymes either into the membrane vacuole containing a phagocytosed microorganism or into the extracellular environment, potentially causing tissue damage, for example, glomerulonephritis. Granule fusion and lysis with the phagosome integrates the functions of phagocytosis and degranulation. Movement of the granule to the phagocytic vacuole rapidly follows phagocytosis and involves the complex interaction of a microtubule system and perhaps contractile proteins, but the interrelationship is still largely undefined.

The marked increase in the respiration of the stimulated neutrophil has led to the definition of an oxidative microbicidal mechanism. The activation of the respiratory burst associated with phagocytosis is the focus of intense investigation in phagocyte biochemistry. The enzyme responsible for producing toxic oxidative species is the NADPH-oxidase, which utilizes electrons from a reduced pyridine nucleotide generated by the hexose monophosphate shunt (5). The enzyme is dormant until activated, probably by phosphorylation control (6). The dramatic increase in oxygen consumption is nonmitrochondrial and results from activation of a plasma membrane-associated oxidase that generates a free radical, superoxide (O_2^-). In order to tolerate the production of potent oxygen free radicals, the ubiquitous and essential enzyme for aerobic life, superoxide dismutase, must dismute O_2^- to form hydrogen peroxide (H_2O_2). H_2O_2 is also a powerful oxidant and mediates oxidative microbial killing with the lysosomal enzyme, myeloperoxidase. Because peroxides are toxic to the cell, they are, in turn, metabolized to water by the glutathione system and catalase. Other highly reactive species may serve as potent mediators of tissue damage (5). Of note, the inability of phagocytes to generate these toxic oxidative species results in recurrent bacterial infections in afflicted patients (2). It is of interest that phagocytes of invertebrates lack this oxidative apparatus, thus relying on nonoxidative degradative mechanisms. The phylogenetic origin of the vertebrate respiratory burst of phagocytosis is unknown; despite recent cloning of some of its various protein constituents, the relationship of this metabolic activity kinship to other oxidative-reductive enzyme systems has not as yet been established.

Phagocyte Physiology

Chemotaxis, phagocytosis, degranulation, and oxidative metabolism share common determinants and interrelated biochemical pathways. Integration of a variety of phagocyte activities is required for normal cellular function, and an abnormality of one activity may be reflected as a disorder in another function (7). In order to establish the interrelationship of these four parameters, an organization of sequential events or hierarchical pattern is necessary. Complete physiological response would involve the initiation of chemotaxis followed by phagocytosis and stimulation of the respiratory burst and degranulation of lysosomal enzymes. Biochemical analysis has allowed further dissection of this functional model. It is of growing interest, however, to extend this model back to Metchnikoff's original observation: he witnessed amoeboid (phagocytic) cells surround an intruder (a thorn) too large to ingest. His first studies, in fact, were directed at physiological inflammation in which he was interested in establishing the endogenous scavenging function of the phagocyte (recall the studies of the metamorphosis of the tadpole wherein the regression of the tail was accomplished by the phagocytes' devouring behavior). The same bactericidal mechanisms are employed both against pathogens too large to ingest (e.g., eosinophils attacking schistosomula) and as vehicles of inflammation directed against sterile targets. The cases of autoimmune diseases (e.g., rheumatoid arthritis) or immune complex disease (e.g., glomerulonephritis) result from activation of phagocytes by uncontrolled host factors. In the case of autoimmune diseases with an acute inflammatory component, immunoglobulin is directed at host tissue (e.g., synovial membrane) and the neutrophil sees only the complexed antibody. In so-called frustrated phagocytosis, the phagocyte attempts to engulf the tissue and in the process elaborates toxic oxygen-derived free radicals, degradative enzymes, and acid. Tissue destruction ensues and the targeted tissue is treated as a pathogen, a target injury. Again, we must note that the basic mechanism Metchnikoff described for the senile process is perfectly applicable to the vast variety of inflammatory conditions we now recognize.

Metchnikoff was, in fact, even more prescient in defining the normal physiological role of the phagocyte in the aging process. An excellent example is the case of the human erythrocyte, which lives but 120 days. The red cell surface moieties change over this period and eventually become recognized as different from younger cells. The so-called senescent antigen is recognized by the splenic macrophage that engulfs the marked erythrocyte and destroys it. Macrophages phagocytose and eliminate blood cells that are no longer functional, leaving mature viable cells unharmed, a process that requires the ability to distinguish between "self" and "senescent self." Earlier hypotheses related a decrease in the net surface charge or increased density of aged erythrocytes in the recognition process; however, more recently, the macrophage appears to recognize antibody bound to newly exposed senescent antigens, derived from band 3, the erythrocyte transporter (8). Whether the neo-antigen is a proteolyzed or oxidized product or a newly formed dimer of a native protein is not known. The senescent antigen, in addition to being found on the erythrocyte, has been demonstrated on the surface of lymphocytes, neutrophils, platelets, embryonic kidney cells, and adult liver cells (9). In this case, the neo-antigen is recognized by immunoglobulin, and the original proviso of antibody independent reactions is not met. However, altered physicochemical plasma membrane structures may be recognized by phagocytes (10), thus the relative importance of immune (i.e., antibody) versus nonimmune recognition mechanisms of phagocyte targets is of central interest.

The phagocyte also functions in antibody-independent mediated immune reactions. Three noninfectious models that have received recent attention are tumoricidal systems, wound healing, and postischemic injury. Several studies have indicated that neutrophils develop in vitro and in vivo tumoricidal activity (11), which has been shown to occur on stimulation with phorbol esters during phagocytosis and both in association with antibody-dependent cellular cytotoxicity and in the presence of lectins (12). Recent studies using flow cytometric analysis have demonstrated that activated murine neutrophils effectively kill tumor cells within the first twenty-four hours of coculture with target tumor cells (13). This model clearly represents an antibody-independent mechanism, but the recognition apparatus has not been defined, a recurrent problem in deciphering the biology of these processes. Without defining the phagocyte receptor and its ligand, the phenomenology remains elusive.

The same issue is noted in another example, the remodeling of tissue, first described by Metchnikoff in the metamorphosis of the tadpole; in the modern context, it has focused on experimental cutaneous wound repair. Wounds are almost always immediately invaded by neutrophils, where they persist for days, being replaced by macrophages (14); newly synthesized fibronectin and a fibrinogen-derived peptide are neutrophil chemoattractants and promote neutrophil adherence (15), but the specific roles of neutrophils in resorptive or synthetic processes of wound repair have not been established as shown in the monocyte/macrophage in bone resorption (16).

A more compelling example is the recent appreciation that the neutrophil mediates cardiac destruction subsequent to ischemia and reperfusion (17). In this case, blood-derived neutrophils target damaged ischemic tissue as an inflammatory locus, enhancing the primary damage by a secondary assault. Mechanisms of neutrophil-mediated injury include toxic oxidative radical formation, lipid peroxidation, elastase release, and leukocyte capillary plugging (18). Similar neutrophil-mediated injury after ischemic damage has been shown in the lung (19), kidney (20), and colon (21). As in each of these models, the mechanism(s) of phagocyte recognition have not been defined.

Models of wound-healing, postischemic injury and tumor killing are presumably examples of routine phagocyte function as it scavenges dead or damaged cells, both normal and malignant, to maintain vigorous and fully functional organic behavior; the most important examples include tissue injury of all kinds (i.e., ischemic, traumatic, thermal) and tumor surveillance. The deleterious effects of the colon not withstanding, the sea of carcinogens, tumor promotors, environmental and dietary toxins, and external insults lead the phagocyte to multiple recuperative functions aside from protection of the host from invading pathogens, and Metchnikoff recognized its fundamental role in "harmonizing" bodily function. We have however made little progress in defining the nonimmune recognition process by which phagocytic cells recognize or fail to detect damaged or malignant cells. The control mechanisms by which normal tissue is processed—for instance, in bone resorption, an ongoing normal process by macrophage-derived osteoclasts—is largely unexplored.

Phylogenetic Considerations

We will now briefly consider more general issues of phagocyte function, that is, its role as discerned by phylogenetic comparison. In Metchnikoff's early debate on constructing the first metazoan, mechanistic issues of development were foremost in argument (i.e., development by introgression versus emboly), but implicit was the basic construction of differentiated function between somatic and gametic investment, and the phagocyte was defined as the entity that preserved the integrity of the individual. (That first multicellular individual functioned similarly to the colonial flagellate *Volvox aureus,* which has generally lost the totipotential to produce new colonies (as in *Gonium* or *Pandorina*), and true cellular differentiation occurs between germ and somatic cells.) And it is here, in the poorly defined nether world of invertebrate immunity, that Metchnikoff's epic hypothesis took root and eventually flourished into the complexity of function found in vertebrates. In *Lectures on the Comparative Pathology of Inflammation* (22) Metchnikoff traced the phylogenetic development of phagocytes. He clearly differentiated "intracellular digestion" in Rhizopoda and Infusoria from protozoan "osmotic absorption" (22, p. 2), and used the infusorian, *Protospongia* as the closest extant species to bridge protozoan and metazoan organization. This two-layered animal with flagellated ectoderm and an inner mass containing amoeboid cells is the phylogenetic precursor to the sponge, with true three-layer organization, one of which, the mesohyl is the primitive home of the specialized phagocyte (23). Sponges defend themselves by several mechanisms: (a) separation of dying or diseased tissue with a callouslike wall, (b) generation of antibiotic substances, (c) phagocytosis by choanocytes or amebocytic cells found on canal walls and archeocytes of the mesohyl, and (d) agglutinating factors that appear to enhance phagocytosis, which may well be the most primitive humoral recognition factors of nonself markers. (These substances are distinct from aggregation factors that mediate self-recognition in syngeneic and allogenic interactions [see later].) It is of interest that sponges tolerate an extensive interaction with commensals and symbionts in a stable relation that appears to form a dynamic mutual exchange of metabolites. In certain sponges, bacteria may occupy up to forty percent of the mesohyl volume. There is an implicit assumption that the sponge is able to control the density and composition of its internal symbiont community, but it is of interest from this perspective how Metchnikoff incorporated divergent data into his grand scheme choosing to ignore the problem of distinguishing defensive from nutritive functions.

It was in the coelenterates that he found a more orthodox defensive phagocyte. Ameboid cells are found in all three cell layers, but Metchnikoff did not differentiate between the nonphagocytic interstitial cells of the Hydrozoa class and the true phagocytes, called amebocytes in modern parlance, that appear in Scyrhozoa (jellyfish) and Anthozoa (anemones, corals) (24). Although interstitial cells of hydrae may participate in graft rejection and wound healing, they are not required. In contrast, the amebocyte participates in healing, tissue reorganization, and phagocytosis of foreign tissue. True parasites are uncommon, although coelenterates have not been found to generate agglutinins, bactericidins, or antibodylike substances, they utilize antibiotics, the stolon armed with nematocytes (stinging cells), and mucus for noncellular defense. The different classes have distinct phagocytic responses: hydrozoans do not have an inflammatory reaction because only stationary, endodermal cells phagocytose. In scyphozoans and anthozoans, infiltration occurs, but a basic difference is observed between the response to foreign invasion and feeding, which involve two different cell types. Truly not much is known beyond Metchnikoff's first observations published in his *Lectures* of how a splinter injected into a jellyfish is surrounded within twenty-four hours by numerous amebocytes, but it was this observation and similar descriptions in phyla extended to vertebrates that enabled Metchnikoff to erect a grand scheme of host defense. It was truly an extraordinary intuitive grasp of an underlying biological process.

Again, it is in primitive organisms, that principles of allorecognition and the development of the immune system may be sought and possibly extrapolated to vertebrate immunity. Fusion between individuals with different commitments to somatic function results in parasitism; and mechanisms to prevent indiscriminate fusion must closely follow the evolution of cellular differentiation. It is at this level of phylogenetic development that the origins of active host response by primitive immune cells must be found. Leo Buss writes:

> The coupling of historecognition with intraspecific competition strongly implies that the fusion/rejection loci of clonal invertebrates are genes which act to control the units of selection. Fusion results in competition between cell lineages, and rejection results in competition between individuals. The decision to fuse or to reject is a decision to compete at the level of the cell or at the level of the individual. (25, p. 150)

Although colonials exhibit this parasitism (e.g., when *Hydractinia echinata* [a colonial hydroid] male and female colonies fuse, the male component dominates the production of gametes), all major sessile, colonial taxa (Porifera, Cnidaria) have genetic mechanisms to restrict fusion to close (compatible) kin. This is a form of allorecognition that is also found in annelids, but primitive mobile organisms (mollusks, nematodes, arthropods) generally have less-developed allorecognition systems. But these metazoans are still at risk for somatic parasitism and have both elaborate systems of historecognition to define self and defensive systems that have xenorecognition capacities to establish and maintain host integrity. The issue is well reviewed in N. A. Ratcliff and E. L. Cooper (26). Although we can readily explain the development of an immunological defensive system, the basis of a complex allorecognition system (mixed histocompatibility complex [MHC]) in vertebrates and echinoderms is not so obvious. The enigma of transplant rejection in vertebrates as an evolutionary phenomenon is a persistent problem. Did the vertebrate immune system evolve as a convergent system or is it homologous to clonal invertebrates and thus adapted for xenorecognition?

> The vertebrate immune system may represent a convergent evolution of allorecognition, one which arose as a nonadaptive byproduct of sophisticated modes of xenorecognition. Alternatively, the immune systems of vertebrates and echinoderms may

be homologous with those found in clonal invertebrates, only to have subsequently become adopted as a mechanism of xenorecognition. The latter hypothesis is supported by the fact that several primitive echinoderms (which are presumed ancestral stock for the chordates) were sedentary, potentially clonal, organisms. Thus, vertebrate ancestors may well have encountered fusion as a naturally occurring event and developed allorecognition as a response to the threat of somatic cell parasitism following fusion. Further support is found in the fact that vertebrate recognition of foreign tissue still requires simultaneous self-recognition (i.e., antigens presented on macrophages result in the release of interleukins only to T-cells which match the antigen in the context of appropriate self-markers). Hence the primitive system, though no longer required for fusion once mobility was acquired, was nevertheless required in xenorecognition and, accordingly, not lost in the course of evolution. (25, pp. 151–152; see also [27].)

Based on recent definition of a molecular suprafamily of recognition proteins that include immunoglobulin, MHC, and cell adhesion molecules (CAMs) (28), we might tentatively conclude that xenorecognition arose out of specialized function of the more primitive invertebrate allorecognition system. Our view of these issues are more fully explored elsewhere (29).

Notes and References

Abbreviations used in these notes:

AC   *Academic Collection of Works* (*Akademicheskoe sobranie sochinenii*), Vols. I–XVII. Moscow: Academy of Medical Sciences of USSR.

SBW *Selected Biological Works* (*Izbrannye biologicheskie proizvedeniya*), B. A. Dogel & A. E. Gaisinovich, eds. Moscow: Academy of Science of USSR, 1950.

Preface

1. Chernyak, L. and Tauber, A. I. "The Idea of Immunity: Metchnikoff's Metaphysics and Science." *J. Hist. Biol.:* 23:187–249, 1990.
2. Chernyak, L. and Tauber, A. I. "The Birth of Immunology: Metchnikoff, the Embryologist." *Cell. Immunol.:* 117:218–233, 1988.
3. Tauber, A. I. and Chernyak, L. "The Birth of Immunology: II. Metchnikoff and His Critics." *Cell. Immun.:* 121:447–473, 1989.
4. Tauber, A. I. and Chernyak, L. "Metchnikoff and a Theory of Medicine." *J. Royal Soc. Med.:* 82:699–701, 1989.
5. Tauber, A. I. "Metchnikoff, the Modern Immunologist." *J. Leuk. Biol.:* 47:560–566, 1990.

Chapter 1

1. Carter, K. C. "The Koch-Pasteur Dispute on Establishing the Cause of Anthrax." *Bull. Hist. Med.:* 62:42–57, 1988.
2. Brock, T. D. *Robert Koch: A Life in Medicine and Bacteriology.* Madison, WI: Science Tech Publishers, 1988, pp. 179–182.
3. Metchnikoff's career has been extensively documented, the most widely used source has been the biography by his wife, published in France in 1919 and translated into English, German, and Russian (O. Metchnikoff. *The Life of Elie Metchnikoff.* English translation by E. R. Lankester. London: Constable and Boston: Houghton Mifflin, 1921). / The most important Russian sources are Metchnikoff's collection of autobiographical essays, *Stranicy vospominanii* [*The Pages of Memory*]. A. E. Gaisinovich, ed. Moscow: Academy of Science of USSR, 1946—the Russian academic edition of his opus; Metchnikoff's correspondence:

a. I. I. Metchnikoff. *Pis'ma* [*The Letters*], *1863–1916,* A. E. Gaisinovich and B. V. Levshin, eds. Moscow: Nauka, 1974.

b. I. I. Metchnikoff: *Pis'ma k O. N. Metchnikovoi,* Vol. 1 (1876–1899); Vol. 2 (1900–1914), A. E. Gaisinovich and B. V. Levshin, eds. Moscow: Nauka, 1978, 1980.

c. "Metchnikoff's letters to A. P. Bogdanov" in *Rukopisnye materialy I. I. Metchnikova,* G. A. Kniazev and B. E. Raikov, eds. Moscow–Leningrad: Arkhiv Akademiia nauk SSSR 1960, pp. 53–67.

And various comprehensive biographies written by Russians, e.g.:

a. B. Mogilevskii. *Il'ja Il'ich Metchnikoff.* Moscow: Molodaya Guardinya, 1958. This biography is typical of a genre in Soviet literature; it is a volume in a popular Russian series *The Life of Remarkable People.* Written in a fictional style, it does not have references or any traces of research in the history of science. All biographical matters are presented in clichéd oppositions: conservative versus progressive, Western versus Russian, religious versus scientific. Of course, Metchnikoff represents the enlightened view of world struggle.

b. D. F. Ostrjakin. *I. I. Metchnikof in His Struggle for a Materialistic Weltanschauung.* Kiev, Vysshanya Shkola 1977. As Ostrjakin states:

This book is not a result of studies of Metchnikoff's scientific activity. The author has limited himself by more narrow goals to clarify that critique of different kinds of philosophical idealism, religion and extra-religious mysticism presented by this prominent Russian scientist. (p. 3)

How little this approach might elucidate Metchnikoff's philosophical positions we recognize, as did Metchnikoff himself, for his general philosophical beliefs developed in immediate interactions with the development of his scientific problems. In addition, we note that Ostrjanin's own philosophical erudition is limited by the most trivial declarations of Soviet orthodoxy in "dialectical and historical materialism." Lenin is quoted in the book almost as frequently as Metchnikoff.

c. Semen Resnik's *Metchnikoff.* Moscow: Molodaya guardiya, 1973, was written in the genre of a psychological biography. Resnik sees as the most striking feature of Metchnikoff's personality his complete and ardent preoccupation with the eternal question of life and death. Metchnikoff's relation to Leo Tolstoy and their meeting in 1909 is the dynamic axis of the book: two great thinkers claiming their possession of the final answer of the intellectual/spiritual challenge of the nineteenth century, and each, respectively, rejecting the alternative way (science or religion) to approach the mystery of human existence. The book does not provide any new orientation or information concerning the history of the development of immunological theory, but the comparison with Tolstoy is interesting because it provides support to our belief that we cannot comprehend the intellectual framework of Metchnikoff's personality out of context of the "metaphysical extremism" of the Russian culture of his time.

d. Another adoring commentary that closely follows Olga's biography, with minor supplemental material, is S. Zalkind's *Ilya Mechnikov: His Life and Work.* English translation by X. Danko: Moscow: Foreign Languages Publishing House, 1959. Its particular feature of interest is its photographic presentations.

There are numerous articles in English describing Metchnikoff's work: G. H. Brieger. "Introduction" in *Immunity in Infective Diseases* by E. Metchnikoff. Trans F. G. Binnie. New York: Johnson Reprint Corp., 1968, pp. ix–xxxi; A. G. Elftman. "Metchnikoff as a Zoologist" in Victor Robinson Memorial Volume. New York: Froben Press, 1948, pp. 49–60; L. J. Rather. Review of the English translation of Metchnikoff's *Lectures* and *Immunity. Med. Hist.:* 14:409–412, 1970; R. B. Vaughn. "The Romantic Rationalist: A Study of Elie Metchnikoff." *Med. Hist.:* 10:201–215, 1965; D. J. Bibel. "Sternberg, Metchnikoff and the Phagocytes." *Milit. Med.:* 147:550–553, 1982; idem. "Elie Metchnikoff's Bacillus of Long Life." *ASM News:* 54:661–665, 1988; idem. "Centennial of the Rise of Cellular Immunology: Metchnikoff's Discovery at Messina." *ASM News:* 48:558–560, 1982; M. L. Karnovsky. "Metchnikoff in Messina: A Century of Studies on Phagocytosis." *N. Engl. J. Med.:* 304:1178–1180, 1981; J. G. Hirsch. "Immunity to Infectious Diseases: Review of Some Concepts of Metchnikoff." *Bacteriol. Rev.:* 23:48–60, 1959; E. Bendiner. Metchnikoff: "Prophet and 'Daemon of Science.'" *Hosp. Pract.* 12:99–110, 1977; L. Heifets. "Centennial of Metchnikoff's Discovery." *J. Reticuloendothel. Soc.:* 31:381–391, 1982; L. R. Cahn. "The Twelfth Ernest Joke Oration: Outsiders and Their Contributions." *Aust. Dent. J.:* 11:1–8, 1966. / Also subjects of chapters in various books: P. de Kruif. *Microbe Hunters.* New York: Harcourt, Brace, 1926; E. Burnet. *Microbes and Toxins.* Translated by C. Broquet and W. M. Scott. New York: Putnam's, 1912; E. E. Slosson. *Major Prophets of Today.* New York: Universal Series Publishing Co., 1914; D. J. Bibel. *Milestones in Immunology: A Historical Exploration.* Madison, WI: Science Tech Publishers, 1988, pp. 119–124, 170–173; and E. Mardus's book (*Man with a Microscope.* New York: Messner, 1968). These largely represent well-documented chronicles of Metchnikoff's life, but none deal with probing the structure of his concepts or the development of his biological ideas. / Concerning the establishment of the phagocytosis theory, Bibel, "Sternberg," op. cit.; idem, "Bacillus of Long Life," op. cit.; C. G. Craddock. "Defenses of the Body: The Initiators of Defense, the Ready Reserves, and the Scavengers" in *Blood, Pure and Eloquent,* ed. M. M. Wintrobe. New York: McGraw-Hill, 1980; and Brieger, op. cit. have addressed the predecessors who approximated Metchnikoff's seminal studies, but again, a detailed analysis of how Metchnikoff arrived at his phagocytosis theory is not developed. The comprehensive history of the phagocyte as a component of inflammation is found in L. J. Rather's *Addison and the White Corpuscles: An Aspect of Nineteenth-Century Biology.* London: Wellcome Institute of the History of Medicine, 1972. As we mentioned, earlier observations of phagocytes did not contain a broad intellectual construct/theory nor a research program dedicated to elucidating the impact of the phagocytic event.

Of the French general studies there are A. Besredka's *Histoire d'une idee: L'oeuvre de E. Metchnikoff.* Paris: Masson, 1921. English translation by A. Rivenson and R. Gestreicher. *The Story of an Idea: E. Metchnikoff's Work.* Bend, OR: Maverick Publications, 1979; and P. Lepine's *Elie Metchnikoff et l'immunologie* (Vichy: Seghers, 1966). But these are only supplementary to Olga Metchnikoff's biography and are essentially uncritical recounts. / Recent shorter French essays include A. Delaunay. "Elie Metchnikoff, 1845–1916." *Lett. Cent. Inst. Pasteur,* no. 5, February 1987; and R. M. Fause. "Dans Le Sillage de Metchnikoff." *Lett. Cent. Inst. Pasteur,* no. 5, February, 1987. / In German, the most notable reference is Heinz Zeiss's *Elias Metschnikow: Leben und Werk.* Jena: Verlag von Gustav Fischer, 1932—a book that extensively catalogues Metchnikoff's academic opera; literature pertinent to his work, including correspondence; secondary studies, and various footnotes of interest in a rather general and uncritical biographical study. / An important contribution made in placing the phagocytosis theory in historical perspective is Robert Herrlinger's "Die historische Entwicklung des Begriffes Phagocytose." *Ergeb. Anat. Entwicklungsgesch:* 35:343–357, 1956.

The most relevant works for our purpose are those that attempt to define the development of immunology and the placement of Metchnikoff's contribution within that context. Metchnikoff's development of the phagocytosis theory as an evolutionist is comprehensively considered in Daniel P. Todes's *Darwin Without Malthus: The Struggle for Existence in Russian Evolutionary Thought.* Oxford and New York: Oxford University Press, 1989, especially pp. 82–103, which we will discuss in detail. The most complete single analysis of immunology's early debate is that of A. M. Silverstein: "Cellular Versus Humoral Immunity: Determinants and Consequences of an Epic 19th Century Battle." *Cell. Immun.:* 48:208–221, 1979; and idem. "Development of the Concept of Immunologic Specificity: I–IV." *Cell. Immun.:* 67:396–409, 71:183–195, 78:174–190, 80:416–425, 1982–1983. These papers are included in a comprehensive history of immunology: A. M. Silverstein: *A History of Immunology.* New York: Academic Press,

1989. Silverstein recognized that "there was little or no context of immunologic thought in which to fit the Metchnikovian theory." He places the phagocytosis theory initially in the context of elucidating the inflammatory reaction. He notes how Metchnikoff challenged the accepted dogma of the very nature of inflammation (viewed as deleterious), and as a nonpathologist, nonphysician, and a Russian, he was viewed with more than reserved circumspection. Silverstein, like some others, carefully and usefully chronicles the early debate, but he is particularly sensitive to the political and social aspects of the scientific conflict. (The debate is further detailed in a report of the huge 1890 medical congress (held in Berlin) in P. M. H. Mazumdar's "Immunity in 1890." *J. Hist. Med.:* 27:312–324, 1972.) In this regard, Silverstein recognized Thomas Kuhn's paradigm construct, and he implicitly uses a strategy effectively employed by Ludwig Fleck (*Genesis and Development of a Scientific Fact.* Chicago: University of Chicago Press, 1979). Silverstein's treatment is tantalyzingly brief in regards to the complexity of the cellularlist-humoral debate. He does not treat (neither do other historians) the issues of central concern to our endeavor: (a) the metaphysical structure of Metchnikoff's theory, (b) the placement of immunity within the issues of teleology and vitalism debated in late-nineteenth-century biology, and (c) concepts of pathology in the context of evolutionary debate.

4. Bernstein H. *With Master Minds.* New York: Universal Series Publishing Co., 1913, pp. 50–71.

5. Olga Metchnikoff wrote (apparently expressing her husband's belief), "He was able to stop the publication of this article, the first he ever wrote, and it never appeared" (*Life,* op. cit., p. 33). But it did appear:

> The paper was published, not in the "Bulletin [of the Moscow Society of Naturalists]" but in [the] "Herald of Natural Sciences," a popular-scientific journal published by the Society of the Researchers of Nature. The publication probably remained unknown to Metchnikoff because it appeared not only in another journal [the "Herald"] but also much later, in 1865. More bizarre, it was published in the last issue of the journal ["Herald"] for 1860, which was issued with a delay of almost five years. In numbers 47–52 of the journal, we find the paper, "Some Facts from Infusoria Life, a Paper of Il'ya Metchnikoff of Kharkov" (pp. 1564–1569). At the end of the paper, the date is noted: "November, 1862." Thus, the paper is Metchnikoff's first scientific publication, whose existence had remained unknown to the author himself. (A. E. Gaisinovich, in *Stranicy vospominanii,* op. cit., pp. 192–193, fn. 19).

6. de Kruif, op cit., p. 209.

7. Metchnikoff, E. "Untersuchungen Ueber den Stiel der Vorticellen." *Arch. Anat., Physiol. wiss. Med.* pp. 180–186, 1863.

8. Metchnikoff, E. "Nachtraegliche Bemerkungen ueber den Stiel die Vorticoelinen." *Arch. Anat., Physio. wiss. Med.* pp. 291–302, 1864.

9. Metchnikoff, E. "Ueber die Entwicklung von *Ascaris nigrovenosa.*" *Arch. Anat. Physiol. wiss. Med.,* 4:409–420, 1865. Leuckart answered Metchnikoff in the same journal ("Zur Entwickelungsgeschichte der *Ascaris nigrovenosa:* Zugleich eine Erwiderung gegen Herrn Candidat Mecznikow." 6:641–658, 1865). In his turn, Metchnikoff sent a letter to the editor, DuBois-Reymond, in which he promised to answer Leuckart in a special publication, which appeared in Goettingen as a brochure in 1866, "Engegnung auf eine Erwiderung des Herrn Prof. Leuckart in Gissen in Betreff der Frage ueber die Nematodenentwicklung, Von Elias Metschnikoff in Charkow."

10. Metchnikoff, E. "Vospitanie s antropologicheskoi tochki zrenia." *Vestnik Evropy.* 1871, 1:205–236. (Reprinted in *Sorok let iskania racional'nogo mirovozzrenia.* Moscow: Scientific Word, 1913, pp. 23–48.)

11. Metchnikoff, E. *The Nature of Man: Studies in Optimistic Philosophy.* English translation by P. C. Mitchell. New York: Putnam's, 1903.

12. Metchnikoff, E. *The Prolongation of Life: Optimistic Studies.* English translation by P. C. Mitchell. London: Heinemann, 1907.

13. Metchnikoff formulated the general task of comparative embryology inductively but, to obtain productive conclusions from this approach, concurrence regarding principles of comparison was required; in order to appreciate variations, necessary presuppositions are made about that which is varying. So, comparative embryology itself requires some phylogenetic assumptions. But these assumptions, in their turn, arise from reconstruction on the basis of embryological observations, not on a universal and metaphysical scheme. For many embryologists of the first post-Darwinian generation, reconstruction of different phylogenetic lines was recognized as a scientific goal. But as soon as this process began, the inevitable reversal of goal and means changed their respective places, and inner difficulties of comparative embryology turned into special problems that required new phylogenetic hypotheses for their solution. Precisely in this manner, Metchnikoff's comparative studies of two embryonic layers were not a mere means to establish phylogeny, but constituted a direct problem in their own right. This was his scientific preoccupation for the next fifteen years.

14. Metchnikoff, E. "Ueber Geodesmus bilineatus (Fascicola terrestris O. Fr. Mueller?) eine europaeische Landplanarie." *Bulletin de l'academie des sciences de St. Petersbourg:* 5:433–447, 1866.

15. Metchnikoff, E. *Lectures on the Comparative Pathology of Inflammation.* English translation by F. A. Starling and E. H. Starling. London: Kegan Paul, Trench, Trübner, 1893. Reprinted by Dover Publications, New York, 1968.

16. Metchnikoff, E. *Immunity in Infective Diseases.* English translation by F. G. Binnie. Cambridge: Cambridge University Press and New York: Macmillan, 1905. Reprinted by Johnson Reprint Corp., New York, 1968.

17. Metchnikoff E. "Issledovanija nad proiskhozhdeniem antitoksinov. O vlijanii organizma na toksiny." *Russkii arkhiv patologii, klinicheskoi mediciny i bakteriologii:* 4(4):26–33, 1897.

18. Metchnikoff, E. *The New Hygiene: Three Lectures on the Prevention of Infective Diseases.* Translated by E. R. Lankester. London: Heinemann, 1906.

19. Metchnikoff, O. *Life,* op. cit.

20. Metchnikoff, E. *Stranicy vospominanii,* op. cit.

21. Dogel, V. A. and Gaisinovich, A. E. "Osnovnye cherty tvorchestva I. I. Metchnikova kak biologa" in *SBW* (1950), pp. 677–725.

22. Nekrasov, A. D. "Raboty I. I. Metchnikova v oblasti embryologii" in *AC,* Vol. 3, pp. 401–437.

23. Belkin, R. I. "Embryologicheskie issledovanija I. I. Metchnikova v ocenke ego sovremennikov" in *AC,* Vol. 3, pp. 438–479.

24. Metchnikoff, E. "Neskol'ko slov o sovremennoi teorii proiskhozhdeniya vidov" (1863). Published for the first time in I. I. Metchnikoff. *Izbrannye biologicheskie proizvedenia.* Moscow: Academy of Science of USSR, 1950.

25. Metchnikoff, E. "O razvitii nizshikh rakoobraznykh v yaice." *Naturalist:* 2:65–72, 1866. (Reprinted in *AC,* Vol. 2, p. 33.)

26. About disagreements between E. Metchnikoff and A. Kowalevsky at that time, see V. A. Dogel, "A. O. Kowalevskii." pp. 38–45; Gaisinovich, op. cit., in "Footnotes" to *Stranicy vospominanii,* op. cit., fn. 2; Nekrasov, op. cit.

27. Metchnikoff, E. "Sovremennoe sostoyanie nauki o razvitii zhivotnykh." *Zhurnal ministerstva narodnogo prosvescheniya:* 158–186, March 1869. (Reprinted in *AC,* Vol. 2, pp. 254–276.)

28. We would not infer that Metchnikoff lacked a quick temper or ambition; quite the opposite, he had them in abundance, which Karl Ernst von Baer easily perceived. He wrote to young Metchnikoff in 1868:

I rejoice about your energy and talents and hope you will be an honor to your fatherland. Be some credit to the old man who, having already completely achieved his own ambitions, expresses the wish that you would go into polemics less frequently.... New discoveries and soundness of work make by themselves their own way. (*Stranicy vospominanii,* pp. 180–181)

29. Pre-Metchnikoff theories are reviewed in general histories of microbiology, e.g., W. Bulloch. *The History of Bacteriology.* London: Oxford University Press, 1938; A. Catiglioni. *A History of Medicine.* New York: Knopf, 1947; W. D. Foster. *A History of Medical Bacteriology and Immunology.* London: Heinemann, 1970; and most specifically by L. J. Rather, *Addison and the White Corpuscles: An Aspect of Nineteenth-Century Biology.* London: Wellcome Institute of the History of Medicine, 1972.

30. Neuburger M. *Die Lehre von der Heilkraft der Natur in Wandel der Zeiten.* Stuttgart: Verlag von Ferdinand Enke, 1926. English translation *Doctrine of the Healing Power of Nature Throughout the Course of Time,* by L. J. Boyd. New York: 1932.

31. Neuburger, op. cit., writes:

It states in the book, de natura hominis, by nature is to be understood the combination of the four cardinal humors. These constitute the nature of the body and through them it becomes sick and well. "The body of man contains within itself blood and phlegm and two kinds of bile, that is, yellow and black. And these (four elements) constitute in him the nature of the body and because of them he is ill or well."

In the same sense, mixture of the four fundamental constituents of the body, the word *physis* is also used in many places, yet not uniformly in the entire Corpus Hippocraticum. Because of this, Galen states (in Hipp., de acutor, morb. victu., Comm. II.31) that *physis* by Hippocrates signifies different things. "Accordingly, the word 'physis' of itself signifies many things." Many times by *"physis"* is to be understood *the four qualities* (warm, cold, moist, dry), many times *the four cardinal humors in their combined effect.* Occasionally it is the *innate heat, the final cause of all natural effects.* (Galen, de placit. Hipp. et Plat. Lib. VIII, cap 7.) In the book, de carnibus, one finds the famous citation borrowed from Heraclitus that warmth is the original basis of all things: "It is my opinion that what we call warmth is immortal and perceives and sees and hears and knows all, both that which is and that which is to be." ... "Natur" is for Hippocrates at one time, *lawfulness,* at another *essence* and *substance;* he extends the conception of the power even farther. (p. 7, fnn. 1 and 2 [1932])

32. Ibid.:

The chief founder of the Stoic physical theology, Chrysippos, sought in the fourth book of this work "On Providence" also to answer the question how the unspeakable misery of bodily distress and diseases could be reconciled with purposefulness in the cosmos, with providence: "whether the ills of man arise in accordance with nature." From Gellius, Noct. Atticae VIII (VI), 1, we learn the attempted solution of the question from the philosopher: It is in no way intended by the creative power which joins defects and ailments with so many excellencies and uses, the direct work of nature, but it yields itself only by inference, as the unavoidable secondary consequence. Because as for example nature occupies itself with the shaping of the human body, it requires the higher view and the most ultimate purposeful direction in union with its creative work so that the head will be composed of the most delicate and finest bones. But this viewpoint of higher purpose, useful direction, had a certain disadvantage directly as a result, since indeed the head possessed only a weak defense from the outside and relatively slight shocks and impacts against it show it to be very slightly resistant: "in a like manner also diseases and illnesses have been caused while health was being secured." (p. 10, fn. 3 [1932])

33. Rhazes, *A Treatise on the Small-Pox and Measles.* English translation by W. A. Greenhill. London: Sydenham Soc., 1848.

34. Fracastorius, H. *De Contagione et Contagiosis Morbis et eorum Curatione* (1546). English translation *Contagion, Contagious Diseases and their Treatment* by W. C. Wright. New York: Putnam's, 1930, pp. 60–63.

35. Pasteur, L. "Sur Les Maladies virulentes et en particulier sur la maladie appelee vulgairement cholera des poules," *Compt. Rend. Acad. Sci.* 90:239–248, 1880.

36. Salmon, D. E. and T. Smith. "On a New Method of Producing Immunity from Contagious Diseases." *Proc. Biol. Soc. Wash.*, 3:29–33, 1884–1886.

37. Behring, E. and S. Kitasato. "Ueber das Zustandekommen der Diphtherie-Immunitat und der Tetanus-Immunitat bei Thieren." *Deutsche Med. Wchnschr.* 16:1113–1145, 1890.

38. Pasteur's musing on the topic of possible active self-protection apparently never surpassed this old metaphysical circle of self-supporting "nature", which he expressed as "life prevents life." Emile Duclaux wrote (*Pasteur, the History of a Mind.* Translated by E. F. Smith and F. Hedges. Philadelphia and London: Saunders, 1920):

> Pasteur, who in his heart was indifferent to theories and asked of them only that they suggest experiments to him, held for a long time a purely cellular conception of microbial disease. It was by a struggle between the red blood corpuscles and the bacteridium that he explained in 1878 the resistance of the living fowl to anthrax, and we see him at every instant, in that period, having recourse to vital resistance, and saying: "Among the lower forms of life, still more than in the higher species of plants and animals, life prevents life." Again, it was this same sentiment which guided him in the experiments which we have seen him making, to prevent the development of the anthrax bacteridium by inoculating at the same time with some common bacteria. (p. 317)

Duclaux continued:

> The theory of Metchnikoff had, moreover, for [Pasteur's] mind, this satisfying aid that it equalized the competitive forces. There is something disproportionate in a bacteridium which kills an ox. One understands better a localized struggle between the leucocytes of the ox and the invading microbes, which perish if they are too feeble, or too few in number, but which take possession of everything if they are the stronger, because they have the power of multiplication in their favor. (p. 318)

Why is there something disproportionate in a bacteridium that kills an ox? Obviously, the self-protective properties of the macroorganism are equalized (intuitively) here with the organism as a whole. On the other hand, the satisfaction of equalizing the competitive forces (the phagocytes and bacteria) completely corresponds to the belief that "among the lower forms of life, still more than in the higher species of plants and animals, life prevents life." This belief may explain why Pasteur regarded Metchnikoff's views sympathetically; it cannot account for the intellectual origin of Metchnikoff's theory.

39. "The metaphorical idea of 'warfare against disease' waged by the forces of the body is not predominant in the Hippocratic–Galenic tradition, if indeed it occurs at all" (Rather, *Addison*, op. cit., p. 188). Elsewhere Rather writes of the metaphorical war against disease waged by the forces of the human body (See "On the Source and Development of Metaphorical Language in the History of Western Medicine" in *A Celebration of Medical History*, ed. Lloyd G. Stevenson. Baltimore and London: Johns Hopkins University Press, 1982, pp. 135–153. See also Peter H. Niebyl's commentary, which follows Rather's paper, pp. 154–156.):

> The notion is, however, relatively new. It has little part in the Hippocratic–Galenic tradition. . . . The idea that disease is or is caused by something that can be "cast out" is, of course, an ancient and ubiquitous one, but I am speaking here of official academic medicine in the West. (Rather, p. 142)

40. Coleman, W. *Biology in the Nineteenth Century.* Cambridge: Cambridge University Press, 1971.

41. Rather, L. J. "On the source and development . . .", op. cit.:

> Riches of metaphor and analogy abound in the medical literature of Germany throughout the Romantic period and far into the first half of the nineteenth century. . . . In 1845, long before the bacteriological era, Carl Heinrich Schultz (1795–1871), a many sided naturalist and physi-

cian, continued—in what was by that time an outmoded fashion frowned on by scientific physicians such as Jacob Henle and Rudolf Virchow—to formulate much of his pathophysiology in terms of the metaphorical "battle against disease" *(Krankheitskampf)* and "defensive processes" *(Wehrprozesse)* of the body. The two key terms in Schultz's metaphorical construct are *Heerde* and *Keim,* respectively the "focus" of the body and the "germ" of the disease. The "germ" is a hostile force of undermined nature; it is not, of course, a bacterial organism. . . . *Heerde* is the German word for "hearth," the seat of warmth and life of the home, the sun of its little microcosm, a force in its own right. (pp. 143–144)

And Rather continues:

To physicians of the postromantic school of strict science such language was almost anathema, and its use was vigorously opposed by Henle, Virchow, Gabriel Andral, Rudolph Lotze, and many others. (p. 144)

Rather cites Virchow:

We no longer regard the pus corpuscles as gendarmes ordered by the police state to escort over the border some foreigner or other who is not provided with a passport. (p. 145)

42. Rather writes in *Addison,* op. cit.:

Addison interpreted inflammation as a healing and protective response, mediated in some way by cell activities, on the part of the organism. As far as the first part of his thesis was concerned, it was well within the medical tradition and was no doubt shared by a large number of his colleagues in England. In Germany on the other hand, attempts to explain biological events in terms of ends and purposes—so called teleological explanations—had fallen into disrepute among scientifically minded physicians. The essentially teleological interpretation of the inflammatory process as a "defense reaction" had to a considerable extent come under this ban. (p. 180)

43. Metchnikoff, E. *Sorok let iskania,* op. cit.
44. Metchnikoff, E. "Zakon zhizni: Po povodu nekotorykh proizvedenii gr. L. Tolstogo," *Vestnik Evropy,* 1891, 9:228–260. (Reprinted in *Sorok let iskania,* op. cit., pp. 216–247.) In order to comprehend how far Metchnikoff had deserted the optimism of Haeckel's "biogenetic law," we might compare his opinion with Arthur Keith's (*The Construction of Man's Family Tree.* London: Watts, 1934, p. 10) summary of Haeckel's point of view: the apes are but "abortive attempts at man-production." Concerning the introduction of juvenile features into adult descendants as a topic of nineteenth-century discussions of the "biogenetic law," see S. J. Gould, *Ontogeny and Phylogeny.* Cambridge: Harvard University Press, 1977, pp. 177–184. Here Gould cites Edward Cope (1883) ("America's foremost recapitulationist"):

As these characters result from a fuller course of growth from the infant, it is evident that in these respects the apes are more fully developed than man. Man stops short in the development of the face, and is in so far more embryonic. The prominent forehead and reduced jaws of man are characters of "retardation." (p. 179)

It is obvious how much more disharmonic and "monstrous" is Metchnikoff's vision of man.

45. Metchnikoff, E. "Mirovozzrenie i medicina" ("Weltanschauung and Medicine"). *Vestnik Evropy* 1910, 1:217–235. (Reprinted in *Sorok let iskania,* op. cit., pp. 274–291, p. 274.)
46. Metchnikoff, E. "Vospitanie s antropologicheskoi tochki zrenia," *Vestnik Evropy.* 1871, 7:205–235. (Reprinted in *Sorok let iskania,* op. cit., pp. 23–48.)
47. Metchnikoff, E. "Vozrast vstupleniya v brak: Antropologicheskii ocherk." *Vestnik Evropy,* 1874, 1:232–283. (Reprinted in *Sorok let iskania,* op. cit., pp. 48–98.)

48. Metchnikoff, E. "Ocherk vozzreniya na chelovecheskuju prirodu"—*Vestnik Evropy,* 1877, 4:532–560. (Reprinted in *Sorok let iskania,* op. cit., pp. 99–121.)

49. Metchnikoff, E. "Bor'ba za suschestvovanie v obshirnom smysle." *Vestnik Evropy,* 1878, 7:9–47; 8:437–483. (Reprinted in *Sorok let iskania,* op. cit., pp. 122–200.)

Chapter 2

1. Metchnikoff E. "Sovremennoe sostoyanie nauki o razvitii zhivotnykh." *Zhurnal ministerstva narodnogo prosvescheniya.*:158–186, March 1869. (Reprinted in *AC,* Vol. 2:254–276.)

2. Pander, C. *Beytraege zur Entwickelungsgeschichte des Huehnchens im Eye.* Wuerzburg: 1817; and *Dissertatio inauguralis, sistens historiam metapmorphoseos, quam ovum incubatum prioribus guinue diebus subit.* Wuerzburg: 1817.

3. Pander, C. *Beytraege,* op. cit., pp. 11–12. Quoted from J. M. Oppenheimer. *Essays in the History of Embryology and Biology.* Cambridge: MIT Press, 1967.

4. Pander. *Dissertatio,* op. cit., pp. 26–27.

5. von Baer, K. E. *Ueber Entwicklungsgeschichte der Thiere: Beobachtung and Reflection.* Koenigsberg: Borntraeger, 1828–1837.

6. Oppenheimer, op. cit.

7. See, for example, B. A. Dogel and A. E. Gaisinovich. "Osnovnye cherty tvorchestva I. I. Metchnikova kak biologa" in *SBW* (1950), pp. 677–725.

8. Obeying the temptation to reconstruct history "logically," Metchnikoff wrote in his essay "Alexandr Onufrievich Kowalevsky: Ocherk iz istorii nauki v Rossii" that "Fritz Mueller's little book served as the starting point for a great number of works in the history of development of lower animals, among which the studies of Kowalevsky occupy first place." E. Metchnikoff. "Alexandr Onufrievich Kowalevsky. An essay from the History of Science in Russia." *Vestnik Evropy,* 12:772–799, 1902. (Reprinted in *Stranicy vospominanii,* Academy of Science of USSR, 1946, pp. 14–44). A. E. Gaisinovich commented on Metchnikoff's essay:

> The question about the influence of F. Mueller's book on the beginning of Kowalevsky's embryologic studies is quite unsettled. First of all, Metchnikoff himself points further (p. 21, 1946) that during his sojourn in Tuebingen Kowalevsky drew up for himself an extensive plan of independent works. However, it is known Kowalevsky was in Tuebingen in 1862 and returned to Russia in 1863. Mueller's book was published, apparently, in the beginning of 1864 (the introduction was written in South America in September 7, 1863). It is doubtful whether Kowalevsky could know of it before his arrival to Naples in October, 1864. But even independently from these facts, the plan of Kowalevsky's works (taking even the choice of his objects of research) does not reveal any influence of Mueller's book. As is well known, Mueller based his opinions exclusively on the crustaceans. Meanwhile, Kowalevsky writes "during my visit to Naples in 1864 my first concern was to study the history of Amphixus' development." And later, Kowalevsky did not work on the embryology of crustaceans. The choice of his first research objects obviously reveals some other peculiar reason. Gaisinovich, op. cit., pp. 194–195.

9. Mueller, F. *Fuer Darwin.* Leipzig: W. Engelmann, 1864. English translation by W. S. Dallas, *Facts and Arguments for Darwin.* London: John Murray, 1869.

10. Huxley, T. H. "On Anatomy and Affinity of the Family of the Medusae." *Philos. Trans. R. Soc. Lond.* John Churchill & Sons 139. 413–434, 1849. Oppenheimer writes that Huxley, as early as 1849, "had appreciated the fundamental relationship between the body-layers of invertebrates and the embryonic layers of vertebrates," but in Huxley's work of 1869 (*Introduction to the Classification of Animals . . .*) he does not mention any relation between coelenterate ectoderm and entoderm on the one hand and embryonic serous and mucous layers on the other. Oppenheimer concludes, "Yet twenty years later he and all other investigators were still awaiting to utilize the generalization in any way, even for pedagogic reasons" (Oppen-

heimer, op. cit., p. 264). As a generalization, the idea was well suited for its time and need not have waited for the Darwinian era for its utilization. Zaddach received support from Huxley in the 1850s and 1860s. It seems as if Huxley's modesty in 1869—in respect to the idea he first expressed in 1849—is most easily explained by the results of August Weismann and Metchnikoff's research that began in 1864 and 1865 and that brought forth a skepticism in respect to the naturphilosophical form of the idea of a parallelism between ontogeny and phylogeny and in respect to the naturphilosophical intention to order the animal realm in a unilinear way. On the other hand, it is our usual historical aberration that when dealing with a pre-Darwinian idea concerning an affinity of organic forms, we are inclined to consider the idea as something that surpassed its time.

11. Metchnikoff, E. "Embryologische Studien an Insecten." *Z. wiss. Zool.:* 16(1):388–500, 1866. Metchnikoff's first research in embryology was immediately provoked by Nikolay Wagner's discovery of the phenomenon that was later defined by von Baer as pedogenesis—parthenogenetic reproduction by insect larvae structurally unable to copulate. (See E. Metchnikoff. "Ueber die Entwicklung der Cedidomyenlarven aus Pseudoovum." *Archiv. Naturgeschichte: (Berlin):* 1:304–310, 1865. See also Metchnikoff's letter to von Baer, "Issledovanija o dvukrylykh nasekomykh" in *Zapiski akademii nauk:* (Saint Petersburg): 10(1):78–84, 1866, (Reprinted in *AC,* Vol. 2, pp. 56–60) and von Baer's answer—"About Professor Wagner's Discovery of Asexual Reproduction of Larvae." *Zapiski akademii nauk:* (Saint Petersburg): 10(1):app., 1–77, 1866. Note that Metchnikoff began his embryological study with the phenomenon that later played a role in undermining the strict parallelism between ontogeny and phylogeny.

There are some interesting parallels and contrasts in the scientific biographies of Metchnikoff and Weismann. Both started as embryologists having Leuckart as their mentor. At the beginning of their careers, Weismann attempted to reject any similarity of vertebrate and arthropod embryology (at least in respect to the germ-layers doctrine); Metchnikoff endeavored the opposite. The study of pedogenesis, as evidence of a discrepancy between ontogenetic and phylogenetic order, was Metchnikoff's first step in that long path that finally led him to the phagocytosis theory. The first insight leading Weismann to the germ-plasm theory was also related to his embryological studies of the problem of sex; those studies were embedded in his comprehension of the germ-layer concept and ontogenetic-phylogenetic parallelism. (See F. B. Churchill, "Weismann, Hydromedusae, and the Biogenetic Imperative: A Reconsideration" in *A History of Embryology,* ed. T. J. Horder, J. A. Witkowski, C. C. Wylie. Cambridge: Cambridge University Press, 1985, pp. 7–33.) Weismann's first reference to the continuity of germ-cell protoplasm also took place in 1883 when Metchnikoff first announced the protective function of amoeboid mesodermic cells. Weismann's germ-plasm theory prepared the twentieth-century revolution in heredity theory, but it also gave scientific support to the ancient metaphysical understanding of ontogeny as realization of a "plan," and it correspondingly contributed to the restricted view of evolution as "the evolution of adults." (See L. W. Buss. Princeton, N.J., *The Evolution of Individuality,* 1987) Metchnikoff's understanding of heredity was closer to nineteenth-century intuitions (heredity is the similarity between parents and their offsprings), but his concept of ontogeny was quite untraditional and oriented toward the problem of the responsibility that ontogeny assumes for phylogeny.

12. Zaddach, E. G. *Untersuchungen ueber die Entwicklung und den Bau der Gliederthiere.* No. 1: Die Entwicklung des Phryganiden-Eies. Berlin: G. Reimer 1854.

13. Huxley, T. H. "On the Agamatic Reproduction and Morphology of Aphis. *Linn. Soc.:* 22:193–220, 221–236, 1858.

14. Leuckart, R. "Fortpflanzung und Entwicklung den Pupiparen und Beobachtung an Melophagus ovinus." *Abh. Nat. Gesell. Halle:* 4:145–226, 1858.

15. Weismann, A. "Die Entwicklung der Diptera im Ei, nach Beobachtungen an Chironomus Speciosus, Musca vomitoria und Pulex canix." *Z. wiss. Zool.*: 13:107–220, 1863; idem, "Die nachembryonale Entwicklung der Musciden nach Beobachtungen an Musca vomitoria und Sarcophaga carnaria." *Z. wiss. Zool.* 14:187–336, 1864; idem, *Die Entwicklung der Dipteren.* Leipzig: W. Engelmann, 1864.

16. Metchnikoff, E. "Ueber die Entwicklung der Cecidomyenlarven" *Archiv. Naturgeschichte (Berlin).* 7:304–310, 1865.

17. Metchnikoff, E. "Issledovanija o dvukrylykh nasekomykh." *Zapiski akademii nauk.* (Saint Petersburg): 10(1):78–84, 1866. (Reprinted in *AC,* Vol. 2, pp. 56–60.)

18. von Baer, K. E. op. cit., *Zapiski akademii nauk,* (Saint Petersburg): 10(1):1–77, 1866.

19. Metchnikoff, E. "Untersuchungen ueber die Embryologie der Hemipteren." *Z. wiss. Zool.*: 16(1):128–132, 1866.

20. Metchnikoff, E. "Embryologische Studien an Insecten," op. cit.

21. Metchnikoff, E. *Embryologische Studien an Medusen. Ein Beitrag zur Genealogie der Primitivorgane.* Vienna: A. Hoelder, 1886. (Reprinted in Russian in *SBW* [1950], pp. 271–472.)

22. In his paper of 1849, Huxley used the old terminology: *the serous layer* and *the mucous layer.* Apparently, the terms *ectoderm* and the *entoderm* were coined in 1853 by George Allman in his paper "On the Anatomy and Physiology of Cordylophora." The term *mesoderm* was introduced by T. H. Huxley in 1871 in his *A Manual of the Anatomy of Vertebrated Animals.* London: J. A. Churchill 1871; New York: D. Appleton, 1872. (See pp. 10–11 [1872].) On this topic, see also Oppenheimer, op. cit., pp. 262–263.

23. Spencer, H. "The Social Organism." In *Illustrations of Universal Progress. A Series of Discussions.* New York: D. Appleton, 1889.

24. Metchnikoff quoted von Koelliker, A. *Icones Histiologicae oder Atlas der Vergleichenden Gewebelehre.* Leipzig: W. Engelmann, 1864–1865. (pt. 2, p. 90):

> However, in any case a conformity in the structure of hydroids and young fetuses of vertebrates is striking and, undoubtedly, further studies of the question followed by research in structure and histology of development of many animals will lead to discovery of a simple law of development." (21, p. 420, 1950)

25. Metchnikoff, E. "Alexandr Onufrievich Kowalevsky," op. cit. (Reprinted in *Stranicy vospominanii,* op. cit., pp. 14–44.)

26. Metchnikoff complained about his friend Kowalevsky in *Embryologische Studien an Medusen,* op. cit.:

> Kowalevsky writes [*Embryol., Studien an Wuermer u. Arthropoden. Mem. de l'Acad. Sciences de S. Petersburg,* Vol. XVI, N12, 1871, p. 5]: 'The embryonic layers, which I accept, have only in common with those described by Metchnikoff, in that they are embryonic layers.' The unfairness of these harsh words are evident when our data is compared. In recent times Kowalevsky himself studied the scorpion and became convinced that our respective descriptions of the embryonic layers coincide completely. The situation in which my participation in the question of the embryonic layers is usually completely disregarded, ascribed to the incorrect interpretation of my data by Kowalevsky. (*SBW* [1950], p. 422)

27. This discovery of alternating generations in *Ascaris* was the cause of a quarrel between Metchnikoff and Leuckart. Metchnikoff made the observation by applying his own method during a holiday absence of Leuckart from the laboratory. Leuckart proposed that Metchnikoff continue the research in collaboration, but then published the results under his own name just mentioning Metchnikoff's "help." Outraged, Metchnikoff began a public polemic against Leuckart. The older scientist argued that Metchnikoff worked in his laboratory according to the senior's plan. He further argued that Metchnikoff had, indeed, observed the fact, but only

in the same sense in which Columbus's cabin boy first noticed land from the mast and then might lay claim to have discovered America.

28. Nekrasov, A. D. "Raboty I. I. Metchnikova v oblasti embriologii" in *AC*, Vol. 3, pp. 401–437.

29. Metchnikoff, E. "O razvitii nizshikh rakoobraznykh v yaice." *Naturalist:* 2:65–72, 1866. (Reprinted in *AC*, Vol. 2, pp. 33–44.)

30. Kowalevsky, A. O. *Pis'ma A. O. Kovalevskogo k I. I. Metchnikovu [Letters of Kowalevsky to E. Metchnikoff]*. Moscow–Leningrad. 1955.

31. Kowalevsky, A. O. "Entwicklungsgeschichte des *Amphioxus Lanceolatus,"* *Mém. de L'acad. de St. Pétersbourg:* Vlle Série, T. 16, No. 12, 1867.

, 32. Metchnikoff, E. Dissertation for master's degree in zoology. University Saint Petersburg, 1867. (Reprinted in *AC*, Vol. 2, pp. 145–177.)

33. Metchnikoff, E. Dissertation for a doctorate degree in zoology. *Zapiski akademii nauk.* (Saint Petersburg): 13(1):app. 1, pp. 1–48. 1868. (Reprinted in *AC*, Vol. 2, pp. 178–207.)

34. Metchnikoff, E. "Embryologie des Scorpions." *Z. wiss. Zool.:* 21:204–232, 1871. (Submitted to journal in 1869.

35. Nekrasov, A. D. *AC*, Vol. 3, fn. 143, p. 492.

36. Kowalevsky, A. O. "Entwicklungsgeschichte der einfachen Ascidien." *Mém. de L'acad. de St. Pétersbourg*, 1866.

37. Metchnikoff, E. "Entwicklungsgeschichtliche Beitraege." *Bulleten akademii nauk.:* 13:709–732, sec. "Melages biologiques," 1869. (Submitted to the journal in 1868.) (Reprinted in *AC*, Vol. 2, pp. 239–250.)

38. Metchnikoff, E. "Zur Entwicklungsgeschichte der einfacher Ascidien." *Z. wiss. Zool.:* 12:339–347, 1872.

39. Metchnikoff, E. "Embryologie der doppelfluessigen Myriapoden." *Z. wiss. Zool.:* 24:253–283, 1874. (Submitted to the journal in 1873.)

40. Haeckel, E. *Generelle Morphologie der Organismen: Allegemeine Grundzuege der organishen Formen-Wissenschaft Mechanisch Begruendet durch die von Charles Darwin Reformierte Deszendenz-Theirie, Vol. 2.* Berlin: Reimer, 1866.

41. Semper, C. *Reisen in Archipel der Philippen*, pt. 2, Vol. 1, no. 5. Leipzig: 1868.

42. Metchnikoff, E. "Ocherk voprosa o proiskhozhdenii vidov." ["Essay on the Question About Origin of Species"]. *Vestnik evropy* 1876, 3:68–136; 4:715–747; 5:117–149; 7:158–197; 8:567–606. (Reprinted in *SBW* [1950] pp. 7–238, and in *AC*, Vol. 4, pp. 155–327.)

43. Unwilling to use Haeckel's terms *phylogeny* and *ontogeny,* Metchnikoff referred to *genealogy* and *individual development* (or *history of individual development*), respectively.

44. It was von Baer himself who recommended that Metchnikoff submit his work "Embryologische Studien an Insecten" (n. 11) to the contest for the Saint Petersburg Academy Prize, which was established by von Baer and carried his name. Metchnikoff shared the prize with A. O. Kowalevsky. In his letter to Metchnikoff von Baer wrote, "I rejoice over your energy and talent and hope that you will be a credit to your fatherland." (von Baer, Letter to Metchnikoff in *Stranicy vospominanii*, pp. 180–181).

45. von Baer. *Entwicklungsgeschichte der Thiere*, op. cit., p. 258.

46. About von Baer's attitude toward the idea of evolution, see B. E. Raikov. *Karl Ernst von Baer 1792–1876: Sein Leben und sein Werk.* Leipzig: J. A. Barth, 1968.

47. Gould, S. J. *Ontogeny and Phylogeny.* Cambridge: Harvard University Press, 1977.

Chapter 3

1. Metchnikoff, E. "Pozvonochnaya teoriya cherepa." *Zapiski novorossiiskogo universiteta:* 7:3–20, 1871. (Reprinted in *AC*, Vol. 1, pp. 189–199.)

2. Metchnikoff, E. "Studien ueber die Entwicklung der Medusen u. Siphonophoren." *Z. wiss. Zool.:* 24:15–83, 1874.

3. Haeckel, E. *Zur Entwicklungsgeschichte der Siphonopheren.* Utrecht: C. van der Post, Jr., 1869.

4. Nekrasov, A. D. notes:

The extensive material upon which the studies were conducted (seven species), the care for the siphonophorus larvae, and the presentation of their development . . . all this is sufficient to prize the work as classical. Although eighty years have passed since publication of the "Studies," the drawings are still presented in zoology and embryology textbooks, and they are referred to in all researches related to the phylogeny of the siphonophores. It is true, there are now not many supporters of Metchnikoff's view that the siphonophores were descended from the medusas. (*AC,* Vol. 3, p. 421)

5. Metchnikoff, E. *Uchenie ob organicheskikh formakh, osnovannoe na teorii prevrascheniya vidov.* Saint Petersburg: A. Zalenskii, 1869. (Reprinted in *AC,* Vol. 4, pp. 23–107.)

6. Metchnikoff, E.:

The more the [morphological] material is accumulated . . . the more the lack is felt of a carefully thought-out plan that would reduce this multitude of unrelated facts to a unity, not to a scientific abstraction, but to one that, as far as possible, would coincide with living reality. That is what Haeckel has undertaken relying on Darwin's theory. (*AC,* Vol. 4, pp. 23–24)

7. Haeckel, E. *Die Kalkschwaemme: Eine Monographie.* Vol. 1, Berlin: G. Reiner 1872.

8. At that time, only two layers were recognized in the sponges. Haeckel believed that the external one (the syncytium), which formed the skeleton, was the ectoderm and that the inner layer of the ciliated cells was the entoderm. Metchnikoff considered the external layer that formed the skeleton as the mesoderm, partially because he always observed the formation of the needles in Echinodermata in the larva's mesoderm. ["Thus, for instance, we see that the bare amoeboid cells of the skeletonogenic layer in echinoderm larvae are wandering in the body's cavity and as a result of active motions they gather in certain places, for instance, upon the stone canal" Metchnikoff, E. "Zur Entwicklung der Kulkschwamme," *Z. wiss. Zool.:* 24:1–4 1874.] Haeckel believed that the adult sponges had only two layers—the mesoderm and the entoderm. F. E. Schultze ("Ueber den Bau und die Entwicklung von Sycandra rapharus Haeckel." *Z. wiss. Zool.:* 25:247–280, 1875) established that there was in sponges a true external (third) layer that had been unrecognized by previous researchers. Metchnikoff agreed with Schultze in his paper "Beitrage zur Morphologie der Spongien." (*Z. wiss. Zool.:* 27:275–286, 1876.)

9. Metchnikoff, E. "Zur Entwicklung der Kalkschwaemme," pp. 1–14. (Reprinted in *AC,* Vol. 3, pp. 30–39.)

10. Metchnikoff, E., "Beitrage zur Morphologie der Spongien," op. cit.

11. Metchnikoff, E. "O pischevaritel'nykh organakh presnovodnykh turbellarii." *Zapiski novoross. ob. est.:* 5(1):1–12, 1877. (Reprinted in *AC,* Vol. 1, pp. 252–259.)

12. E. Metchnikoff wrote in "Spongiologische Studien." *Z. wiss. Zool.:* 33:349–387, 1879. [Submitted to journal in 1878.]:

In the early autumn of 1874 my colleague A. Kowalevsky obtained several specimens of natural larvae of the species *Halisarca,* closely related to *H. Dujardinii,* which I am calling *H. pontica.* Because I had been studying the development of sponges for a long time, Professor Kowalevsky proposed that I join him to study the material. . . . My friend's sharing [in the work] was much more important than my own as a secondary worker." (pp. 349–350)

13. Lieberkuehn, N. "Beitraege zur Anatomie der Spongien," *Muellers Archiv.:* pp. 376–403, 1857.

14. Lieberkiehn, N. "Beitraege zur Entwickelungsgeschichte der Spongillen." *Muellers Archiv.:* pp. 1–19, 399–414, 496–514, 1856.

15. Metchnikoff, E. "Issledovanie o razvitii planarii." *Zapiski novoross. ob. est.:* 5:1–16, 1877 (Reprinted in *AC,* Vol. 3, pp. 51–60.) In Metchnikoff's time, the term *planarians* was used for all turbellarias.

16. Metchnikoff, O. *Life of Elie Metchnikoff.* English translation by E. R. Lankester. Boston: Houghton Mifflin, 1921 and London: Constable, 1921.

17. Metchnikoff, E. *Embryologische Studien an Medusen. Ein Beitrag zur Genealogie der Primitivorgane.* Vienna: A. Holder 1886. (Reprinted in Russian in *SBW* [1950] pp. 271–472.)

18. Balfour, F. M. *Embryological Studies.* London: Adlard, 1880–1883; *idem, Handbuch der Vergleichenden Embryologie.* Jena: G. Fischer, 1880.

19. Buetschli, O. Bemerkungen zur Gastraea-Theorie. *Morphol. Jahrb.:* 9:415–425, 1883–1884.

20. Metchnikoff, E. "Vergleichend-embryologische Studien. 3 Ueber die Gastrula einiger Metazoan." *Z. wiss. Zool.,* 37:286–313, 1882. In relation to this, it is worthy to notice that Haeckel himself recognized his debt to Kowalevsky, quoted in *Mueller–Haeckel. The Basic Biogenetic Law.* Moscow, 1940

> For me the special value presented the outstanding studies of ontogeny of different lower animals published by A. Kowalevsky for the last seven years and which, in my opinion, are the most important and the most fruitful among all modern works in the field of ontogeny. p. 201.

On the other hand, there is an apparent misunderstanding in the historical literature where sometimes Kowalevsky is said to be Haeckel's disciple. Thus, in Erik Nordenskioeld's *The History of Biology* (New York: Tudor, 1928) we can read, "Alexander Kowalewsky (1844–1901), an academician of St. Petersburg, worked in the spirit of Haeckel, encouraged by his commendation" (p. 529). The information is quite misleading and beside this we can add that A. Kowalevsky was five years older than Metchnikoff and he was born not in 1844, but in 1840.

21. Buetschli, O. "Entwicklungsgeschichtliche Beitraege." *Z. wiss. Zool.:* 29:216–256, 1877.

22. Hatschek, B. "Beitrage zur Entwicklungsgeschichte u. Morphologie der Anneliden." *Wien, Akad. Sitzber:* 74:443–461, 1877.

Chapter 4

1. Metchnikoff, O. *Life of Elie Metchnikoff* (English translation by E. R. Lankester. London: Constable and Boston: Houghton Mifflin, 1921).

2. It is interesting to note similar reassessments by Darwin. "The study of Darwin's paper is now revealing how careful we need to be in our assessment of his autobiographical account of the discovery" (Bowler, P. J. *Evolution: The History of an Idea.* Berkeley: University of California Press, 1984, p. 21.)

3. Todes, D. P. "Mechnikov, Darwinism, and the Phagocytic Theory" in *Darwin Without Malthus: The Struggle for Existence in Russian Evolutionary Thought.* Oxford and New York: Oxford University Press, 1989, pp. 82–103.

4. Bowler, op. cit., p. 233.

5. Stebbins, R. E. "France," in *The Comparative Reception of Darwinism,* ed. T. F. Glick. Chicago: University of Chicago Press, 1974.

6. For instance, Todes, op. cit., writes:

> Beginning in the early 1890s Mechnikov's comments about Darwin's theory (but not "Darwinism" or "Darwinists") grew increasingly friendly. The striking change in the content and tone of his remarks permits us to speak with but slight exaggeration of two Mechnikovs.

The first was a Russian zoologist writing in the 1860s and 1870s. This Mechnikov was passionately concerned with evolutionary theory per se and wrote constantly about it, drawing on his own work in embryology and zoology. For him Darwin's theory was a powerful but tainted hypothesis, and the social milieu in which he lived encouraged scientific alternatives to its dubious Malthusian aspects.

The second Mechnikov was a pathologist working in France at the turn of the century. He was interested in evolutionary theory primarily for its relationship to phagocytosis. He did not write a single article about evolutionary theory per se, nor did he mention it, except in passing, in his copious letters to his wife. The intellectuals of his adopted home had never welcomed even those aspects of Darwin's theory that he had always found compelling, and an alarming number of them endorsed what Mechnikov considered to be antiscientific alternatives to it.

This second Mechnikov embraced the selection theory and proudly identified his phagocytic theory with it. For him, Darwin had provided the best available response to those pathologists who dismissed the phagocytic theory as teleological and to those philosophers who denied science's capacity to explain the seemingly purposeful qualities of nature. Scattered comments reveal that Mechnikov retained his earlier reservations about Darwin's theory, but these had become quite secondary.

The first Mechnikov did not associate his phagocytic theory with Darwin's ideas. In his initial, confident communication of 1883, he linked it simply with an "evolutionary point of view." Eight years later the second Mechnikov first invoked Darwin's name when responding to his critics in *Lectures on the Comparative Pathology of Inflammation.* (p. 98–99)

7. Baumgarten, P. "Referat." *Berl. Klin. Woch.:* 21:802–804, 818, 1884.

8. Metchnikoff, E. "Ueber den Kampf der Zellen gegen Erysipelkokken: Ein Beitrag zur Phagocytenlehre." *Arch. Pathol. Anat.:* 107:209–249, 1887.

9. Baumgarten, P. "Zur Kritik der Metschnikoff'schen Phagocytentheory." *Z. Klin. Med.:* 15(1, 2):1–41, 1889.

10. The essay "Neskol'ko slov o sovremennoi teorii proiskhozhdeniya vidov" ["A Few Words About the Modern Theory of Origin of Species"] was published first only in 1950 in *SBW,* pp. 655–672. The essay was written for a magazine *Vremya* [*Time*] but either was not sent or was not published. (The magazine was closed by censorship in 1863, but it resumed publication the next year.)

11. Vucinich, A. "Russia: Biological Sciences" in Glick, *The Comparative Reception of Darwinism,* op. cit., pp. 227–255.

12. Metchnikoff, E. "Alexandr Onufrievich Kowalevsky: Ocherk iz istorii nauki v Rossii." ["A. O. Kowalevsky: Essay on the History of Science in Russia"]. *Vestnik Evropy.* 1902, 6(12):772–779. (Reprinted in *AC,* Vol. 14, pp. 9–32.)

13. Metchnikoff, E. "K istorii biologii v Rossii za istekauschee pyatidesyatiletie po lichnym vospominaniyam." ["On the History of Biology in Russia for the Last Fifty Years (Personal Recollection)"]. *Russkie vedomosti.* January 1, 1914. (Reprinted in *AC,* Vol. 14, pp. 50–58.)

14. About von Baer's attitude toward the idea of evolution, see Metchnikoff in *SBW* (1950), pp. 63–71; B. E. Raikov, *Karl Ernst von Baer 1792–1876: Sein Leben und sein Werk.* Leipzig: J. A. Barth, 1968; and T. Lenoir, *The Strategy of Life. Teleology and Mechanics in Nineteenth-Century German Biology.* Dordrecht: D. Reidel Publishing Co., 1982, pp. 246–275.

15. Scude, F. M. and M. Acanfora. "Darwin and Russian Evolutionary Biology," in *The Darwinian Heritage,* ed. D. Kohn. Princeton, N.J.: Princeton University Press, 1985, pp. 731–752.

16. Vucinich, op. cit., writes:

Darwin's works that followed the *Origin* were received with equal enthusiasm. In August, 1867, Darwin wrote to [Sir Charles] Lyell that he was visited by a young Russian who is translating my new book into Russian [Francis Darwin, ed. *The Life and Letters of Charles Darwin,* 2 vols. (New York: Basic Books, 1959), Vol. 2, p. 256.] The book was the *Variation of Animals and*

Plants Under Domestication and the young Russian was Vladimir Kovalevsky [the younger brother of Alexander O. Kovalevsky], who subsequently became a well-known evolutionary paleontologist. At that time, the *Variation* was not yet published, and it seems most probable that the translation was made from a set of proofs given to Kovalevsky by Darwin. Thanks to Kovalevsky's rapid work, the first section of the Russian translation of the *Variation* was published several months prior to the publication of the English original. Darwin's *The Descent of Man* was published in 1871, and by 1872, not less than three translations of this work were published in Russia. Darwin's *Expression of the Emotions in Man and Animals* was published in England in November, 1872, and in Russian in December, 1872. (p. 235)

Further, Scudo and Acanfora, op. cit., noted:

Unlike other countries such as France, in which a similar debate [on ways in which natural selection would be an essential complement to the already accepted mechanisms of evolution] was resolved mostly against natural selection. . . . [I]n Russia the essential causative role of natural selection in evolution started being seriously questioned only in the 1930s, by Lysenkoism. Also uniquely, in Russia the debate continued to be centered on Darwin himself and on all his theories. Little attention was paid to various other forms of Darwinism, and Weismannism was mostly—and usually very distinctly—rejected. (p. 732)

17. The sentiment today closely approximates Metchnikoff's position and is best summed up by Gould when he states that Darwin's theory of natural selection "explodes any concept of inherent progress" (Gould, S. J. "Darwin's Big Book." *Science* 188:824–826, 1975). Also see, "The process results in a series of adaptive reactions to ecological opportunities, so the evolution of evolutionary potential is a more valid way of comparing exploitive and reproductive strategies." (P. W. Price. *Evolutionary Biology of Parasites.* Princeton, N.J.: Princeton University Press, 1980. p. 14).

18. Metchnikoff, E. *Uchenie ob organicheskikh formakh, osnovannoe na teorii prevraschenija vidov.* Saint Petersburg: A. Zalenskii 1869. (Reprinted in *AC,* Vol. 4, pp. 23–107.)

19. Haeckel, E. *Generelle Morphologie der Organismen: Allgemeine Grundzuege der organishen Formen-Wissenschaft Mechanisch Begruendet durch die von Charles Darwin Reformierte Deszendenz-Theorie,* Vols. 1 and 2. Berlin: Reimer, 1866.

20. Metchnikoff, E. "Sovremennoe sostoyanie nauki o razvitii zhivotnykh." *Zhurnal ministerstva narodnogo prosvescheniya:* 158–186, March 1869. (Reprinted in *AC,* Vol. 2, pp. 254–276.)

21. Bowler, P. J. *The Non-Darwinian Revolution: Reinterpreting a Historical Myth.* Baltimore: Johns Hopkins University Press, 1988.

22. Hull, P. L. "Darwinism as a Historical Entity: A Historiographical Proposal," in Kohn, *The Darwinian Heritage,* pp. 773–812.

23. Mivart, Saint G. J. *On the Genesis of Species.* London: Macmillan, 1871.

24. Actually, Bowler might be understood as saying that the morphologist thesis of linear evolution is but a natural product of the disciplinary construct: morphology must describe different developmental patterns that reflect the underlying unity of living beings. Bowler has not argued that the construct of linear development dominated nineteenth-century studies of evolution *and* developmental morphology; to do so would imply that the approach has its historical boundaries defined by some intellectual or cultural tradition allowing other approaches to both types of study. What Bowler argues is that the morphological notion of linear development dominated nineteenth-century comprehension of Darwinism and more generally evolutionary thinking—to its detriment. See Bowler, *Evolution,* op. cit.

25. Metchnikoff, E. "Zadachi sovremennoi biologii." *Vestnik evropy.* Vol. 2, pp. 742–770, 1871. (Reprinted in *AC,* Vol. 4, pp. 109–132.)

26. Metchnikoff alludes here to Fritz Mueller's criteria as found in *Facts and Arguments for Darwin.* English translation by W. S. Dallas, London: John Murray, 1869:

Which of the different modes of development at present occurring in a class of animals may claim to be that approaching most nearly to the original one. . . . *The primitive history of a species will be preserved in its developmental history the more perfectly, the longer the series of young states through which it passes by uniform steps; and the more truly, the less the mode of life of the young departs from that of the adults, and the less the peculiarities of the individual young states can be conceived as transferred back from later ones in previous periods of life, or as independently acquired.* (pp. 120–121.)

27. Bowler writes in *Non-Darwinian Revolution,* op. cit.:

It is worth remembering that evolution was originally used to denote the growth of the embryo and that Darwin himself seldom referred to his theory by that name. The increased use of evolution to denote the theory of transmutation followed the adoption of the name by progressionist writers such as Herbert Spencer and its use in the translations of Haeckel's works, such as *Evolution of Man.* There is thus a sense in which the very name of the evolution theory represents a violation of Darwinian principles, reflecting an effort to promote individual growth as a model for the development of life on the earth. The popularity of the term indicates the popularity of the progressionist and almost teleological interpretation of living development that Haeckel was promoting. (p. 88)

See also, P. J. Bowler, "The Changing Meaning of 'Evolution.'" *J. Hist. Ideas:* 36:95–114, 1975.

28. Metchnikoff, E. *The Nature of Man: Studies in Optimistic Philosophy.* English translation by P. C. Mitchell. New York: G. P. Putnam, 1903, pp. 1–16, 166–199.

29. Metchnikoff, E. *The Prolongation of Life: Optimistic Studies.* English translation by P. C. Mitchell. London: Heinemann, 1907.

30. Metchnikoff, E. "Vospitanie s antropologicheskli tochki zrenia" *Vestnik Evropy.* 1871, 1:205–235. (Reprinted in *Sorok let iskania racional'nogo mirovozzrenia.* Moscow: Scientific Word, 1913, pp. 23–48.)

31. Metchnikoff, E. "Vozrast vstupleniya v brak: Antropologicheskii ocherk." *Vestnik Evropy,* 1874, 1:232–283. (Reprinted in *Sorok let iskania,* op. cit., pp. 48–98.)

32. It is interesting that in some respects the opposition influenced even Marxism through Hegel's *Phenomenology of Spirit* and his writings on "Philosophy of Nature"; concerning the principal equality of the terms *spirit* and *life* in Hegel's philosophy [see Herbert Marcuse *Hegels Ontologie und die Grundlegung einer Theorie der Geschichtlichkeit,* 1932; see also Herbert Marcuse. *Hegels Ontologie und die Theorie der Geschichtlichkeit.* Frankfurt on Main: Vittorio Klostermann, 1968 (unrevised edition of 1932 work). [English translation by S. Benhabib. *Hegel's Ontology and the Theory of Historicity.* Cambridge: MIT press, 1987]. Opposing bourgeois society and its traditional predecessors, Karl Marx saw in the latter the dominance of the same "vegetative" activity, an attachment to a traditional object (to Aristotelians, natural place) and the anti-innovative, basically *reproductive* nature of production. (See K. Marx. "Formen die der Kapitalistischen Produktion Vorhergehn," *Grundrisse der Kritik der Politischen Ökonomia* [*Formations Preceding Capitalism*], 1857. Frankfurt: Europäische Verlagsanstalt, 1967, pp. 375–413.) In this sense, we can say that the concept of progress as it functioned in Marx's historical materialism was supported by the same ancient opposition of the vegetative activity and the animal activity.

33. Buss, L. W. *The Evolution of Individuality.* Princeton, N.J.: Princeton University Press, 1987.

34. Several of Metchnikoff's examples: The family Terebellidae belongs to the class Annelida. All genera of the family have well-developed systems of blood vessels, the only exception being the genus *Polycirrus.* The latter, similar to the other genera even in small detail, does not possess a blood system. The difference cannot be explained as an adaptation to special conditions because the *Polycirrus* lives in the same environment with other representatives of the

class. On the other hand, this peculiarity can not be explained by deviation of inherited transmission. As Metchnikoff writes:

> The latter explanation would force us, together with "the neo-Darwinians," to assume that the vessel system of Annelida is not essential as an adaptive device and has been transmitted to them as a useless heritage. But this cannot be the case, since the Annelida blood system plays an active role, connected in some genera with special gills.

> Some facts from the history of animal reproduction and development are especially demonstrative. We see quite often that two animals, which are so similar that it is difficult to find between them any difference pertaining to distinction between species, are essentially different in respect to reproduction. For instance, the polyp *Clytia cilindrica* produces a special medusa by means of a bud; but another species, *Clytia intermedia,* being very similar to the first, produces instead of medusa, peculiar sex-buds. Nothing can be explained here by the difference in external conditions because both species live in the same environment and the very similarity between them testifies to that similarity of conditions.

35. Metchnikoff, E. "Ocherk voprosa o proiskhozhdenii vidov" ["Essay on the Question About Origin of Species"]. *Vestnik Evropy,* 1876, 3:68–134; 4:715–747; 5:117–149; 7:158–197; 8:567–606. (Reprinted in *SBW* [1950], pp. 7–238; and in *AC* Vol. 4, pp. 155–327.)

36. Jenkin, F. "The Origin of Species." *N. Br. Rev.:* 46:277–318, 1867. (Reproduced in D. L. Hull. *Darwin and His Critics.* Chicago: University of Chicago Press 1973, pp. 303–344.

37. This collectivistic picture of the struggle for existence has been considered in recent Metchnikovian studies as the true paradigm for his future phagocytosis theory (which allegedly reflected the idea of interspecies struggle). Todes cites (op. cit.) the rejection of the Malthusian metaphor as the most characteristic feature of Darwin's reception and reinterpretation in nineteenth-century Russia. He argues that Russians, in contrast to Darwin himself, were inclined to consider those forms of struggle and competition that took place between different species or between organisms and abiotic environments as more essential than the forms of struggle and competition between individuals of the same species. However, this very interesting and productive observation has its own limits. We are not concerned with the trivial exceptions from such a generalization, but rather its specific internal contradictions. The typical Russian attitude toward Darwinism had its parallel in a more general paradigmatic opposition of Russia and Western Europe. Among "progressive" and "conservative" groups of Russian society, it was equally broadly believed that Russian collectivistic essence opposed the individualistic essence of Western Europe. It was broadly believed that Russian collectivism *(sobornost')* was rooted in the organic-synthetic mentality of Russians as opposed to the individualism and analytic-rational mentality of Westerners. The old Slavophiles who formulated this paradigmatic opposition asserted that Russians inherited this organic mentality from the Eastern fathers of the Church. Ironically, the very opposition of the analytic-rational and the organic-synthetic spiritualities was borrowed from German Romanticism, in which the opposition supposedly expressed two extremes of Western culture. Identifying the uniqueness of the Russian historic being with the latter pole, the Slavophiles worked within the intellectual framework of Western culture and thus inadvertently incorporated it. Arguing for Russian uniqueness, these Russian intellectuals revealed within themselves their European souls (as, e.g., Fyodor Dostoyevsky, who considering himself as heir of the old Slavophiles's idea, recognized, at the same time, Western Europe as "our second motherland"). The paradox was one of the central subjects of Russian philosophy and literature in the nineteenth century. The same kind of paradox is found in Russian collectivistic reinterpretations of Darwinism. First of all, as the theoretical paradigm of the Slavophiles's *sobornost'* can be found in German romanticism's elaboration of such concepts as "nature," "tradition," "nation," exactly in the same way the theoretical paradigm of Russian unwillingness to accept Darwinian individualism, incorporated in (and manifested by) the Malthusian metaphor, can be found in Western criticism of Darwin's ideas.

Among those collectivistic critics can be counted most of Darwin's morphologist opponents with whom Metchnikoff dealt at length in the *Essay.*

38. Naegeli, K. W. "Verdraengung der Pflanzenformen durch ihre Mitbewerber." *Muenchen, Akad. Sitzber.:* 4:109–164, 1874.

39. Naegeli, K. W. "Du Development des espèces sociales." *Arch. des Sci. Phys. Nat.:* 53:211–236, 1875.

40. Todes, D. P. "Darwin's Malthusian Metaphor and Russian Evolutionary Thought, 1859–1917." *Isis:* 78:537–551, 1987.

41. Bronn, H. G. *Untersuchungen ueber die Entwickelungs-Gesetze der organischen Welt waehrend der Bildungs-Zeit unserer Erd-Oberflaeche.* Stuttgart; E. Schweizerbart, 1858.

42. Bonner, J. T. *Size and Cycle: An Essay on the Structure of Biology.* Princeton, N.J.: Princeton University Press, 1965.

43. von Baer, K. E. *Ueber Entwickelungsgeschichte der Thiere: Beobachtung und Reflecxion.* Koenigsburg: Erster Theil, 1828. An essential collection of translated fragments from the work are found in *Scientific Memoirs: Selected from the Transactions of Foreign Academies of Science and from Foreign Journals,* ed. Arthur Henfrey and T. H. Huxley. London: Natural History, 1853. (Reprinted New York: Johnson Reprint Corp., 1966.)

44. Metchnikoff was interested in the problems of anthropology (both in its biological and philosophical aspects of the "nature of man") since his youth (see M. A. Gremiackii, "Metchnikoff kak antropolog" [Metchnikoff as the Anthropologist] in E. Metchnikoff. *AC,* Vol, 16, pp. 355–364; R. I. Belkin and M. A. Gremiackii, "Kommentarii k stat'iam po antropologii i etnografii" [Commentaries to the papers on Anthropology and Ethnology] in *AC,* Vol. 16, pp. 365–384). This interest continued throughout his life and his late writings on the topic of the nature of man have been translated into the major European languages and are well known. The main theme of these works is to establish an optimistic Weltanshauung through surmounting biological disharmonies by means of "rational life" (i.e., through orthobiosis). Thus, throughout his life, Metchnikoff continued to consider the human organism as basically disharmonious and imperfect. His anthropological works of the 1870s are less well known, some pertaining more to general philosophical questions and to the foundation of Metchnikoff's (pessimistic) Weltanschauung. Certain of these publications are the reports of his research as a field anthropologist: "Zametki o naselenii Kalmykskoi stepi Astrakhanskoi gubernii" [Notices About the Population of the Kalmuk Steppes of the Astrakhan Province] (1873); *AC,* Vol. 16, pp. 9–26; "O stroenii vek u mongolov i kavkazcev" [About the Eyelids' Structure of the Mongols and Caucasians] (1874), ibid. pp. 27–33; "Antropologicheskii ocherk kalmykov kak predstavitelei mongol'skoi rasy" [Anthropological Essay on the Kalmuks as the Representatives of the Mongolian Race] (1876), ibid. pp. 67–77. In these works, as he states himself, Metchnikoff attempted to apply to the field of anthropological research the same comparative methods he used in embryological studies. He tried to demonstrate that at least one of the reasons for differences between human races is the retardation of development conditioned by the time shifts of sexual maturation. In addition, Metchnikoff published a special essay, "Anthropology and Darwinism" (*Vestnik Evropy,* 1875, pp. 159–195. Reprinted in *AC,* Vol. 16, pp. 27–66), in which he discussed application of the Darwinian concept of natural selection and sexual selection in relation to man. The principles of the discussion, its main ideas and anti-Darwinian objections, are essentially the same as we encountered in the "Essay on the Question About the Origin of Species," (ref. 35).

45. Mueller, H. *Die Befruchtung der Blumen durch Insecten und die gegenseitigen Anpassungen beider,* Leipzig: W. Engelmann, 1873.

46. Unlike many modern historians of science (see, e.g., R. W. Burkhardt, Jr., "Lamarck: Evolution and the Politics of Science." *J. Hist. Biol.:* 3:275–296, 1970) who see Lamarck's

eclipse as due to the influence of his main rival, Cuvier, Metchnikoff sees the immediate result of Lamarck's weakness:

> On the one hand, it was very much damaged by its deductive method of organization, and on the other hand, it failed because it was impossible to enliven and assign it a practical meaning in science. We saw that Lamarck established "the laws", "the zoological principles", "the axioms", and he drew inferences from them, but all this only on a purely theoretical basis. Lamarck does not give a factual confirmation even in those cases when it would be possible to give [such a confirmation], and he disdains reality to such a degree which befits perhaps only a mathematician or a supranaturalist. On the other hand, we see, that as soon as Lamarck starts on the proper scientific soil, studying and distributing facts, he appears to be exactly the same zoologist and systematician as all the others: speaking about species, he gives to the concept the same meaning as do the other zoologists. . . . The introduction in *Natural History of Invertebrates* appears to be a code of the *a priori* formulated laws, but the *Natural History* itself is such an exclusively systematic book that it earned for its author the title of "the French Linnaeus." (35, *SBW,* pp. 43–45)

This discrepancy between Lamarck's generalizations and his scientific practice explains (Metchnikoff argues) why Lamarck's teaching could not be taken seriously by naturalists and under which conditions (i.e., in the situation of revitalized interest in evolutionary ideas that was provoked by the scientific sophistication of its presentation in Darwin's *Origin*) Lamarck's theoretical generalizations could receive appropriate evaluation. Metchnikoff concluded that despite the theory being highly remarkable, it hardly had any influence in its time.

47. Metchnikoff, E. "Bor'ba za suschestvovanie v obshirnom smysle." *Vestnik Evropy,* 1878, 7:9–47; 8:437–483. (Reprinted in *Sorok let iskania,* op. cit., pp. 122–200.)

48. Darwin and Metchnikoff's relation to the ideas of Wilhelm Roux's book *Der Kampf der Theile im Organismus.* Leipzig: W. Engelmann, 1881 will be discussed in chapter 5.

Chapter 5

1. As noted, Metchnikoff began his formal studies of infectious diseases in the summer of 1880, while on vacation in the country. He encountered an epidemic of beetles *(Anisoplia austriaca)* that had infected the grain crop. Remembering an observation the year before of a dead fly enveloped with a fungus, he applied the struggle of species to a practical solution: create a fungus *(muscardine)* epidemic to limit the beetle infestation. He succeeded in infecting healthy *Anisoplia,* then an application was attempted in the field by others (success not reported).

2. The extensive literature on fermentation and the development of the germ theory is summarized in several excellent secondary sources: W. Bulloch. *The History of Bacteriology.* Oxford: Oxford University Press 1938, pp. 41–66; J. B. Conant, ed. *Pasteur's and Tyndall's Study of Spontaneous Generation.* Cambridge: Harvard University Press, 1953; R. Dubos. *Louis Pasteur: Free Lance of Science.* New York: Scribner's, 1960; W. D. Foster. *A History of Medical Bacteriology and Immunology.* London: Heinemann, 1970.

3. Bastian, H. C. *The Beginning of Life: Being Some Account of the Nature, Modes of Origin and Transformation of Lower Organisms.* London: Macmillan, 1872.

4. Summarized by J. Tyndall. *Essays on the Floating Matter of the Air in Relation to Putrefication and Infection,* London: 1881; New York: D. Appleton, 1888.

5. An excellent survey account is E. H. Ackeknecht, "Anticontagionism Between 1821 and 1867." *Bull. Hist. Med.:* 22:562–593, 1948.

6. Crellin, J. K. "The Dawn of the Germ Theory: Particles, Infection and Biology," in *Medicine and Science in the 1860s,* F.N.L. Poynter, ed. London: Wellcome Institute of the History of Medicine, 1968, pp. 57–76. See also K. D. Keele. "The Sydenham–Boyle Theory

of Morbific Particles." *Med. Hist.:* 18:240–248, 1974; P. A. Richmond. "Some Variant Theories in Opposition to the Germ Theory of Disease." *J. Hist. Med.:* 9:290–303, 1954. It is ironic that Henle in defending the contagious etiology of infectious disease and writing forty years before Metchnikoff, also used a thorn as his putative model, which is similar to the famous Messina experiment that was designed for a related, but distinctly different, purpose. See Jacob Henle. *On Miasima and Contagion: Pathologische Untersuchungen.* Berlin: August Hirschwald Verlag, 1840. (Trans. by T. D. Brock. in *Robert Koch: A Life in Medicine and Bacteriology.* Madison, WI: Science Tech Publishers, 1988):

> Consider the case of a thorn which has been thrust into a finger and causes inflammation . . . if the thorn is removed it can be stuck into the finger of another person, and cause the same disease a second time. It is not the disease which is being transferred, but the cause of the disease. Now suppose that the thorn could reproduce itself in a diseased body, or that every small part of the thorn could turn into a new thorn. Then, through the transfer of each small part of the thorn, one could cause the same disease in others. The thorn, not the disease, is the parasite. . . . The contagion, as we consider it, is similar to the thorn. The contagion is not itself the disease, but the inducer of the disease. . . . As an example, when a needle is immersed in a solution containing a small amount of smallpox vaccine, this is sufficient to cause an infection. This effect by such a small dose depends on the ability of the agent to reproduce itself. . . . This is therefore further proof that the contagion is alive. (p. 28)

7. Richardson, B. W. "On the theory of zymosis." *Trans. Epidem. Soc.:* 1:20–30, 1860; and *On the Poisons of the Spreading Diseases: Their Nature and Mode of Distribution.* London: 1867; see also A. S. MacNalty. *A Biography of Sir Benjamin Ward Richardson.* London: 1950.

8. Beale, L. S. *Disease Germs: Their Real Nature.* Philadelphia: Lindsay & Blakiston, 1870; idem. *Disease Germs: Their Supposed Nature.* London: Harrison and Sons, 1879; idem. *Bioplasm: An Introduction to the Study of Physiology and Medicine.* London. John Churchill and Sons, 1872.

9. Sanderson, J. B. "Introductory Report on the Intimate Pathology of Contagion." App. to the *Twelfth Report on the Medical Officer of the Privy Council, 1869.* London: 1870, pp. 229–256.

10. Ross, J. *The Graft Theory of Disease: Being an Application of Mr. Darwin's Hypothesis of Pangenesis to the Explanation of Phenomena of the Zymotic Diseases.* London: John Churchill and Sons, 1872.

11. Drysdale, J. *Germ Theories of Infectious Disease.* London and Liverpool: 1878.

12. Koch, R. "Die Aetiologie der Milzbrand-Krankheit, begrundet auf die Entwicklungsgeschichte des Bacillus Anthracis." *Beitr. Biol. Pflanzen:* 2:277–310, 1877.

13. Koch, R. "Die Aetiologie der Tuberculose." *Berl. Klin. Woch.:* 19:221–230, 1882. (Based on a lecture to the Physiological Society of Berlin given on 24 March 1882). Idem. *Ueber die Aetiologie der Tuberculose.* (Verhandlungen des Congresses fur Innere Medicin, Erster Congress.) Wiesbaden: J. F. Bergmann, pp. 56–66, 1882.

14. Koch, R. "Zur Untersuchung von pathogenen Organismen." *Mittheilungen an der Kaiserlichen Gesundhesitsamte:* 1:1–48; plates 1–14 (84 figs.) 1881. *New York Times,* 3 May 1882.

15. Pasteur, L. "Memoire sur la fermentation appelee lactique. (Extrait par l'auteur)." *Compt. Rend. Acad. Sci.:* 45:913–916, 1857; idem. "Memoire sur la fermentation alcoolique." *Ann. Chim. Phys.,* (3rd ser.) 58:323–426, 1860; idem. "Animalcules infusoires vivant sans gaz oxygène libre et déterminant des fermentations." *Compt. Rend. Acad. Sci.:* 52:344–347, 1861; idem, "Influence de l'oxygène sur le développement de la levure et la fermentation alcooloque." *Bull. Soc. Chim. (Paris),* 28 June 1861, pp. 79–80 (resumé); idem, "Memoire sur les corpuscles organises qui existent dans l'atmosphere: Examen de la doctrine des générations spontanées." *Ann. Sci. Nat:* (4th ser.) 16:5–98, 1861. J. Lister. "On a New Method of Treating

Compound Fracture, Abscess, Etc.; With Observations on the Conditions of Suppuration." *Lancet:* 1:326, 357, 387; 2:95, 1867; idem. "On the Antiseptic Principle in the Practice of Surgery." *Br. Med. J.:* 2:246–248; Lister and Pasteur's (translated) articles are collected in T. D. Brock. *Milestones in Microbiology.* Englewood Cliffs, N.J.: Prentice-Hall, 1961. F. F. Cartwright, "Antiseptic Surgery" in Poynter, op. cit., pp. 77–103; J. Shepard. "Lister and the Development of Abdominal Surgery," in Poynter, op. cit., pp. 105–116; see especially Metchnikoff's tribute: Metchnikov, I. I. *The Founders of Modern Medicine: Pasteur, Koch, Lister,* trans. D. Berger. New York: Walden, 1939.

16. Ackerknecht, E. H. *Rudolf Virchow: Doctor, Statesman, Anthropologist.* Madison: University Wisconsin Press, 1953, pp. 105–118. This source contains extensive references to Virchow's work.

17. Virchow, R. "i. Krankheitswesen und Krankheitsursachen." *Arch. Pathol. Anat.:* 79:1–19 (esp. see p. 10), 1880.

18. Virchow, R. "i. Krankheitswesen und Krankheitsursachen." *Arch. Pathol. Anat.:* 79:185–228 (esp. see p. 195), 1880.

19. Virchow, R. "Der Kampf der Zeilen und der Bakterien." *Arch. Pathol. Anat.:* 101:1–13, 1885.

20. As cited by Ackerknecht (ref. 16, p. 115), based on Robert Koch's unpublished letters to Carl Fluegge in the H. B. Jacobs Collection of the Johns Hopkins Institute of the History of Medicine.

21. Metchnikoff, E. *Lectures on the Comparative Pathology of Inflammation* (1891). English translation by F. A. Starling and E. H. Starling. London: Kegan Paul, Trench, Trübner, 1893, and New York: Dover, 1968.

22. Metchnikoff, E. *Immunity in Infective Diseases* (1901). Trans. F. G. Binnie, Cambridge, 1905. New York: Johnson Reprint Corp., 1968.

23. Rather, L. J. *Addison and the White Corpuscles: An Aspect of Nineteenth-Century Biology.* London: Wellcome Institute of the History of Medicine. 1972.

24. Brieger, G. H. "Introduction" in E. Metchnikoff, *Immunity in Infective Disease,* op. cit., pp. ix–xxxi.

25. Bulloch. *History of Bacteriology,* op. cit., pp. 255–283.

26. Foster, op. cit., pp. 92–126.

27. Craddock, C. G. "Defenses of the Body: The Initiators of Defense, The Ready Reserves and the Scavengers," in *Blood: Pure and Eloquent,* ed. M. M. Wintrobe. New York: McGraw-Hill, pp. 417–456, 1980.

28. Ecker, A. "Ueber die Veraenderungen, welche die blutkorperchenhaltige Zellen in der Milzerleiden." *Z. Ration. Med.:* 6:261–265, 1847.

29. Virchow, R. "Ueber blutkoerperchenhaltige Zellen." *Arch. Pathol. Anat.:* 4:515–540, 1852.

30. Jones, T. W. "Report on the Changes in Blood in Inflammation and on the Nature of the Healing Process." *Br. For. Med. Rev.:* 18:225–280, 1844.

31. Haeckel, E. "Ueber die Gewebe des Flusskrebses." *Muellers Arch.:* pp. 469–568, 1857.

32. Haeckel, E. *Die Radiolarien.* Berlin: George Reimer, 1862.

33. Von Recklinghausen, F. D. "Ueber Eiter und Bindegewebeskoerperchen." *Arch. Pathol. Anat.:* 28:157–197, 1863.

34. Preyer, W. "Ueber amoeboide Blutkoerperchan." *Arch. Pathol. Anat.:* 30:417–441, 1864.

35. Frey, H. *Handbuch der Histologie and Histochemie des Menchen.* Leipzig: W. Engelmann, 1867.

36. Stricker, S. *Handbuch der Lehre von den Geweben der Menschen und der Tiere,* Vol. 1. Leipzig: W. Engelmann, 1871.

37. Kusnezoff, A. "Ueber Blutkoerperchenhaeltige Zellen der Milz." *Wien, Akad. Sitzungsb.* 67(3):58–67, 1873.

38. Klebs, E. *Beitrage zur pathologische Anatomie der Schusswunden.* Leipzig: Vogel, 1872.

39. Koch, R. "Untersuchungen ueber die Aetiology der Wundinfectionskrankheiten." Leipzig: Vogel, 1878.

40. Panum, P. L. "Das putride Gift, die Bakterien, die putride Infection oder Intoxication und die Septicaemie." *Arch. Pathol. Anat.:* 60:301–352, 1874.

41. Grawitz, P. "Beitraege zur systematischen Botanik der pflanzlichen Parasiten mit experimentellen Untersuchungen ueber die durch sie bedingten Krankheiten." *Arch. Pathol. Anat.:* 70:546–548, 1877.

42. Herrlinger, R. "Die Historische Entwicklung des Begriffes Phagocytose." *Ergeb. Anat. Entwicklung Geschichte,:* 35:334–357, 1956.

43. Muellendorf, J. "Ueber Ruckfallstyphus nach Beobachtungen im staedtischen Krankenhaus zu Dresden, 1879." *Dent. Med. Wochen.* 5:620–622, 630–632, 642–644, 1879.

44. Bibel, D. J. "Sternberg, Metchnikoff and the Phagocytes." *Milit. Med.:* 147:550–553, 1982.

45. Sternberg, G. M. "A Contribution to the Study of the Bacterial Organisms Commonly Found upon Exposed Mucous Surfaces and in the Alimentary Canal of Healthy Individuals." *Johns Hopkins Univ. Biol. Stud.* 2:157–181, 1883. This paper was presented in August 1881 at the Cincinnati meeting of the American Association for the Advancement of Science. The published version contained the cited quotation as a note; the paper was also published in *Proc. Am. Assoc. Adv. Sci.* 30:83–94, 1881–1882.

46. Sternberg, G. M. *Immunity: Protective Inoculations in Infectious Diseases and Serum Therapy.* New York: William Wood, pp. 14–16, 1895.

47. Sternberg, G. M. "The Metchnikoff Theory." JAMA: 63:779–780, 1914.

48. Besredka, A. *The Story of an Idea: E. Metchnikoff's Work: Embryogenesis, Inflammation, Immunity, Aging Pathology, Philosophy.* Preface by L. Gross. English translation by A. Rivenson and R. Gestreicher, Bend, OR: Maverick Publications, 1979.

49. Metchnikoff, O. *The Life of Elie Metchnikoff.* English translation by E. R. Lankester. London: Constable and Boston: Houghton Mifflin, 1921.

50. Metchnikoff articulated his frustration of lacking medical credentials in reference to his final departure from Russia for the Pasteur Institute. This was the result of the failed vaccination program that he could not control because he was regarded as a biologist with no medical expertise. (Hutchinson, J. F. "Tsarist Russia and the Bacteriological Revolution." *J. Hist. Med.:* 40:420–439, 1985).

51. Canguilhem, G. *The Normal and the Pathological.* Trans. C. R. Fawcett in collaboration with R. S. Cohen. Originally published by D. Reidel, Dordrecht, The Netherlands, in 1978. Reissued by Zone Books, New York, 1989.

52. von Aesch, A. G. *Natural Sciences in German Romanticism.* New York: AMS Press, 1966.

53. Rather, L. J. "On the Source and Development of Metaphorical Language in the History of Western Medicine," in *A Celebration of Medical History,* ed. L. G. Stevenson. Baltimore and London: Johns Hopkins University Press: pp. 135–153, 1982.

54. Besredka actually asks a rhetorical question. He attempts to make Metchnikoff's conversion explicable:

> What appeared at first sight a fanciful turning point of ideas was, in reality, nothing but the relentless pursuit of the same theme without a single break. (see n. 48, p. 9)

Besredka believed that the phagocytosis idea arose from the question:

> For what purpose [do] mesodermal cells, usually found in the depth of the organism and sep-
> arated from the environment by the ectoderm and from the body cavities by the entoderm,
> have the ability to engulf and digest solid particles? (48, p. 12)

Because, as Besredka believed, this question had originated in Metchnikoff's embryological
and evolutionary studies, turning to protective phagocytosis was "nothing but the relentless
pursuit of the same theme without a single break". But this question, omitting the pathological
context of Metchnikoff's preceding biological studies, does not contain in itself anything that
could possibly explain the reorientation of his thought from normal biology to pathology. We
discussed earlier that the idea of a protective mechanism is not self-obvious and is hardly compatible with that intuition of organism that takes organismic integrity as something immediately guaranteed. The teleological question—For what purpose do mesodermal cells engulf and
digest solid particles?—does not ask *what* is the organismic integrity that authorizes a structure
to serve a certain purpose and does not express any doubt in such a guaranteed integrity. The
question does not imply a disharmonious, pathological vision of an organism's nature, for
integrity, which the question apparently implies, harmony is normal. The question that allegedly reflected Metchnikoff's central intuition actually presented an old Hippocratic idea of the
self-sustaining integrity (i.e., the idea of the whole acting as a physician on behalf of its own
parts). Why then could the question lead to the thought about a particular structure that would
possibly serve as a physician on behalf of the whole? Why would the integrity, which was understood as the natural power healing and harmonizing the parts of the whole (actually *making*
them part of the whole), include a special subsystem (a special part) whose *normally* performed
function is as a personal physician of integrity? Is the subsystem, then, active as *a part* of the
whole, when the whole is absent (so, when the part is not a part)? Is the *norm* under which the
healing subsystem is active reflect the state of the organism's disintegration? If so, the phagocytosis idea could not originate in the question about a possible purpose of mesodermic cells
if the question had been taken without the pathological context of Metchnikoff's biological
ideas. Besredka misses the context completely and in his account of the biological prehistory
of the phagocytosis theory, he repeats Metchnikoff's late rationalization reflecting his optimistic appeasement. Besredka writes:

> His mighty mind . . . never really had deviated from his single and continuous idea—yet, what
> a deep and fertile idea! This guilding idea of Metchnikoff is the concept that the morphological
> elements develop in the animal kingdom, according to a single plan. (See n. 48, p. 3)

We saw how far he wandered from the real state of affairs. Besredka does not explain actually
how the idea of the protective phagocytosis was born. He only attempts to explain how the
idea could be linked to the set of associations presented by Metchnikoff's preceding works.

55. Coleman, W. *Biology in the Nineteenth Century.* Cambridge: Cambridge University
Press, 1971.

56. Cohnheim, J. *Vorlesungen ueber allgemeinen Pathologie: Ein Handbuch fuer Aerzte und
Studirende.* Berlin: 1877–1880, 2 vols. Vol. 1, 1877, 2nd ed., 1882. [*Lectures on General
Pathology: A Handbook for Practitioners and Students*]. Translated from the second German
edition by Alexander B. McKee and M. B. Dub. London: New Sydenham Society, 1889.

57. Henle, J. "Bericht ueber die Arbeiten im Gebiet der rationellen Pathologie seit Anfang
des Jahres 1839." *Z. rationelle Med.:* 2:1–433, 1844. Inflammation, pp. 34–287; idem. *Handbuch der rationellen Pathologie.* Braunschweig: F. Vieweg,1846–1853, Vol. 2, p. 417. B. Still-
ing. *Physiologische pathologische und medicinisch-praktische Untersuchungen ueber die Spin-
alirritation,* Leipzig: O. Wigand, 1840.

58. Virchow, R. "Ueber die akute Entzundung der Arterien." *Archiv. Pathol. Anat.:* 1:272–
378, 1847; idem. "Ueber parenchymatose Entzundung." *Archiv. Pathol. Anat.;* 4:261–324,
1852, "Handb. d. Spec. Pathol., 1:46; idem. "Cellularpathologie." 4(1):365–458, 1971.

59. Virchow, R. "Cellular-Pathologie." *Arch. Pathol. Anat.:* 8:1–39, 1855.

60. Virchow, R. *Die Cellularpathologie in ihrer Begruendung auf physiologische und pathologische Gewebelehre.* Berlin: Hirschwald, 1858; 2nd ed. 1859. Frank Chance's English translation (*Cellular Pathology as Based Upon Physiological and Pathological Histology*) of the 2nd ed. was published in 1860 (London: John Churchill & Sons), in 1863 (Philadelphia: Lippincott), and in 1971 (New York: Dover).

61. Cohnheim, J. "Ueber Entzuendung und Eiterung", *Arch. Pathol. Anat.:* 40:1–79, 1867,

62. Pagel, W. "The Speculative Basis of Modern Pathology: Jahn, Virchow and the Philosophy of Pathology." *Bull. Hist. Med.:* 18(1):1–43, June 1945.

63. Freudian longing for death and longing for life are, of course, not the only late echo of this Romantic approach to the nature of life. Metchnikoff's instinct of life and instinct of death present another example of these late reverberations. From Metchnikoff's point of view, the dominance of the instinct of death in adolescents, when the organism has not yet achieved the harmonious equilibrium characteristic of the mature organism, determines youthful pessimism. Optimism is characteristic of maturity because the harmony of the mature organism releases the instinct of life. And finally, the healthy life *(orthobiosis)* satiates the instinct of life and, at old age, releases the instinct of death—the instinctive longing for death as the final rest. Metchnikoff's idea of mature harmony may be quite naturally considered as a late analogy of the naturphilosophical "egoistic" pole, this is associated with the idea of organism's acme— the state of complete development and self-sustaining self-equality. Because any deviation from the state reflects the "cosmic" tendency, (i.e., the movement toward death), it references the pathological side of life. If the fully developed organism is the normal, then the deviation from the norm (i.e., the earlier stages in individual development or preceding links in the genealogical chain) must be considered in relation to the norm as the pathological. And vice versa what seems to be a pathological phenomenon could be interpreted as a return to an earlier stage of development. Not only the naturphilosophers of the first decades of the nineteenth century, but Virchow in his *Cellular Pathology* readily used this speculative trope (see, e.g., ref. 60, p. 90, 1971). Hence, Metchnikoff's opposition of the disharmonious (pathological) immature human organism and harmonious (healthy) mature organism seems to consistently fit this Romantic tradition. In any case, we will argue that however close the connections with this tradition may be found in Metchnikoff's intellectual machinery, there was something of radical novelty in his approach to organismic integrity.

64. It was not specifically Virchow's belief; G. Canguilhem, op. cit.:

In the course of the nineteenth century, the real identity of normal and pathological vital phenomena, apparently so different, and given opposing values by human experience, became a kind of scientifically guaranteed dogma, whose extension into the realms of philosophy and physiology appeared to be dictated by the authority biologists and physicians accorded to it. This dogma was expounded in France by Auguste Comte and Claude Bernard, each working under very different circumstances and with very different intentions. (See n. 51, p. 43)

65. Virchow fits well into the teleomechanistic tradition, whose commitment to following the integration offered by an organizing principle of teleological origin, found itself wedged between the Romanticism of *naturphilosophie* (which also invoked Kantian principles) and the emerging chemomechanical reductionists, with whom Cohnheim would more likely find compatibility. The teleomechanistic school is well described by Timothy Lenoir (*The Strategy of Life: Teleology and Mechanics in Nineteenth-Century German Biology.* Dordrecht, The Netherlands: Reidel, 1982. Reissued by the University of Chicago Press in 1989).

66. Neuburger, M. *Die Lehre von der Heilkraft der Natur in Wandel der Zeiten.* Stuttgart: Verlag von Ferdinand Enke, 1926. English translation *Doctrine of the Healing Power of Nature Throughout the Course of Time,* by L. J. Boyd. New York: 1932.

67. Pagel, W. *Virchow und die Grundlagen der Medizin des XIX. Jahrhunderts.* Jena: 1930.

68. Pagel writes:

When elaborating the "seat" of the physiological and pathological phenomena in the ultimate units of the organs and tissues Jahn speaks of the autonomous life of the "Fibres," true to Hallerian tradition. In addition he mentions (a) cells as "tissue-globules" such as described by the immediate forerunners of cellular histology, for example [Rene] Dutrochet, [Henri] Milne-Edwards, [Lorenz] Oken and others. Jahn also evolves (b) the concept of the "cell", i.e., the unit of primitive undifferentiated myxoid tissue, as the ultimate seat of disease. This "cell" represents a primitive vesicle, a minute "hydatid" and is, no doubt, meant in a similar sense as the "modern" cell. It is, however, a pre-Schleiden–Schwann concept. . . . In the earlier times of cellular histology, but before the appearance of Virchow as a scientific author in 1843, Jahn replaced the vague "globules" and minute "hydatids" by the cells proper . . . Then he quite clearly declares them to be the ultimate units of normal and pathological life and thereby anticipates cellular pathology in its theoretical foundations. (ref. 62, pp. 16–17)

69. This kind of similarity in no way can be considered as a sufficient proof for the basic identity of intellectual patterns. The Romantic literature preserved the notion of the "natural brotherhood of all people" that was so characteristic of the Enlightenment. But for the latter, the fact that "all people are relatives" is a source of optimism: estrangement presents only external aspects of social life but not its essence. This belief structured the subject of the foundling as one of the most popular in Enlightenment literature. But in Romantic literature, the same cliché—"all people are relatives"—introduced the theme of gloomy underground forces of Nature. This theme was structured on the symbol of incest, the forces of the primordial unity that erases all culturally established distinctions and articulations. The intellectual figure, which within one culture presented the primary harmonizing force of social life, turned within another, into a symbol of the inherited depravity of human nature and by extension of human society. Similarly, coexistence of two systems of organs—those of the vegetative life and those of the animal life—were asserted for centuries as the manifestation of a hierarchical harmonized unity of organism, but this was adopted in Metchnikoff's works in a very different format by the concept of inherited disharmonies.

70. This idea of cell sovereignty was to find further support and development in its Darwinian reinterpretation. After all, Darwin's theory was perceived by too many as another expression of the typical Victorian idea—harmony could be expressed and achieved only through struggle. (In some way, the idea was but a British analogy for the German idea of harmony as expressed by "polarity" or the Hegelian notion that established self-equality in the splitting the self and in self-contradiction.)

71. Roux, W. *Der Kampf der Thile im Organismus.* Leipzig: W. Engelmann, 1881.

72. Metchnikoff, E. "Bor'ba za suschestvovanie chastei zhivotnogo organizma" [The Struggle for the Existence of Parts of the Animal Organism] in: *Pomosch golodajuschim: Nauchno-literaturnyi sbornik.* Moscow: 1892, pp. 321–326. Reprinted in *AC*, Vol. 4, pp. 364–374.

73. Metchnikoff, E. "Ocherk voprosa o proiskhozhdenii vidov" [Essay on the Question Concerning the Origin of Species]. *Vestnik evropy,* 1876, 3:68–136; 4:715–747; 5:117–149; 7:158–197; 8:567–606. (Reprinted in *SBW* [1950], pp. 7–238; and in *AC,* Vol. 4, pp. 155–327.)

74. Darwin, C. Letter to G. F. Romanes, 16 April, 1881. *Life and Letters,* ed. F. Darwin, Vol. 3. London; John Murray, p. 244, 1887. Darwin notes that G. H. Lewes had a strong affinity to Roux, "viz., that there is a struggle going on within every organism between the organic molecules, the cells and the organs."

75. The oppositions in Heraclitus aphorisms are those most ancient oppositions of mythology: top and down, right and left, warm and cold, male and female, and so on.

76. Metchnikoff, E. *The Nature of Man. Studies in Optimistic Philosophy.* English translation by P. C. Mitchell. New York: Putnam's, 1903.

77. Diepgen, P. *Unvollendete: vom Leben und Wirken fruehverstorbener Forscher und Aerzte aus anderthalb Jahrhunderten.* Stuttgart: Thieme, 1960.

78. Maulitz, R. C. "Rudolf Virchow, Julius Cohnheim and the Program of Pathology." *Bull. Hist. Med.*: 52:162–182, 1978.

79. Cohnheim, J. *Neue Untersuchungen ueber die Entzuendung,* Berlin: A. Hirschwald 1873.

80. Samuel, S. "Ueber Entzuendung und Brand." *Arch. Pathol. Anat.*: 51:41–99, 178–209, 1870.

81. Ziegler, E. *Lehrbuch der allgemeinen und speciellen pathologischen Anatomie und Pathogenese,* 2nd ed. Jena: Fischer, 1882. See also the English translation of the first part *(General Pathological Anatomy)* made on the basis of the first German edition: *A Text-Book of General Pathological Anatomy and Pathogenesis.* Translated and edited by D. Macalister, New York: William Wood, 1883.

82. Virchow, R. "Der Kampf der Zellen und der Bakterien." *Arch. Pathol. Anat.*: 101:1–13, 1885.

83. Metchnikoff, E. "Ueber den Kampf der Zellen gegen Erysipelkokken. Ein Beitrag zur Phagocytenlehre." *Arch. Pathol. Anat.*: 107:209–249, 1887.

84. Rather, L. J., Review of the reprinted editions of Metchnikoff's *Lectures on the Comparative Pathology of Inflammation* and *Immunity in Infectious Diseases. Med. Hist.*: 14:409–412, 1970.

85. Todes, D. P. "Mechnikov, Darwinism, and the Phagocytic Theory," in *Darwin Without Malthus: The Struggle for Existence in Russian Evolutionary Thought.* Oxford and New York: Oxford University Press, 1989, pp. 82–103.

86. Metchnikoff, E. "Obschii ocherk paraziticheskoi zhizni," *Priroda:* b. 2, pp. 33–82, 1874. (Reprinted in *AC,* Vol. 1, pp. 200–234.)

87. The thought was one of the most important expressions of Metchnikoff's actual pessimism of that time. He explicitly discusses the relation between his interpretation of the struggle for existence and his pessimistic Weltanschauung in his essay "The Struggle for Existence in a General Sense" ["Bor'ba za suschestvovanie v obshirnom smysle," *Vestnik evropy,* 1878, 7:9–47; 8:437–483. (Reprinted in I. I. Metchnikoff. *Sorok Let Iskania Racional'nogo Mirovozzrenia.* Moscow: 1913, pp. 122–200.)

88. Metchnikoff, E. "Bolezni lichinok khlebnogo zhuka." Odessa: 1879; (Reprinted in *AC,* Vol. 4, pp. 339–360.)

89. Metchnikoff, E. "Materialy k ucheniju o vrednykh nasekomykh juga Rossii" ["Materials to the Teaching About the Harmful Insects of Russian South"]. *Zapiski novoross. ob. est.:* 6(1):1–10, 1880. (Reprinted in *AC,* Vol. 1, pp. 269–274); idem, "Zamechaniya na sochinenie g. Lindemana o khlebnom zhuke" ["Notices to the Treaty of Mr. Lindeman About the Beet Weevil]. *Sel'skoe Khoziaistvo i Lesovodstvo:* sec. 2, pp. 131–149, 1880. (Reprinted in *AC,* Vol. 1, pp. 275–289); idem, "Zur Lehre der Insektenkrankheiten." *Zoologischer Anzeiger,* Vol. 3, pp. 44–47, 1880. It is true that Metchnikoff refers to special measures that could be taken by *man* in order to protect the cultured plants. But we have no more reason to say that the idea of such a protection could play a paradigmatical role for the idea of protective phagocytosis than, for instance, to say that medicine as the social institution (or the police, or the military) was for Metchnikoff the paradigm of his phagocytosis theory.

90. It is of interest that the evolutionary biology of parasites is still a largely neglected area of inquiry, leaving us without a coherent theory. Metchnikoff's parasite argument (i.e., whether more generalized organisms and phylogenies persist more favorably than those more specialized) was followed most notably by Cope in 1896 (E. D. Cope. *The Primary Factors of Organic Evolution.* Chicago: Open Court, 1896) in his proposed law of the unspecialized. Cope believed that evolutionary advance is made from unspecialized forms and specialization leads to dead

ends. (As discussed by Price [P. W. Price. *Evolutionary Biology of Parasites,* Princeton, NJ: Princeton University Press, 1980, pp. 11–12]). This modern version has been often repeated in regards to evolution of parasites, and thus the conclusion was drawn that extinction rates in parasitic taxa is higher than in predatory. But Simpson (G. G. Simpson. *The Major Features of Evolution.* New York: Columbia University Press, 1953) has persuasively argued that the fossil record shows no preference in extinction rates of specialized and generalized clades, and more recently others have addressed the dual issue of (a) whether generalists survive longer than specialists and (b) if the degree of specialization of the focus for the selective processes that induce extinction, and concluded negatively in both cases (K. W. Flessa, K. V. Powers, and J. L. Cisne. "Specialization and evolutionary longevity in the Arthropoda." *Paleobiology* 1:71–81, 1975). If evolutionary success is to be measured by adaptive reactions, the modern verdict is that parasites are unsurpassed, "It is clear that parasitiasm as a way of life is more common than all other feeding strategies combined." (P. W. Price, op. cit., p. 8). Metchnikoff might well feel vindicated!

91. Metchnikoff, E. "Untersuchungen ueber die mesodermal Phagocyten einiger Wirbelthiere." *Bio. Zentralb.,* 3(18):560–565, 1883.

92. Metchnikoff, E. "Materialy k sravnitel'noi patologii vospaleniya" in *Protokoly Obschestva Odesskikh Vrachei,* 5, 1883–1884. (Reprinted in *AC,* Vol. 5, pp. 16–20.)

93. Metchnikoff, E. and Soudakewitch, J. "La phagocytose musculaire." *Ann. l'Inst. Pasteur.:* 6:1–20, 1892.

94. Metchnikoff, E. "Ueber die pathological Bedeutung der intracellulaeren Verdauung," *Fortsch. d. Med.:* 17:558–569, 1884.

95. Metchnikoff, E. "Ueber eine Sprosspilzkrankheit der Daphnien: Beitrag zur Lehre ueber den Kampf der Phagocyten gegen Krankheitserreger." *Arch. Pathol. Anat.:* 96:177–195, 1884.

Chapter 6

1. Sauerbeck, E. *Die Krise in der Immunitatsforschung.* Leipzig: Klinkhardt, 1909.

2. Pasteur, L. "Sur les maladies virulentes et en particulier sur la maladie appelee vulgairement cholera dec poules." *Compt. Rend. Acad.:* 90:239–248, 1880. English translation, "On Virulent Diseases, and in Particular the Disease Commonly Called Fowl Cholera," in *Milestones in Immunology: A Historical Exploration,* by D. J. Bibel, Madison, WI: Science Tech Publishers, 1988, pp. 159–161.

3. Von Nencki, M. "Ueber die Lebensfähigkeit der Spaltpilze bei fehlendem Sauenstoff." *J. Prakt. Chem.:* May 9:337–358, 1879. (Cited in V. N. Sirotinin. "Ueber die entwickelungshemmenden Stoffwechselproducte der Bacterien und die sog. Retentionshypothese." *Z. Hyg.*; 4:262–290, 1888.

4. Chauveau, A. "De la prédisposition et de l'immunité pathologiques: Influence de la provenance ou de la race sur l'apitude des animaux de l'espèce ovine à contracter le sang de rate." *Compt. Rend. Acad. Sc.:* 89:498–502, 1880; idem. "Des Causes qui peuvent faire varier les résultats de l'inoculation charbonneuse sur les moutons algériens: Influence de la quantité des agents infectants." *Applications à la théorie de l'immunité:* Ibid. 90:1526–1530, 1880; idem. "Du Renforcement de l'immunité des moutons algériens: À L'égard du sang de rate, par les inoculations préventives. Influence de l'inoculation de la mère la réceptivite du foetus." Ibid. 91:148–151, 1880.

5. Lewis, T. R. and Cunningham, D. D. "Microscopial and Physiological Researches into the Nature of the Agent or Agents Producing Cholera." *8th Ann. Rep. Sun-Comm. Gov. of India (1871).* Calcutta: 1872, app. C, pt. 2, p. 159.

6. Traube, M. and Gscheidlen, R. *Ueber Faulniss und den Widerstand der lebenden*

Organismen gegen dieselbe Jahrescber d. schlesischen: Gesellsch. f. Vaterland Cultur (1874). Breslau: 1875, pp. lii, 179.

7. Grohmann, W. *Ueber die Einwirkung des zellenfreien Blutplasma auf einige pflanzliche Microorganismen, (Schimmel, Spross-, pathogene und nicht pathogene Spaltpilz): Eine Untersuchung aus dem physiol.* Institut zu Dorpat: Kruger, 1884.

8. Von Behring, E. "Ueber die Ursache der Immunitaet von Ratten gegen Milzbrand." *Gentrabl. Klin. Med. (Leipzig):* 9:681–690, 1888.

9. Von Behring, E. "Untersuchvenger ueber das Zustandekommen der Diptherie-Immunitat ber Thieren." *Deut. Med. Woch.:* 16:1145–1148, 1890. English translation "Studies on the Mechanism of Diptheria in Animals" in T. D. Brock, *Milestones in Microbiology.* Englewood Cliffs, NJ: Prentice-Hall, 1961, pp. 141–144.

10. Baumgarten, P. "Der gegenwaertige Stand der Bacteriologie." *Berl. Klin. Woch.:* 27:585–588, 1900; 28:615–618, 1900.

11. Salmon, D. E. and Smith, T. "On a new method of producing immunity from contagious disease." *Proc. Biol. Soc. Wash.:* 3:29–33, 1884–1886.

12. Fodor, J. "Bakterien im Blute lebender Thiere." *Arch. Hyg.:* 4:129–148, 1886.

13. Wyssokowitsch, W. "Ueber die Schicksale der ins Blut injizierten Mikroorganismen im Koerper der Wirbelthiere." *Z. Hyg.:* 3–46, 1886.

14. Fodor, J. "Die Fahigkeit des Blutes Bakterien zu vernichten." *Dtsch. Med. Woch.:* 8:745–747, 1887.

15. Nuttall, G. "Experimente ueber die bacterienfeindliches Einfluesse des thierischen Koerpers." *Z. Hyg.:* 4:353–394, 1888. English excerpted translation, "Experiments on the Antibacterial Influence of Animal Substances," in H. A. Lechevalier and M. Soltorovsky, eds., *Three Centuries of Microbiology.* New York: McGraw Hill, 1965, pp. 211–215, and D. J. Bibel, op. cit., pp. 161–166. Note these translations differ from our own and convey an altered meaning.

16. Buechner, H. "Ueber die bakterientodtende Wirkung des Zellenfreien Blutserums." *Centralb. Bakteriol. Parasistenk.:* 5:817–823; 6:1–11, 1889.

17. Von Behring, E. and Nissen, F. "Ueber bacterienfeindliche Eigenschaften verschiedener Blutserumarten; ein Beitrag zur Immunitutsfrage." *Z. Hyg.:* 8:412–433, 1890.

18. Von Behring, E. and Kitasato, S. "Ueber das Zustandekommen der Diphtheire-immunitut und der Tetanus-Immunitat bei Thieren." *Dtsch. Med. Woch.:* 16:1113–1114, 1890. English translation, "The Mechanism of Immunity in Animals to Diptheria and Tetanus" in Brock, T. D. *Milestones in Microbiology.* Op. cit., pp. 138–140.

19. Behring, E. and Wernicke, E. "Ueber Immunisirung und Heilung von Versuchstieren bei der Diphtherie." *Z. Hyg.* 12:10–44, 1892.

20. Silverstein, A. M. "Cellular Versus Humoral Immunity: Determinants and Consequences of an Epic 19th-Century Debate." *Cell. Immunol.:* 48:208–221, 1979. (Republished in similar form in A. M. Silverstein, *A History of Immunology.* New York: Academic Press, 1989, pp. 38–58.)

21. Mazumdar, P.M.H. "Immunity in 1890." *J. Hist. Med.:* 27:312–324, 1972.

22. Buechner, H. *Centralb. Bacteriol. Parasitenk.:* 6:561–565, 1889.

23. Metchnikoff, E. *Immunity in Infective Diseases.* Translated by F. G. Binnie, 1905. New York: Johnson Reprint Corp., 1968.

24. Metchnikoff, E. "Untersuchung ueber die intracellulare Verdauung bei wirbellosen Thieren," in *Arbeiten aus dem Zoologischen Institut zu Wien,* Vol. 5, pt. 2, pp. 141–168, 1884 [proof in 1883]; the same in Russian. *Russkaya Medicina:* 4:59–61, 1884; 4:83–84; 5:107–110; 6:131–132 (Reprinted in "Izbrannye biologicheskie proizvedenya" pp. 239–270, 1950.) English translation in *Q. J. of Microscop. Sc.:* n.s. 24; pp. 89–111, 1884.

25. Koch, R. "Die Aetiologie der Milzbrand-Krankheit, begrundet auf die Entwicklungsgeschichte des Bacillus anthracis." *Beitr. Z. Biol. Pflanzen.* 2(2):277–310, 1876. English trans-

lation, "The Etiology of Anthrax Based on the Developmental Cycle of *Bacillus anthracis*," in H. A. Lechevalier and M. Solotorsky, op. cit., 69–79.

26. Metchnikoff, E. "Ueber eine Sprosspilzkrankheit des Daphnien: Beitrag zur Lehre ueber den Kampf des Phagozyten gegen Krankheitzerreger." *Arch. Pathol. Anat.*: 86:177–195, 1884. English translation, "A Yeast Disease of Daphnia: A Contribution to the Theory of the Struggle of Phagocytes Against Pathogens Fungus," in Lechevalier and Solotorsky, op. cit., pp. 188–195; and Brock, op. cit., pp. 132–138.

27. Baumgarten, P. "Referte." *Berl. Klin. Woch.* 21:802–804, 818, 1884.

28. Metchnikoff, E. "Ueber die Beziehung der Phagocyten zu Milzbrandbacillen." *Arch. Pathol. Anat.*: 97:502–526, 1884. English translation by D. Magasanik and A. H. Coons. "Concerning the Relationship Between Phagocytes and Anthrax Bacilli." *Rev. Inf. Dis.* 6:761–770, 1984.

29. Metchnikoff, E. "Ueber den Kampf der Zellen gegen Erysipelkokken." *Arch. Pathol. Anat.*: 107:209–249, 1887.

Because my critics are interested in the wounding of the unhappy animal, I can state that my assistant strongly constricted its neck to stop its resistance (during the taking of the last sample). Because at that time I did not have a laboratory and worked at a private apartment, all my research was conducted under conditions which were far from favorable. I do not have any reason to be sorry about the publication of my sole (in the explained way) experiment because results have proven to be correct. (p. 244)

When Metchnikoff had the opportunity to repeat the experiment, he obtained the same results.

30. Metchnikoff, E. "Ueber die pathologische Bedentung der intracellularen Verdauung." *Fortschr. Med.*: 17:558–569, 1884.

31. Limoges, C. "Natural Selection, Phagocytosis, and Preadaptation: Lucien Cuenot, 1886–1901." *J. Hist. Med.*: 31:176–214, 1976.

32. Metchnikoff, E. "Ueber den Phagocytenkamf beim Rueckfalltyphus." *Arch. Pathol. Anat.*: 109:176–192, 1887.

33. Metchnikoff, E. "Ueber die phagocytaere Rolle der Tuberkelriesenzellen." *Arch. Pathol. Anat.*: 113:63–94, 1888.

34. O. Metchnikoff. *Life of Elie Metchnikoff.* London: Constable, and New York: Houghton and Mifflin, 1921.

35. von Christmas-Dirckinck-Holmfelu, : "Ueber Immunitaet und Phagocytose." *Fortsch. Med.*: 5:401–411; 5(18):583–586, 1887.

36. Emmerich, R. "Die Heilung des Milzbrandes." *Archiv. Hyg.*: 6(4):442–501, 1887.

37. Emmerich, R., and di Mattei, E. "Vernichtung von Milzbrandbacillen im Organismus." *Fortschr. Med.*: 5(20):653–663, 1887.

38. Pawlowsky, A. D. "Die Heilung des Milzbrandes durch Bacterien und das Vehalten der Milzbrandbacillen in Organismus: Ein Beitrag zur Lehre der Bakteriotherapie." *Arch. Pathol. Anat.*: 108:494–521, 1887.

39. Lowy, I. "Immunology and Literature in the Early Twentieth Century: *Arrowsmith* and the *Doctor's Dilemma*." *Med. Hist.*: 32:314–332, 1988.

40. Fluegge, C. "Studien ueber die Abschwaechung virulenter Bacterien und die erworbene Immunitaet." (G. Smirnow, V.N. Sirotinin, H. Bitter, G. Nuttall). *Z. Hyg. (Leipzig)*: 4:208–230, 1888.

41. Baumgarten, P. "Zur Kritik der Metschnikoff' schen Phagocytentheorie." *Z. Klin. Med.*: 15(2):1–41, 1889.

42. Weigert, C. "Referat: Metschnikoff. Ueber den Phagocytenkampf beim Rueckfalltyphus." *Fortschr. Med. (Berlin)*: 5:732–735, 1887.

43. Weigert, C. "Bemerkung zu dem Verstehenden." *Fortsch. Med. (Berlin)*: 6:83–86; 6:809–821, 1888.

44. Ziegler, E. "Ueber die Ursache und das Wesen der Immunitaet des menschlichen Organismus gegen Infectionskrankheiten. *Beitr. zur Pathol.*: 5:417–439, 1889.

Chapter 7

1. Silverstein, A. M. "Cellular Versus Humoral Immunity: Determinants and Consequences of an Epic 19th-Century Debate." Cell. Immunol.: 48:208–221, 1979; and idem. *A History of Immunology.* New York; Academic Press, 1989.

2. Mazumdar, P.M.H. "Immunity in 1890." *J. Hist. Med.*: 27:312–324, 1972.

3. Fodor, J. "Bakterien im Blute lebender Thiere." *Arch. Hyg.*: 4:129–148, 1886.

4. Nuttall, G. "Experimente ueber die bacterienfeindliches Einfluesse des thierischen Koerpers." *Z. Hyg.*: 4:353–394, 1888. English translations in H. A. Lechevalier and M. Soltorovsky, op. cit., pp. 211–215; and D. J. Bibel, op. cit., pp. 161–166.

5. Metchnikoff, E. "Sur L'attenuation des bacteridies charbonneuses dans le sang des moutons refractaires." *Ann. Inst. Pasteur* (Paris): 1:42–44, 1887.

6. Metchnikoff, E. *Immunity in Infective Diseases* (1901). Translated by F. G. Binnie, 1905. New York: Johnson Reprint Corp., 1968.

7. Denys, J. and Leclef, J. "Sur Le Mécanisme de l'immunité chez le lapin vaccine contre le streptocoque pyogène." *La Cellule* (Lierre and Louvain): 11:177–221, 1895.

8. Mennes, Fr. "Das Antipneumokkoen-Serum und der Mechanismus der Immunität des Kaninchens gegen den Pneumococcus." Z. Hyg. (Leipzig): 25:413–438, 1897.

9. Marchand, L. "Étude sur la phagocytose des streptocoques attenues et virulents." *Arch. Méd. Exp.*: 10:253–294, 1898.

10. Wright, A. E. and Douglas, S. R. "An Experimental Investigation of the Role of the Blood Fluids in Connection with Phagocytosis." *Proc. R. Soc.*: 72:357–370, 1903.

11. Behring, E. and Kitasato, S. "Ueber das Zustandekommen der Diphtheire-immunitut und der Tetanus-Immunitat bei Thieren." *Dtsch. Med Woch.*: 16:1113–1114, 1890. English translation in Brock *Milestones in Microbiology,* op. cit., pp. 138–140.

12. Behring, E. "Untersuchvenger ueber das Zustandekommen der Diptherie-Immunitat ber Thieren." *Dtsch. Med. Woch.*: 16:1145–1148, 1890. English translation in T. D. Brock, op. cit., pp. 141–144.

13. Pasteur, L., Chamberland, C., and Roux, E. "Compte rendu sommaire des experiences faites a Pouilly-le-Fort, pres Melun, sur la vaccination charbonneuse." *Comp. Rend. Acad. Sci.*: 92:1378–1383, 1881.

14. Sewall, H. "Experiments on the Preventive Inoculation of Rattlesnake Venom." *J. Physiol.*: 8:203–210, 1887.

15. Virchow, R. *Die Cellularpathologie,* 4th ed. Berlin: A. Hirschwald 1871, pp. 530–531.

16. Metchnikoff, E. "Études sur l'immunité, 5th memoire: Immunité des lapins vaccines contre le microbe du Hogcholéra." *Ann. Inst. Pasteur:* 6:289–320, 1892.

17. Pfeiffer, R.F.J. "Studien zur cholera-aetiologie." Z. Hyg.: 16:268–286, 1894.

18. Pfeiffer, R.F.J. "Weitere Untersuchungen ueber das Wesen der cholera immunitat und ueber specifische baktericide process." Z. Hyg.: 18:1–16, 1894. English translation and commentary, "Further Investigations on the Nature of Immunity to Cholera and Specific Bactericidal Processes" in Bibel, op. cit., pp. 197–200.

19. Lister, J. "Discussion of Immunity." *Br. Med. J.*: 2:378–380, 1891.

20. Metchnikoff, E. *Lectures on the Comparative Pathology of Inflammation.* (1891) translation by F. A. Starling and E. H. Starling. New York: Dover, 1968.

21. Metchnikoff, E. "Études sur l'immunité. Sixième memoire: Sur La Destruction extracellulaire des bactéries dans l'organisme." *Ann. Inst. Pasteur:* 9:433–461, 1895.

22. Bordet, J. "Les leucocytes et les proprietes actives du serum chez les vaccinés." *Ann. Inst. Pasteur:* 9:462–506, 1895. English translation and commentary, "Leukocytes and the Active Property of Serum from Vaccinated Animals," in Brock, op. cit., pp. 144–148.

23. Bordet, J. "Sur Le Mode d'action des serums prévéntifs." *Ann. Inst. Pasteur:* 10:104, 193, 1896. "On the Mode of Action of Preventive Sera." *Studies in Immunity* (collected and translated by F. P. Gay). New York: Wiley, 1909, pp. 81–103.

24. Bordet, J. "Sur l'agglutination et la dissoltuion des globules rouges par le serum d'animaux injectés de sang defibriné." *Ann. Inst. Pasteur:* 12:688–695, 1898. English translation and commentary "On the Agglutination and Dissolution of Red Blood Cells by the Serum of Animals Injected with Defibrinated Blood," in Bibel, op. cit. pp. 200–204; and *Studies in Immunity,* op. cit., pp. 134–141.

25. Buechner, H. "Ueber die Schutzstoffe des Serums." *Verhandl. Congresses Innere Med.* (Weisbaden): 11:268–275, 1892.

26. Ehrlich, P. and Morgenroth, J. "Ueber haemolysine" *Berl. Klin. Woch.:* 37:453–458; 681–687, 1900.

27. Marshall, M.S. "The concept of immunity." *Cent. Rev.:* 3:95–113, 1959.

28. Silverstein, A. M. "Development of the Concept of Immunologic Specificity: I." *Cell. Immunol.:* 67:396–409; 71:183, 1982; *idem. A History of Immunology,* op. cit., pp. 87–123.

29. Metchnikoff in *The Nature of Man: Studies in Optimistic Philosophy.* Translated by P. C. Mitchell. New York: Putnam's, 1903, writes:

> Morality should be based not on human nature in its existing vitiated condition, but on human nature, ideal, as it may be in the future. Before all things, it is necessary to try to amend the evolution of the human life, that is to say, to transform its disharmonies into harmonies (Orthobiosis). This task can be undertaken only by science, and to science the opportunity of accomplishing it must be given. (p. 289)

30. In addition to diphtheria and tetanus antitoxins, Ehrlich himself had shown that antibodies could be formed against the plant toxins ricin and abrin. (See P. Ehrlich, "Experimentelle Untersuchungen über Immunität. I. See Ueber Ricin." *Dtsch. Med. Wschr.* 17:976–979, 1891 and "Experimentelle Untersuchungen über Immunität. II. See Ueber Abrin." *Dtsch. Med. Wschr.:* 17:1218–1219, 1891.)

31. Ehrlich, P. "Die Wertbemessung des Diphtherieheilserums und deren theoretische Grundlagen." *Klin. Jahrb.:* 60:299–326, 1897. English translation, "The Assay of the Activity of Diptheria-curative Serum and Its Theoretical Basis in *The Collected Papers of Paul Ehrlich,* vol. 2. Comp. and ed. F. Himmelweit, M. Marquardt, and H. Dale. London: Pergamon, 1957, pp. 107–125; and the German ed., pp. 86–106.

32. Weigert, C., Neue Fragestellungen in der patholgischen Anatomie." *Verh, Ges. Dtsch. Naturforsch. Aerzte:* 68(1):121–139, 1896.

33. The historical development of the modern clonal selection theory up to 1970 is discussed in detail by Silverstein, *A History of Immunology,* op. cit., pp. 77–81.

34. Ibid, pp. 66–75.

35. Landsteiner K. and M. Reich. "Ueber Unterschiede zwischen normalen und durch Immuniesierung entstandenen Stoffen, des Blutserums." *Centralbl. Bakteriol.:* 39:712–717, 1905.

36. Ehrlich, P. and Morgenroth, "Ueber Haemolysine, Zweite Mittheilung." *Berl. Klin. Woch.* 36:481–486, 1899. English translation, "On Hemolysis, Second Communication in *Collected Papers,* vol. 2, op. cit., pp. 165–172; German ed., pp. 156–164.

37. Bordet's early studies are most accessible in the English translation, *Studies in Immunity.* New York: Wiley, 1909. The debate with Ehrlich is summarized there in "A General Resume of Immunity," pp. 496–530.

38. Bordet, J. "On the Mode of Action of Cytolytic Sera, and on the Unity of the Alexin in a Given Serum" in Bordet, op. cit., pp. 228–240. Originally published as "Sur le mode d'action des sérums cytolytique et sur l'unité de l'alexine dans un même sérum." *Ann. Inst. Pasteur:* 15:303–318, 1901.

39. Fleck L. in *Genesis and Development of Scientific Fact* (first published by Benno Schwabe, Basel, 1935; English translation by F. Bardley and J. T. Trenn, University of Chicago Press, 1979) writes:

If bacteria (antigen 1) are mixed with the corresponding inactivated immune serum (1) (that is, the bacteriolytic amboceptor), as well as with the complement, bacteriolysis will occur. If one now adds to this a mixture of blood corpuscles (antigen 2) and the corresponding immune serum (2) that is, the hemolytic amboceptor), no hemolysis will occur, because the complement has been used up in the first process (bacteriolysis) and is no longer available for the second (hemolysis). . . . Because it is visible to the naked eye, hemolysis can be detected more easily than bacteriolysis, which requires microscopic examination. This complement fixation method has therefore become the most important instrument in serology, since according to this scheme the hemolytic system (the hemolytic amboceptor plus the corresponding blood corpuscles) can be used to indicate the occurrence of bacteriolysis, that is, whether the bacteriolysin used [is the "specific" one for, and thus] reacts with the bacteria used. With this method, if the bacteria are known the bacteriolysin can be diagnosed. Conversely if the serum, that is the bacteriolysin, is known, the bacteria can be diagnosed. In the first case we have a method of recognizing, for instance in the serum of patients, the presence of certain antibodies upon which a diagnosis of the disease can be based. In the second we can determine with very great certainty whether the unknown bacteria belong to the same species as the standard bacteria used for artificial immunization. This complement fixation method according to Bordet and Gengou was soon successfully used by Widal and LeSourd for abdominal typhus and by Wassermann and Bruck for abdominal typhus and meningitis. Many other workers used it later for such diseases as swine pox, cholera, and gonorrhea.

In 1906 "Wassermann and Bruck proceeded to utilize this reaction for the first time for the detection of antigens in human and animal organ extracts. With the aid of specific tuberclebacillus immune sera, they demonstrated the presence of lysed tubercle bacillus substances (tuberculin) in tuberculous organs. With the aid of tuberculin, in turn, they demonstrated the occurrence of a specific antibody in the blood, namely antituberculin". [C. Bruck. *Handbuch der Serodiagnose der Syphilis* 2nd ed. Berlin: Springer, 1924, p. 3.] These experiments were not rated very highly . . . , nevertheless, they were the starting point for Wassermann's syphilis experiments. . . .

In the end an edifice of knowledge was erected that nobody had really foreseen or intended. Indeed, it stood in opposition to the anticipations and intentions of the individuals who had helped build it. For Wassermann and his co-workers shared a fate in common with Columbus. They were searching for their own "India" and were convinced that they were on the right course, but they unexpectedly discovered a new "America." Nor was this all. Their "voyage" was not straight sailing in a planned direction but an Odyssey with continual change of direction. What they achieved was not even their goal. They wanted evidence for an antigen or an amboceptor. Instead, they fulfilled the ancient wish of the collective: the demonstration of syphilitic blood. (pp. 66–70)

40. Portier P. and Richet C. "Nouveaux faits d'anaphylaxie ou sensibilisation aux venins par dóses reitérées. *Compt. Rend. Soc. Biol., Paris:* 54:548–551, 1902.

41. Arthus, M. C.R. Injections répétées de sérum de cheval chez le lapin." *Compt. Rend. Soc. Biol., Paris:* 55:817–820, 1903.

42. Von Pirquet C. and Schick B. *Die Serumbrankheit.* Leipzig and Vienna: Deuticke, 1905. English translation: *Serum Sickness.* Baltimore, MD: Williams and Wilkins, 1951.

43. Donath, J. and K. Landsteiner, "Ueber paroxysmale Hamoglobinurie." *Muenchen. Med. Wchnshr.:* 51:1590–1593, 1904. Other instances of autoimmune hemolytic anemias were

reported a few years later by A. Chauffard and J. Troisier, *Sem. Med. (Paris):* 28:345, 1908; 29:601, 1909.

44. Silverstein, *History of Immunology,* op. cit., pp. 172–175.

45. Ehrlich P. and Morgenroth J. "Über Haemolysine. Sechste Mittheilung." *Berl. Klin. Woch.*: 38:598–604, 569–574, 1901. Reprinted in English translation, "On Hemolysis: Sixth Communication," in *Collected Papers,* op. cit., pp. 278–297; German ed., pp. 256–277.

46. Ehrlich, P. "Über Haemolysine. Fünfte Mittheilung." *Berl. Klin. Woch.*: 38:251–257, 1901. Reprinted in English translation, "On hemolysis: Fifth Communication," in *Collected Papers,* vol. 2, op. cit., pp. 246–255.

47. For discussion of the history of autoimmunity see Silverstein. *History of Immunology,* op. cit.; R. Root-Bernstein, "Self, nonself, and autoimmunity" in *Organism and the Origins of Self,* ed., A. I. Tauber, Dordrecht: Kluwer Academic Publishers, 1991; D. Goltz. Horror Autotoxicus: "Ein Beitrag zur Geschichte und Theorie der Autoimmunpathologie im Spiegel eines vielzitierten Begriffes." Thesis, (Muenster, 1980); A.-M. Moulin, "Histoire du systeme immunitaire: Immunologie et medicine (1880–1980)." Thesis, University of Lyon, 1987; A. Eyquem, "L'immuno-pathologie de l'auto-immunisation 1900–1980" *Arch. Inst. Pasteur* (Tunis) 58:281–295, 1981.

48. Silverstein. *History of Immunology,* op. cit., p. 163.

49. Kossel H. "Zur Kenntnis der Antitoxinwirkung." *Berl. Klin. Woch.*: 35:152, 1898; L. Camus and E. Gley. "Nouvelles recherches sur l'immunité contre le serum d'anguille:" *Ann. Inst. Pasteur (Paris):* 13:779–787, 1899.

50. Bordet, J. "Les sérums hémolytiques, leurs antitoxines et les théories des sérums cytolytiques." *Ann. Inst. Pasteur:* 14:257–297, 1900, in *Studies in Immunity,* op. cit. "Hemolytic Sera and Their Antitoxins and Theories Concerning Cytolytic Sera in General," pp. 186–216.

51. See Silverstein. *History of Immunology,* op. cit., p. 263–265.

52. Besredka, A. "Les antihemolysines naturelles." *Ann. Inst. Pasteur (Paris):* 15:785–807, 1901.

53. Widal, M. M. and Rostaine, P. "Insuffisance d'antisensibilisatrice dans le sange des hemoglobinuriques." *Compt. Rend. Soc. Biol.*: 58:321–324, 372–376, 1905.

54. Ehrlich, P. "Experimental Researches on Specific Therapy. On Immunity with Special Reference to the Relationship Between Distribution and Action of Antigens. First Harben Lecture." *Harben Lectures for 1907 of the Royal Institute of Public Health.* London: Lewis, 1908. (Reprinted in *Collected Papers,* vol. 3, op. cit., pp. 106–117.)

55. Ehrlich, P. "Experimental Researches on Specific Therapy. On Athreptic Functions. Second Harben Lecture." (Reprinted in *Collected Papers,* vol. 3, op. cit., pp. 118–129.)

56. Metchnikoff, E. *The Nature of Man,* op. cit.

57. Ibid, pp. 73–74.

58. Metchnikoff, E. *The New Hygiene: Three Lectures on the Prevention of Infectious Diseases.* Chicago: W. T. Keener, 1906. It is interesting to note that current research of colonic cancer has considered high fecal pH as an important etiological factor, and Metchnikoff is still cited in this regard. See, e.g., W. R. Bruce. "Recent Hypothesis for the Origin of Colon Cancer." *Cancer Res.*: 47:4237–4242, 1987.

59. Metchnikoff, E. *The Prolongation of Life: Optimistic Studies.* Translated by P. C. Mitchell, London: Heinemann, 1907.

60. *A Supplement to the Oxford English Dictionary Vol. 1,* ed. R. W. Burchfield, Oxford: Oxford University Press, vol. 1, p. 144, 1972.

61. As noted in the last chapter, Metchnikoff stressed from his first studies that the phagocyte response was not always sufficient to repel microbial invasion. This was but a specialized case where it was generally understood that

micro-organisms will adapt themselves so far as is permitted by their physiologic peculiarities to the stress of the environment, the exact direction which this adaptation will take being determined by the character of the environment, chemical and physical, and the physical, chemical and physiologic characteristics of the germ involved (P. H. Hiss, Some Problems in Immunity and the Treatment of Infectious Diseases. *Harvey Lectures, 1908–1909,* p. 248)

The modern study of pathogen survival has been particularized to certain microorganisms whose biochemical and immune-evasive techniques are fascinating illustration of interspecies struggle and remain vexing medical problems. (See, e.g., B. B. Finley and S. Falkow, "Common Themes in Microbial Pathogenicity." *Microbiol. Rev.:* 53:210–230, 1989; E. G. Hayunga, "Parasites and Immunity: Tactical Considerations in the War Against Disease—or How Did the Worms Learn About Clausewitz?" *Persp. Biol. Med.:* 32:349–370, 1989; K. A. Joiner, "Studies on the Mechanism of Bacterial Resistance to Complement-Mediated Killing and on the Mechanism of Action of Bactericidal Antibody." *Cur. Top. Microbiol. Immunol.* 121:99–133, 1985. D. J. Krogstad and P. H. Schlesinger, "Acid-vesicle Function, Intracellular Pathogens, and the Action of Chloroquine Against *Plamodium falciparum.*" *N. Eng. J. Med.:* 317:542–549, 1987; J. W. Moulder, "Comparative Biology of Intracellular Parasitism." *Microbiol. Rev.:* 49:298–337, 1985.) The issue most recently has become of central concern in addressing infection with the human immunodeficiency virus (see S. Roy and M. A. Wainberg. "Role of the Mononuclear Phagocyte System in the Development of Acquired Immunodeficiency Syndrome (AIDS)." *J. Leuk. Biol.:* 49:91–97, 1988).

62. Silverstein. *History of Immunology,* op. cit., pp. 173–174.

63. Silverstein. *History of Immunology,* op. cit., p. 38, also cited in "Romantic Researcher" (unsigned article). *MD:* pp. 317–322, June 1966.

64. Well-reviewed by G. B. Mackaness. "The Monocyte and Cellular Immunity." *Sem. Hematol.:* 7:172–184, 1970; and by D. O. Adams, and T. A. Hamilton. "The Cell Biology of Macrophage Activation." *Ann. Rev. Immunol.:* 2:283–318, 1984.

65. Unanue, E. R. "Antigen-presenting Function of the Macrophage." *Ann. Rev. Immunol.:* 2:395–428, 1984.

66. Nathan, C. "Secretory Products of Macrophages." *J. Clin. Invest.:* 79:319–326, 1987.

Chapter 8

1. Roux, W. "Beitrage zur Entwickelungmechanik des Embryo." *Virchows Arch.:* 114:113–153; Reultate 289–291, 1888. "Contributions to the Development Mechanics of Embryo. On the Artificial Production of Half-embryos by Destruction of One of the First Two Blastomeres and the Later Development (Postgeneration) of the Missing Half of the Body," in *Foundations of Experimental Embryology,* ed. B. H. Willier and J. M. Oppenheimer. New York: Hafner—Prentice-Hall, 1964, pp. 2–37.

Appendix A

1. Olson, E. C. "Morphology, Paleontology, and Evolution" in *Evolution After Darwin,* vol. 1, *The Evolution of Life: Its Origin, History and Future,* ed. S. Tax. Chicago: University of Chicago, 1960, pp. 523–545.

2. Smith, J. M. "News and Views." *Nature* (London): 330:516, 1987.

3. Gould, S. J. "Is a New and General Theory of Evolution Emerging?" *Paleobiology:* 6:119–130, 1980.

4. Levins, R. and Lewontin, R. *The Dialectical Biologist.* Cambridge: Harvard University Press, 1985.

5. Grene, M., "II. Sketches" in *Towards a Theoretical Biology,* ed. by C. H. Waddington. Edinburgh: Edinburgh University Press, 1969, pp. 61–69.

6. Grene, M. "Two Evolutionary Theories." *Br. J. Phil. Sci.:* 9:110–127, 185–193, 1958. Reprinted in M. Grene, *The Understanding of Nature: Essays in the Philosophy of Biology.* Dordrecht, The Netherlands: D. Reidel, 1974, pp. 127–153.

7. Mayr, E. "Prologue: Some Thoughts on the History of the Evolutionary Synthesis" in *The Evolutionary Synthesis: Perspectives on the Unification of Biology,* ed. E. Mayr and W. B. Provine. Cambridge: Harvard University Press, 1980.

8. Buss, L. W. *The Evolution of Individuality.* Princeton, NJ: Princeton University Press 1987.

9. Margulis, L. *Symbiosis in Cell Evolution.* San Francisco: Freeman, 1981.

10. Edelman, G. M. *Topobiology: An Introduction to Molecular Embryology.* New York: Basic Books, 1988.

11. Waddington, C. H. *The Strategy of the Genes.* London: Allen & Unwin; New York: Macmillan, 1957, p. 167.

12. Lewontin, R. *The Genetic Basis of Evolutionary Change.* New York: Columbia University Press, 1974; also discussed by E. Sober in *The Nature of Selection: Evolutionary Theory in Philosophical Focus.* Cambridge: MIT Press, 1984, relating phenotypic selection to changes in gene frequency.

13. We further discuss these issues and their possible interpretation in L. Chernyak and A. I. Tauber "The Dialectical Self: Immunology's Contribution" *Organism and the Origins of Self,* ed. A. I. Tauber. Dordrecht: Kluwer Academic Publishers, 1991.

Appendix B

1. Ofek, I. and Sharon, N. "Lectinophagocytosis: A Molecular Mechanism of Recognition Between Cell Surface Sugars and Lectins in the Phagocytosis of Bacteria." *Inf. Immun.:* 56:539–457, 1988.

2. There are many general reviews of phagocyte function, but the two most comprehensive are S. J. Klebanoff and R. A. Clark. *The Neutrophil: Function and Clinical Disorders.* New York: North Holland, 1978; and J. I. Gallin, I. M. Goldstein, and R. Snyderman, eds. *Inflammation: Basic Principles and Clinical Correlates.* New York: Raven Press, 1988.

3. See, e.g., A. G. Ehlenberger and V. Nussenzweig. "The Role of Membrane Receptors for C3b and C3d in Phagocytosis." *J. Exp. Med.:* 145:357–371, 1977.

4. Stossel, T. P. "From Signal to Pseudopod." *J. Biol. Chem.:* 264:18261–18264, 1989.

5. Tauber, A. I. and B. M. Babior. "Neutrophil Oxygen Reduction: The Enzymes and the Products." *Adv. Free Rad. Biol. Med.:* 1:264–308, 1985.

6. See Tauber, A. I., Karnad, A. B., and Ginis, I. "The role of phosphorylation in phagocytic activation," in S. Grinstein and O. D. Rotstein, eds., *Mechanisms of Leukocyte Activation,* New York: Academic Press, 1989. pp. 469–494.

7. Tauber, A. I. "Current Views of Neutrophil Dysfunction: An Integrated Clinical Perspective." *Am. J. Med.:* 70:1237–1247, 1981.

8. Kay, M.M.B., Bosman, J.C.G.M., Johnson, G. J., and Beth, A. H. "Band-3 Polymers and Aggregates, and Hemoglobin Precipitates in Red Cell Aging." *Blood Cells:* 14:275–289, 1988.

9. Kay, M.M.B. "Isolation of the Phagocytosis-inducing IgG-binding Antigen on Senescent Somatic Cells. *Nature* (London): 289:491–494, 1981.

10. Tanaka, Y. and Schroit, A. J. "Insertion of Fluorescent Phosphatidylserine into the Plasma Membrane of Red Blood Cells." *J. Biol. Chem.:* 258:11335–11343, 1983.

11. Morikawa, K., Takeda, R., Yamazaki, M., and Denichi, M. "Induction of Tumoricidal Activity of Polymorphonuclear Leukocytes by a Linear Beta 1, 3-d-Glucan, and Other Immunomodulators in Murine Cells," *Cancer Res.:* 45:1496–1501, 1985.; T. Inoue, and F. Sendo, "In Vitro Induction of Cytotoxic Polymorphonuclear Leukocytes by Supernatant from Concanavalin A-Stimulated Spleen Cell Culture." *J. Immunol.:* 131:2508–2514, 1983; A. K. Lichtenstein, J. Kahle, J. Berek, and J. Zigheboim. "Successful Immunotherapy with Intraperitoneal *Corynebacterium parvum* in a Murine Ovarian Cancer Model Is Associated with the Recruitment of Tumor-lytic Neutrophils into the Peritoneal Cavity." *J. Immunol.:* 133:519–526, 1984; J. Leiboici, A. Borit, U. Sandbank, and A. Wolman. "The Role of Macrophages and Polymorphs in the Levan-Induced Inhibition of Lewis Lung Carcinoma in C57BL Mice." *Br. J. Cancer:* 40:597–607, 1979.

12. K. Morikawa, T. Noguchi, M. Yamazaki, and D. Mizuno. "Calcium-Dependent and -Independent Tumorcidal Activities of Polymorphonuclear Leukocytes Induced by a Linear Beta-1,3-D Glucan and Phorbol Myristate Acetate in Mice." *Can. Res.:* 46:66–70, 1986; S. Tsunawaki, M. Ikenani, M. Denichi, and M. Yamazaki. "Mechanisms of Lectin and Antibody-Dependent Polymorphonuclear Leukocyte-Mediated Cytolysis." *Gan:* 74:265–272, 1983.

13. Ackerman, M. F., Lamm, K. R., Wiegand, G. W., and Luster, M. I. "Antitumor Activity of Murine Neutrophils Demonstrated by Cytometric Analysis. *Cancer Res:* 49:528–532, 1989.

14. Diegelmann, R. F., Kim, J. C., Lindblad, W. J., Smith, T. C., Harriss, T. M., and Cohen, I. K. "Collection of Leukocytes, Fibroblasts and Collagen Within an Implantable Reservoir Tube During Tissue Repair." *J. Leuk. Biol.:* 42:667–672, 1987.

15. Grinnell, F. "Fibronectin and Wound Healing." *J. Cell. Biochem.:* 26:107–116, 1984; W. F. Skogen, R. M. Senior, G. L. Griffin, and G. D. Wilner. "Fibrinogen-Derived Peptide Is a Multidomained Neutrophil Chemoattractant." *Blood:* 71:1475–1479, 1988.

16. Mundy, G. R. "Role of Monocytes in Bone Resorption." *Adv. Exp. Med. Biol.:* 151:401–408, 1982; W. A. Peck, L. Rifas, S. L. Cheng, and V. Shen. "The Local Regulation of Bone Remodeling." *Adv. Exp. Med. Biol.:* 208:255–259, 1986.

17. Romson, J. L., Jolly, S. R., Lucchesi, B. R. "Protection of Ischemic Myocardium by Pharmacologic Manipulation of Leukocyte Function." *Cardio. Rev. Rep.:* 5:690–709, 1984; B. R. Lucchesi, K. M. Mullane. "Leukocytes and Ischemia-Induced Myocardial Injury." *Ann. Rev. Pharmacol. Toxicol.:* 26:201–224, 1986; J. Mehta, J. Dinerman, P. Mehta, T.G.P. Saldeen, D. Lawson, W. H. Donnelly, and R. Wallin. "Neutrophil Function in Ischemic Heart Disease." *Circulation:* 79:549–556, 1989.

18. Engler, R. L. "Free Radical and Granulocyte-Mediated Injury During Myocardial Ischemia and Reperfusion." *Am. J. Cardiol.* 63:19E, 1989.

19. Klausner, J. M., Paterson, I. S., Kobzik, L., Valeri, C. R., Shepro, D., and Hechtman, H. B. "Oxygen Free Radicals Mediate Ischemia-Induced Lung Injury." *Surgery:* 105:192–199, 1989.

20. Hellberg, P.O.A., Kallskog, O., Wolgast, M., and Ojteg, G. "Effects of Neutrophil Granulocytes on the Insulin Barrier of Renal Tubular Epithelium After Ischaemic Damage." *Acta Physiol. Scand.:* 134:313–315, 1988.

21. Shandall, A. A., Williams, G. T., Hallett, M. B., and Young, H. L. "Colonic Healing: A Role for Polymorphonuclear Leukocytes and Oxygen Radical Production." *Br. J. Surg.:* 73:225–228, 1986.

22. Metchnikoff, E. *Lectures on the Comparative Pathology of Inflammation.* English translation F. A. Starling and E. H. Starling. London: Kegan Paul, Trench, Trubner & Co., 1893. Reprinted New York: Dover, 1968.

23. Johnston, I. S. and Hildemann, W. H. "Cellular Defense Systems of the Porifera" in

The Reticuloendothelial System: A Comprehensive Treatise, vol. 3, *Phylogeny and Ontogeny,* ed. N. Cohen and M. M. Sigel. New York: Plenum, 1982, pp. 37–57.

24. Bigger, C. H. and Hildemann W. H. "Cellular Defense System of the Coelenterata," in Cohen and Sigel, *Reticuloendothelial System,* op. cit., pp. 59–87.

25. Buss, L. W. *The Evolution of Individuality.* Princeton, NJ: Princeton University Press, 1987.

26. Ratcliff, N. A. and Cooper, E. L. "Invertebrate Defense Systems: An Overview," in N. Cohen and M. M. Sigel, *Reticuloendothelial Systems,* op. cit., pp. 1–35; Marchallionis, J. J. *Immunity in Evolution.* Cambridge: Harvard University Press, 1977.

27. Buss, L. W. op. cit., pp. 151–152. See also L. W. Buss, and D. R. Green. "Histoincompatability in Vertebrates: The Relict Hypothesis." *J. Comp. Dev. Immunol.:* 9:191–201, 1985.

28. Edelman E. "CAMs and Igs: Cell Adhesion and the Evolutionary Origins of Immunity." *Immunol. Rev.:* 100:9–43, 1987; U. Rutishauser, A. Acheson, A. K. Hall, D. M. Mann, and J. Sunshine. "The neural crest adhesion molecule (NCAM) as a regulator of cell-cell interactions. *Science:* 240:53–57, 1988; T. Matsunaga and N. Mori. "Globulin Superfamily Molecules Are All Related." *Scand. J. Immunol.:* 25:485–495, 1987.

29. Chernyak, L. and Tauber, A. I. "The Dialectical Self: Immunology's Contribution," in *Organism and The Origins of Self,* ed. A. I. Tauber. Dordrecht: Kluwer Academic Publishers. 1991.

Index

DATE DUE

DEMCO 38-297